Occupational Therapy in Australia

This ground-breaking text provides a comprehensive guide to the occupational therapy profession in Australia, from the profession's role in the health care system to the broad scope and nature of its practice.

The book is organised into three sections: the Australian context; professional issues and practice issues. Contributions from 80 Australian occupational therapists working in education, research, policy and practice bring together the most relevant and up-to-date information in this essential book. The authors begin the Australian environment section with an overview of the Australian health care system, a history of occupational therapy in Australia and the role of Australian occupational therapy professional associations and regulatory bodies. The values and philosophy of occupational therapy, ethical and legal aspects of practice and the role of occupational therapy in population health and health promotion are considered next. The professional issues covered in the book include using effective communication skills, client-centred practice principles and a strength-based approach when working with individuals, families, groups, communities, organisations and populations. Additional topics, including occupational science, the education of occupational therapists, research in occupational therapy, evidence-based practice clinical reasoning and occupational therapy models of practice, are also covered in the middle section of the book.

Occupational Therapy in Australia: Practice and Process Issues is established as the essential practice reference for students, practitioners and educators in Australia. This second edition has been revised and updated throughout and includes new chapters on communication skills, environmental aspects of occupational therapy practice and decolonising occupational therapy through a strength-based approach to practice.

Ted Brown is Professor and Undergraduate Course Convenor in the Department of Occupational Therapy at the School of Primary & Allied Health Care, Faculty of Medicine, Nursing and Health Sciences, Monash University—Peninsula Campus, Frankston, Victoria, Australia.

Helen M. Bourke-Taylor is Associate Professor and Research Honours Course Coordinator in the Department of Occupational Therapy, School of Primary & Allied Health Care, Faculty of Medicine, Nursing and Health Sciences, Monash University—Peninsula Campus, Frankston, Victoria, Australia.

Stephen Isbel is Associate Professor & Discipline Lead of Occupational Therapy in the Faculty of Health at the University of Canberra Hospital, Canberra, Australian Capital Territory, Australia.

Reinie Cordier is Professor of Child Mental Health, Welfare and Wellbeing in the Department of Social Work, Education and Community Wellbeing, Faculty of Health and Life Sciences, at Northumbria University, Newcastle upon Tyne, United Kingdom.

Louise Gustafsson is Professor of Occupational Therapy in the School of Allied Health Sciences and the Hopkins Centre, at Griffith University, Nathan Campus, Queensland, Australia.

Occupational Therapy in Australia

Professional and Practice Issues

SECOND EDITION

Edited by
Ted Brown, Helen M. Bourke-Taylor,
Stephen Isbel, Reinie Cordier and
Louise Gustafsson

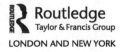

Routledge
Taylor & Francis Group

LONDON AND NEW YORK

Second edition published 2021
by Routledge
2 Park Square, Milton Park, Abingdon, Oxon, OX14 4RN

and by Routledge
605 Third Avenue, New York, NY 10158

Routledge is an imprint of the Taylor & Francis Group, an informa business

First edition published by Allen and Unwin 2017

British Library Cataloguing-in-Publication Data
A catalogue record for this book is available from the British Library

Library of Congress Cataloging-in-Publication Data
Names: Brown, Ted, editor. | Bourke-Taylor, Helen, editor. | Isbel, Stephen, editor. | Cordier, Reinie, editor. | Gustafsson, Louise, editor.
Title: Occupational therapy in Australia : professional and practice issues / Ted Brown, Helen M. Bourke-Taylor, Stephen Isbel, Reinie Cordier, Louise Gustafsson.
Description: Second edition. | Milton Park, Abingdon, Oxon ; New York, NY : Routledge, 2021. | Includes bibliographical references and index. | Summary: "This ground-breaking text provides a comprehensive guide to the occupational therapy profession in Australia, from the profession's role in the healthcare system to the broad scope and nature of its practice"— Provided by publisher.
Identifiers: LCCN 2020042911 (print) | LCCN 2020042912 (ebook) | ISBN 9780367683573 (hardback) | ISBN 9781760877446 (paperback) | ISBN 9781003150732 (ebook)
Subjects: LCSH: Occupational therapy—Textbooks. | Occupational therapy—Australia—Textbooks.
Classification: LCC RM735 .O3417 2021 (print) | LCC RM735 (ebook) | DDC 615.8/515—dc23
LC record available at https://lccn.loc.gov/2020042911
LC ebook record available at https://lccn.loc.gov/2020042912

ISBN: 978-0-367-68357-3 (hbk)
ISBN: 978-1-760-87744-6 (pbk)
ISBN: 978-1-003-15073-2 (ebk)

Typeset in Bembo
by codeMantra

Dedications

Professional Dedication: Australian Occupational Therapy Pioneers

- By 1939, there were three Australians who were qualified occupational therapists: *Ethel Francis, Sylvia Docker* and *Joyce Keam*.
- Ethel May Francis was the first Australian to hold a diploma in Occupational Therapy having graduated from the Philadelphia School of Occupational Therapy in the United States in 1933. She then went on to complete further postgraduate study at Dorset House, the first School of Occupational Therapy in the United Kingdom. Between 1937 and 1939, she worked in Sydney in private practice and mainly worked with patients with psychiatric problems. She started Occupational Therapy departments at the Royal Alexandra Hospital for Children and the Royal Prince Alfred Hospital in Camperdown.
- Sylvia Docker travelled to England in 1934 to train at the London Occupational Therapy School. She returned to Australia in 1938 to work for the Consultative Council of Infantile Paralysis. She pioneered Occupational Therapy Services in Melbourne, working for with the Victorian Crippled Children's Society, School for Crippled Children, and the Austin Hospital from 1939 to 1941. Later she became the first Director of Sydney Occupational Therapy School. In 1959, she was awarded an MBE in 1959 in recognition for her contributions to the Occupational Therapy profession.
- In 1937, Joyce Keam, originally from Tasmania, went to England to study occupational therapy at the Maudsley Psychiatric Hospital, a London University teaching hospital. In 1939, she returned to Australia and worked privately for a group of psychiatrists at the Alencon Private Mental Hospital in Malvern, Victoria. In 1941, she pioneered the establishment of the Occupational Therapy Department at a 2,000-bed army hospital in Heidelberg, Victoria and in 1943 she was promoted to the position of Chief Occupational Therapist at the Australian Army Headquarters in Melbourne and Advisor in Occupational Therapy to the Director of Medical Services.

Dedication to Professor Sylvia Rodger, PhD, MedSt, BOccThy, PhD, FOTARA, FAOTA, AM

Australian Occupational Therapy Clinician, Educator, Researcher, Mentor, and Leader

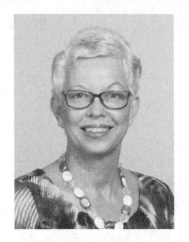

The editorial team met in 2010 at an Occupational Therapy Academic Emerging Leaders Network created by Emeritus Professor Sylvia Rodger (AM). As a leader, Sylvia inspired and challenged us all to make a difference to the occupational therapy profession, and we dedicate this book to her.

Sylvia completed her Bachelor of Occupational Therapy at The University of Queensland (UQ) in 1981 and began her academic career in 1983 at UQ, receiving a Master of Educational Studies in 1987 and PhD in 1996. She was Head of Occupational Therapy at UQ from 2001–2012. Her contributions during this time included development of the Student Practice Evaluation Form-Revised Edition Package© (SPEF-R); Chair of the Australia and New Zealand Council of Occupational Therapy Educators; she led the team that revised the Occupational Therapy Australia Competency Standards in 2010; and she was an Australian Learning and Teaching Fellow.

Sylvia was an occupational therapy innovator and advocate in many contexts and her contributions extended beyond the university education environment. She was instrumental in introducing the Cognitive Orientation to daily Occupational Performance (CO-OP) approach to Australia and she worked with other leaders to conceive and co-found the Autism Cooperative Research Centre (CRC) in 2013, a comprehensive, end-user-focused research centre addressing the needs of people with lived experience of autism across the life span. The Autism CRC was her final professional role and one where her skills in leadership, education and research, and interest in empowering and building others combined and thrived.

Sylvia received over \$3 million in competitive research funding, published four edited books, 22 book chapters and over 190 refereed journal publications. She supervised around 40 postgraduate research students to completion and was the recipient of many awards in recognition of her nationally and internationally acclaimed work as a clinician, academic and researcher including:

- Order of Australia (AM) in January 2015, for services to occupational therapy education and leadership and to the children and their families who are living with Autism Spectrum Disorder;
- Freda Jacob Award from Occupational Therapy Australia in 2014 for professional excellence and significant and exemplary contribution to the profession nationally and internationally particularly related to contribution to occupational therapy education;
- Fellow of the American Occupational Therapy Association Academy of Research in 2013 in recognition of her exemplary and distinguished contributions towards the science of occupational performance;
- Sylvia Docker Lecture in 2011from Occupational Therapy Australia for outstanding contributions to occupational therapy in Australia;

- Mary Rankine Wilson Award for Professional Excellence highlighting her contribution to occupational therapy education and research in 2009.

Sylvia's final award of Fellow of Occupational Therapy Australia Research Academy was presented posthumously at the Occupational Therapy Australia 27th National Conference in 2017 in recognition of her outstanding research achievements and contributions. The award was accepted by her family to a standing ovation from the conference attendees. Sylvia held many different roles in our lives: supervisor, colleague, postgraduate advisor, co-researcher, mentor and friend. We miss her but her legacy continues with us, and many other occupational therapy clinicians, educators, researchers and leaders throughout Australia and the world. How do you honour a career like this? You honour it by continuing to question and challenge, as Sylvia did, and by continuing to enable each person we work with to reach their potential. Sylvia was a true visionary, advocate and champion of occupational therapy.

Editors' personal dedications

Ted Brown

- David Stevens, life partner and constant source of support and patience for the time my academic pursuits take up;
- Sharon Gutman, friend, colleague and co-researcher for her encouragement and collaboration;
- John Waugh and Colin Martin, dear friends who have listened and laughed with me along the way;
- Professor Jane Case-Smith, Professor Jim Hinojosa and Professor Gary Kielhofner, three occupational therapy scholars and visionaries whose contributions to the profession were exceptional and are enduring.

Helen Bourke-Taylor

- I thank my family, Jim, Josie, Catie and Seamus and my parents Des and Judy for endless support and encouragement.

Stephen Isbel

- Dedicated to my family who support me to do what I love doing;
- To my work colleagues who step up each and every time.

Reinie Cordier

- I dedicate the book to Elizabeth Holsten and Anita Bundy who were influential in shaping my academic career, and my family for their unwavering support.

Louise Gustafsson

- Bill and Diane Bender, my parents who provided the opportunities that set me on the path of inquiry and learning;
- Staffan, Hanna and Sofie, my family who provide me with balance and a reminder of what is really important.

Contents

PART II
Professional issues

PART III
Practice issues

Tables

Figures

Boxes

Contributors

Lynne Adamson is Associate Professor of Occupational Therapy in the Faculty of Health at Deakin University, Geelong, Victoria, Australia

Rebecca Allen is a professional advisor of program accreditation with the Occupational Therapy Council of Australia Ltd.

Tammy Aplin is Conjoint Research Fellow in the School of Health and Rehabilitation Sciences, at the University of Queensland and The Allied Health Research Collaborative, The Prince Charles Hospital.

Amy Barrett-Lennard is an orientation and mobility specialist/occupational therapist, working at the Independent Living Services, VisAbility—Perth, Western Australia, Australia

Angela Berndt is Program Director of the Occupational Therapy course at the University of South Australia, Adelaide. Angela is also a Senior Lecturer in the discipline of Allied Health & Human Performance

Michelle Bissett is Senior Lecturer in the discipline of Occupational Therapy in the School of Allied Health Sciences at Griffith University, Southport, Queensland, Australia

Helen Bourke-Taylor is Associate Professor and Research Honours Course Convenor in the Department of Occupational Therapy, School of Primary & Allied Health Care, Faculty of Medicine, Nursing and Health Sciences at Monash University—Peninsula Campus, Frankston, Victoria, Australia

Julie Brayshaw is Chair of the Occupational Therapy Board of Australia, G.P.O. Box 9958, Melbourne, Victoria, 3001, Australia

Jennie Brentnall is Associate Lecturer in the discipline of *Occupational Therapy in the Faculty of Health Sciences at the University of Sydney—Cumberland Campus, Sydney, New South Wales, Australia*

Kieran Broome is Lecturer in the discipline of Occupational Therapy in the School of Health and Sport Sciences, Faculty of Science, Health, Education and Engineering at the University of the Sunshine Coast, Maroochydore, Queensland, Australia

Ted Brown is Professor and Undergraduate Course Convenor in the Department of Occupational Therapy, School of Primary & Allied Health Care, Faculty of Medicine, Nursing and Health Sciences, at Monash University—Peninsula Campus, Frankston, Victoria, Australia

Angus Buchanan is Professor and Head of the School of Occupational Therapy, Social Work and Speech Pathology, Faculty of Health Sciences, at Curtin University, Bentley, Western Australia, Australia

Corrine Butler currently works for The National Aboriginal and Torres Strait Islander Occupational Therapy Network (NATSIOTN)

Rosalind Bye is Director of the Academic Program in Occupational Therapy, in the School of Health Sciences at Western Sydney University, Sydney, New South Wales, Australia

Liana Cahill is Lecturer in the discipline of Occupational Therapy, in the School of Allied Health Faculty of Health Sciences at Australian Catholic University, Melbourne, Victoria, Australia

Libby Callaway is Associate Professor in the Department of Occupational Therapy & Rehabilitation, Ageing & Independent Living Research Centre, School of Primary & Allied Health Care, Faculty of Medicine, Nursing and Health Sciences, at Monash University—Peninsula Campus, Frankston, Victoria, Australia

Ian Cheok is a senior occupational therapist currently working for Lifeworks Occupational Therapy

Marina Ciccarelli is Associate Professor and Discipline Lead in the Department of Occupational Therapy, School of Occupational Therapy, Social Work, and Speech Pathology, Faculty of Health Sciences at Curtin University, Perth, Western Australia, Australia

Lindy Clemson is Professor in the discipline of Occupational Therapy in the Faculty of Medicine and Health at University of Sydney, Sydney, New South Wales, Australia

Reinie Cordier is Professor of Child Mental Health, Welfare and Wellbeing in the Department of Social Work, Education and Community Wellbeing, Faculty of Health and Life Sciences, at Northumbria University, Newcastle upon Tyne, United Kingdom

Michael Curtin is Associate Professor and Head of School of Community Health in the Faculty of Science at Charles Sturt University, Albury, New South Wales, Australia

Anne Cusick is Professor & Chair of Occupational Therapy, and also Head of Occupational Therapy Discipline in the Faculty of Medicine and Health, The University of Sydney. Emeritus Professor, Western Sydney University.

Emma Crawford is Lecturer in Occupational Therapy and Affiliate Lecturer at the UQ Poche Centre for Indigenous Health, School of Health and Rehabilitation Sciences, at The University of Queensland, Queensland, Australia

Susan Darzins is Senior Lecturer in Occupational Therapy in the School of Allied Health, Faculty of Health Sciences at Australian Catholic University, Melbourne, Victoria, Australia

Desleigh de Jonge is Research Fellow at the School of Health and Rehabilitation Sciences, The University of Queensland, Brisbane, Queensland, Australia

Tahnee Elliot is a learning support coordinator and occupational therapist at Gulf Christian College, Normanton, Queensland, Australia. She is also an Adjunct Lecturer, Centre for Rural and Remote Health, James Cook University, Mount Isa Hospital, Mount Isa, Queensland, Australia

Priscilla Ennals is Adjunct Senior Lecturer at the School of Allied Health, Human Services and Sport, La Trobe University Melbourne. She is also an Adjunct Senior Lecturer with the Department of Occupational Therapy, School of Primary & Allied Health Care, Faculty of Medicine, Nursing and Health Sciences at Monash University—Peninsula Campus, Frankston, Victoria, Australia

Louise Farnworth is Adjunct Associate Professor with the Department of Occupational Therapy, School of Primary and Allied Health Care at Monash University—Peninsula Campus, Frankston, Victoria, Australia

Ellie Fossey is Professor, Head of Department and Graduate Research Coordinator with the Department of Occupational Therapy at Monash University—Peninsula Campus, Frankston, Victoria, Australia. Ellie is also Adjunct Professor at the Living with Disability Research Centre, School of Allied Health, Human Services & Sport, La Trobe University, Melbourne, Australia

Jenniffer García is an occupational therapist and MPhil, PhD candidate at the School of Health & Rehabilitation Sciences, The University of Queensland, Brisbane, Queensland, Australia

Emma George is Senior Lecturer at the School of Allied Health Science and Practice, Faculty of Health and Medical Sciences, University of Adelaide, Adelaide, South Australia

Chontel Gibson is Co-founder, Chairperson, Member and Mentor with The National Aboriginal and Torres Strait Islander Occupational Therapy Network (NATSIOTN) and the University of Queensland, Brisbane, Queensland, Australia

Susan Gilbert-Hunt is currently working at the International Centre for Allied Health Evidence, UniSA Allied Health and Human Performance, University of South Australia, Adelaide, South Australia, Australia

Kate Gledhill is Lecturer with the Department of Occupational Therapy, School of Primary & Allied Health Care, Faculty of Medicine, Nursing and Health Sciences at Monash University

Craig Greber is Assistant Professor in Occupational Therapy with the Faculty of Health, University of Canberra Hospital, Canberra, Australian Capital Territory, Australia

Louise Gustafsson is Professor in the Discipline of Occupational Therapy with the School of Allied Health Sciences and the Hopkins Centre, Griffith University, Nathan Campus, Queensland, Australia

Rosamund Harrington is Lecturer in Occupational Therapy with the School of Allied Health Faculty of Health Sciences at Australian Catholic University, Brisbane, Queensland, Australia

Alana Hewitt is Lecturer with the Department of Occupational Therapy, School of Primary & Allied Health Care at Monash University—Peninsula Campus, Frankston, Victoria, Australia

Samantha Hunter is Chief Executive Officer at Occupational Therapy Australia, Fitzroy, Victoria, Australia

Nerida Hyett is Lecturer in Occupational Therapy at La Trobe Rural Health School, La Trobe University, Bendigo Victoria, Australia

Stephen Isbel is Associate Professor & Discipline Lead of Occupational Therapy at the Faculty of Health, University of Canberra Hospital, Canberra, Australian Capital Territory, Australia

Maggie Jamieson is Deputy Chief Executive Northern Territory Health and Adjunct Professor University of Canberra

Annette Joosten is Associate Professor of Occupational Therapy with the School of Allied Health, Faculty of Health Sciences at Australian Catholic University, Melbourne, Victoria, Australia

Ann Kennedy-Behr is Senior Lecturer of Occupational Therapy, Allied Health & Human Performance with the School of Health Sciences, Division of Health Sciences, University of South Australia—City East Campus, Adelaide, South Australia, Australia

Mary Kennedy-Jones is Adjunct Associate Professor of Occupational Therapy with School of Health Sciences at Swinburne University, Melbourne, Victoria, Australia

Lisa Knightbridge is Senior Lecturer with the Department of Occupational Therapy, School of Primary Health Care, Faculty of Medicine, Nursing and Health Sciences at Monash University—Peninsula Campus, Frankston, Victoria, Australia

Aislinn Lalor is Lecturer with the Department of Occupational Therapy with the School of Primary & Allied Health Care, Faculty of Medicine, Nursing and Health Sciences at Monash University—Peninsula Campus, Frankston, Victoria, Australia

Adam Lo is 1st Alternate Delegate (Australia) with the World Federation of Occupational Therapists & Advanced Occupational Therapist, Child and Youth Mental Health Service, Metro South Health, Queensland, Australia

Alexandra Logan is Lecturer with the School of Allied Health, Melbourne Campus at Australian Catholic University, Fitzroy, Victoria, Australia

Lynette Mackenzie is Associate Professor in the Discipline of Occupational Therapy, School of Health Sciences, with the Faculty of Medicine and Health at University of Sydney, Sydney, NSW, Australia

Carol McKinstry is Associate Professor of Occupational Therapy & Head of Rural Department of Allied Health, Rural Health School, College of Science Health & Engineering, Bendigo, Victoria, Australia

Ben Milbourn is Senior Lecturer in the School of Occupational Therapy, Social Work and Social Work with the Faculty of Health Sciences at Curtin University, Bentley, Western Australia, Australia

Matthew Molineux is Professor, and Head of Occupational Therapy with the School of Allied Health Sciences at Griffith University, Queensland, Australia

Monica Moran is Associate Professor of Rural Health at the WA Centre for Rural Health at the University of Western Australia, Geraldton, Western Australia

Claire Morrisby is Lecturer and Graduate Entry Masters Course Coordinator in the School of Occupational Therapy, Social Work and Speech Pathology, with the Faculty of Health Sciences at Curtin University

Lisa O'Brien is Associate Professor in the Department of Occupational Therapy with the School of Primary & Allied Health Care at Monash University—Peninsula Campus, Frankston, Victoria, Australia

Gjyn O'Toole is Senior Lecturer of Occupational Therapy with the Faculty of Health and Medicine at The University of Newcastle, Newcastle, New South Wales, Australia

Dave Parsons is an accredited hand therapist and lecturer with the School of Occupational Therapy, Social Work and Speech Pathology, Faculty of Health Sciences, Curtin University, Bentley, Western Australia, Australia

Annette Peart is Lecturer in the Department of Occupational Therapy with the School of Primary & Allied Health Care, Faculty of Medicine, Nursing and Health Sciences at Monash University—Peninsula Campus, Frankston, Victoria, Australia

Geneviève Pépin is Associate Professor, Discipline Lead, Course Director and Honours Coordinator of Occupational Science and Therapy with the School of Health and Social Development, Faculty of Health at Deakin University, Geelong, Victoria, Australia

Tirritpa Ritchie is Lecturer with the College of Nursing and Health Sciences at Flinders University, Adelaide, South Australia

Andrea Robinson is an occupational therapist at Box Hill Hospital, Eastern Health, Box Hill, Victoria, Australia

Luke Robinson is Lecturer with the Department of Occupational Therapy with the School of Primary & Allied Health Care, Faculty of Medicine, Nursing and Health Sciences at Monash University Peninsula Campus, Frankston, Victoria, Australia

Natalie Roche is Lecturer of Occupational Therapy with the School of Allied Health Faculty of Health Sciences at Australian Catholic University, Melbourne, Victoria, Australia

Jade Ryall is currently working with The National Aboriginal and Torres Strait Islander Occupational Therapy Network, (NATSIOTN)

Ashleigh Ryan is currently working with The National Aboriginal and Torres Strait Islander Occupational Therapy Network (NATSIOTN)

Justin Scanlan is Senior Lecturer and Undergraduate Course Director, Division of Occupational Therapy, Faculty of Health Sciences, University of Sydney—Cumberland Campus, Sydney, New South Wales, Australia

Mandy Stanley is Associate Professor with the School of Medical and Health Sciences at Edith Cowan University, Perth, Western Australia, Australia

Merrill Turpin is Senior Lecturer of Occupational Therapy with the School of Health and Rehabilitation Services at The University of Queensland, Brisbane, Queensland, Australia

Carolyn Unsworth is Professor and Discipline Lead of Occupational Therapy with the Occupational Therapy Department, School of Health, Federation University Australia, Gippsland, Victoria, Australia

Kylie Vogt is Senior Occupational Therapist and Falls Liaison Officer with Southern Community Falls Prevention Team, Southern Adelaide Local Health Network (SALHN), Adelaide, South Australia, Australia

Anita Volkert is National Manager Professional Practice at Occupational Therapy Australia, Fitzroy, Victoria, Australia

Kylie Wales is Lecturer in the Discipline of Occupational Therapy with the School of Health Sciences at The University of Newcastle, Callaghan, New South Wales, Australia

Carolynne White is Participation and Engagement Advisor with Mind Australia Limited, Heidelberg, Victoria, Australia

Gail Whiteford is Strategic Professor and Conjoint Chair with the Department of Allied Health and Community Well-being at Charles Sturt University/NSW Health, Albury, New South Wales, Australia

Alison Wicks is Adjunct Associate Professor at the University of Canberra, Australian Capital Territory, Australia

Sarah Wilkes-Gillan is Lecturer in the Discipline of Occupational Therapy with the Faculty of Medicine and Health at the University of Sydney, Sydney, New South Wales, Australia

Mong-Lin Yu is Lecturer and Fieldwork Program Coordinator (Clinical Placements) & International Student Coordinator with the Department of Occupational Therapy at Monash University—Peninsula Campus, Frankston, Victoria, Australia

Abbreviations

ACAS	Aged Care Assessment Services
ACAT	Aged Care Assessment Teams
ADHD	Attention Deficit Hyperactivity Disorder
ADL	activities of daily living
AHPs	allied health professionals
AHPRA	Australian Health Practitioner Regulation Agency
AHRG	Allied Health Rural Generalist
AIHW	Australian Institute of Health and Welfare
AMPS	*Assessment of Motor and Process Skills*
AOPA	Australian Orthotic Prosthetic Association
AOTCS	*Australian Occupational Therapy Competency Standards*
AOTJ	*Australian Occupational Therapy Journal*
APA	Australian Physiotherapy Association
ARC	Australian Research Council
ARIA+	Accessibility and Remoteness Index
ASD	autism spectrum disorder
ASGC-RA	Australian Standard Geographical Classification—Remoteness Areas
ASOS	Australasian Society of Occupational Scientists
AUSLAN	Australian Sign Language
BADLs	basic activities of daily living
CALD	culturally and linguistically diverse
CAPs	Critically Appraised Papers
CASP	Critical Appraisal Skills Programme
CCMHT	*The Calgary Cambridge Model of History Taking*
CEO	Chief Executive Officer
CIMT	Constraint-Induced Movement Therapy
CINAHL	Cumulative Index to Nursing and Allied Health Literature
CMOP-E	Canadian Model of Occupational Performance and Engagement
COAG	Council of Australian Governments
CO-OP	Cognitive Orientation to Daily Occupational Performance
COPE	Care of People with Dementia in their Environments
COPM	*Canadian Occupational Performance Measure*
COSA	*Child Occupation Self-Assessment*
COSMIN	COnsensus-based Standards for the selection of health Measurement INstruments

CPD	continuing professional development
CPPF	*Canadian Practice Process Framework*
CTT	Classical Test Theory
CUES	Curtin University Empathy Simulator
CVA	cerebrovascular accidents
DALYs	Disability-Adjusted Life Years
DCD	Developmental Coordination Disorder
DIDO	drive in drive out
EBP	Evidence-based practice
ECEI	Early Childhood Early Intervention
FBT	Family Based Treatment
FDM	Fused Deposition Modelling
FIFO	fly in fly out
FIM	*Functional Independence Measure*
FOR	frames of reference
FOTARA	Fellow of the Occupational Therapy Australia Research Academy
GCC	Gulf Christian College
GEM	graduate-entry masters
GP	General Practitioner
HiAP	'Health in All Policies'
HMHF	Healthy Mothers Healthy Families
IALDs	instrumental activities of daily living
ICF	*International Classification of Functioning, Health and Disability*
IEP	Individual Education Plan
IPE	inter-professional practice education
IRT	Item Response Theory
ISOS	International Society for Occupational Science
JCU	James Cook University
LGBTIQ	lesbian, gay, bisexual, transgender, intersex and queer
LHNs	Local Hospital Networks
MICRRH	Mount Isa Centre for Rural and Remote Health
MMM	Modified Monash Model
MOHO	Model of Human Occupation
MOHOST	*Model of Human Occupation Screening Tool*
MRI	Magnetic Resonance Imaging
NATSIOTN	National Aboriginal and Torres Strait Islander Occupational Therapy Network
NDA	National Disability Agreement
NDIA	National Disability Insurance Agency
NDIS	National Disability Insurance Scheme
NHMRC	National Health and Medical Research Council
NHRA	National Health Reform Agreement
NRAS	National Registration and Accreditation Scheme
OECD	Organisation for Economic Co-operation and Development
OLT	Office for Learning and Teaching
O&M	Orientation and Mobility
OPI	occupational performance issue

OPICs	occupational performance issues or challenges
OPMA	Occupational Performance Model (Australia)
OPPM	Occupational Performance Process Model
OTA	Occupational Therapy Australia
OTARF	Occupational Therapy Australia Research Foundation
OTBA	Occupational Therapy Board of Australia
OTC	Occupational Therapy Council of Australia Ltd
OTD	Occupational Therapy Clinical Doctorate
OTIPM	Occupational Therapy Intervention Process Model
OTPF-III	Occupational Therapy Practice Framework—third edition
PADLs	personal activities of daily living
PAR	Participatory Action Research
PEDI	*Pediatric Evaluation of Disability Inventory*
PEDICAT	*Pediatric Evaluation of Disability Inventory Computer Adapted Test*
PEO	Person–Environment–Occupation
PHNs	Primary Health Networks
PICO	Participants, Intervention, Comparison, Outcome
RCT	randomised controlled trial
ROAM	Remote Orientation & Mobility
SCED	Single Case Experimental Design
SLES	School Leaver Employment Supports
SLS	Selective Laser Sintering
SMART	Specific, Measurable, Achievable, Realistic, and Timely
SPI	Structural-Personal Interaction
STC	Sydney Training Centre
TAFE	Technical and Further Education
TCM	Traditional Chinese Medicine
TCP	Transition Care Programs
WFOT	World Federation of Occupational Therapists
WHO	World Health Organization
WWIA	Working with Indigenous Australians
UDRH	University Departments of Rural Health
USC	University of Southern California

Part I
The Australian context

1 An introduction to occupational therapy in an Australian context

Helen Bourke-Taylor, Ted Brown, Stephen Isbel, Reinie Cordier and Louise Gustafsson

Chapter objectives

Upon completion of this chapter, the reader will be able to:

- Describe the structure of this book and the intended purpose and audience.
- Explain the rationale behind an Australian-specific occupational therapy textbook.
- Provide an overview of the relevant Australian population trends related to occupational therapy, according to recent statistical and governmental data.
- Present contemporary workforce trends in occupational therapy.
- Discuss the occupational therapy profession and how this textbook is situated within the Australian context of an evolving, evidence-based responsive profession.

Key terms

occupational therapy; Australia; Australian population; health care

Introduction

You may be an occupational therapy student at the beginning of a degree that will launch your career as a registered occupational therapist. You may be a recent graduate, a practitioner or an overseas trained professional seeking knowledge and skills to practise within the Australian context. You may be an educator charged with responsibilities to create and deliver contemporary curricula within the Australian context. Whoever you are, we invite you to peruse this edited textbook. The book has been designed and written by current experts in the field, both to inform you about the occupational therapy context in Australia and to inspire you!

As defined by the World Federation of Occupational Therapists (WFOT), occupational therapy is a:

> client-centred health profession concerned with promoting health and well-being through occupation. The primary goal of occupational therapy is to enable people to participate in the activities of everyday life. Occupational therapists achieve this outcome by working with people and communities to enhance their ability to engage in the occupations they want to, need to, or are expected to do, or by modifying the occupation or the environment to better support their occupational engagement.
>
> (WFOT, 2012, p. 1)

Occupational therapy is a profession that has evolved in response to the occupational, health and social needs and concerns of Australians across the lifespan. In this chapter we will provide an overview of the order, content and Australian context of the book. After describing the structure of this book, we provide a brief overview of contemporary Australians: who we are and how we live; where we live and work; and how we experience health, ability and disability. Finally, we will present current data about practising occupational therapists in Australia. According to this structure, this chapter is divided into three sections with representative headings.

1. Overview of book structure

This edited book aims to provide an overview of occupational therapy practice and professional issues within an Australian context. This is the second edition of the first comprehensive Australian occupational therapy edited textbook that brings together practice and context issues common to the profession in Australia. The book has been written by Australian authors for use by Australian occupational therapy students and practitioners. The book does not provide in-depth chapters on specific occupational therapy speciality practice areas—such as physical disabilities, paediatrics, mental health, vocational rehabilitation or hand therapy—since comprehensive texts on these topics already exist and are frequently prescribed by educators and academics for use by students. Rather, this book aims to provide a unique Australian perspective on occupational therapy professional and practice issues at an introductory level. It is designed to be a comprehensive text for students to access information about the occupational therapy profession in Australia.

The book is divided into three parts. Each of the parts has chapters written by small teams of authors. Woven throughout the book are chapters and sections of chapters that highlight the unique features of occupational therapy practice and issues pertinent to occupational therapy as a profession in Australia.

The first part addresses foundational issues and includes chapters on the Australian health care and education systems, the history of occupational therapy in Australia, ethical and legal responsibilities of occupational therapy practice, the role of professional associations and regulatory bodies, the scope of practice of occupational therapists in Australia, values and philosophy of occupational therapy, and health promotion and health literacy. The second part focuses on occupational therapy issues of a broad professional nature, including skills for effective communication, client-centred practice, occupational science, education of occupational therapists, evidence-based practice, occupational therapy research, clinical reasoning and commonly used practice models. The third part of the book presents practice issues, including the environment, the occupational therapy practice process, occupation analysis, occupational therapy practice areas, age groups that occupational therapists work with, and clinical practice areas. Activity, task and occupational analysis and specific types of occupation (e.g., self-care, productivity, education, leisure, play, rest, sleep and social participation) will be discussed.

The practice issues section also covers such topics as rural and remote occupational therapy practice, a strengths-based approach for working with Aboriginal and Torres Strait Islander communities, and assessment tools developed by Australian occupational therapists. Other chapters in this part include emerging practice areas in occupational therapy and primary health care, and entrepreneurship, leadership and advocacy in the occupational therapy profession. Each chapter provides an overview, keywords, specific chapter objectives and review questions for the reader to consider. Educators will find the PowerPoints associated with each chapter useful and a good foundation for presentations based on the chapter.

The following section presents an overview of characteristics and defining features of the Australian population. After all, occupational therapy is a profession that has historically served, and will continue to serve, many different people in Australian communities for years to come. The next section addresses questions of interest to occupational therapy practitioners, educators and researchers: *Who are Australians? How and where do they live? What are the main health issues? What occupational therapy services are needed?*

2. Contemporary Australians: Who we are, how we live and work and how we experience health and disability

Who we are

There are over 25.6 million people living in Australia (Australian Bureau of Statistics [ABS], 2020a) with projections estimating that our population size will reach more than 42 million by 2066, (ABS, 2018). Around 3.3 per cent of Australians identify as Aboriginal or Torres Strait Islander, which constitutes around 800,000 people (ABS, 2019a). The three most populous states where Aboriginal and Torres Strait Islanders live are: New South Wales (33 per cent), Queensland (28 per cent) and Western Australia (13 per cent). Although the Northern Territory (NT) is home to 9 per cent of Indigenous Australians, the NT has the highest proportion per regional population of Indigenous Australians (30 per cent) (ABS, 2019a). Aboriginal and Torres Strait Islander people reside mainly in inner and outer regional areas (44 per cent), then cities (37 per cent) and a smaller population in remote and very remote areas (19 per cent) (ABS, 2019a). The occupational therapy profession in Australia is dedicated to an appropriate response to the health, well-being and occupational needs of this important group of first Australians through overt requirements in the Australian Occupational Therapy Competency Standards (AOTCS) implemented in 2019 (Occupational Therapy Board of Australia, 2018).

Australia has diverse family constellations, cultures and dynamics and occupational therapists include the perspectives of Australian families as they engage in family-centred practice in virtually every area of practice. Australia is a diverse nation with 300 ancestries and languages and 100 different religions (ABS, 2017). About 20 per cent of the population were born in Australia, but with one or both parents born overseas (second generation Australian) and 27 per cent of the population were born overseas and residing in Australia (first generation Australians). According to the Australian Bureau of Statistics, first generation Australians come from many countries to live in Australia, the more common being the United Kingdom (15 percent); China (8.3 percent); and India (7.4 percent) (ABS, 2017). With so many Australians born overseas, it is not surprising that one in five Australians speaks a language other than English at home. English remains the most common language, being the primary language in nearly 81 per cent of households. These figures are relevant to occupational therapists due to the need to work with clients who are culturally and linguistically diverse, regardless of whether the person was born overseas or has parents and a family culture that has originated overseas.

In 2016, 49 per cent of families consisted of two adults and children; 21 per cent were couples without children; 12 per cent were single parent families; 9 per cent lived alone; and 4 per cent were adults in a group living arrangement (ABS, 2019b). While about 80 per cent of families with children under 15 years are two–parent homes, 18 per cent have a single mother as head of the household and 3 per cent have a single father as head of the household (ABS, 2019b). The median age of the eldest child was nine, and the median age of the younger child was six (ABS, 2019b). Among both single people and families, over 52 per cent identify as Christian, 8 per cent of the population identify as either Buddhist, Muslim, Hindu or Jewish, and 30 per cent have no religion or did not report it (ABS, 2017). Thus, with Australian citizens coming from such diverse backgrounds, culturally competent occupational therapists, as well as culturally safe interventions, are of the utmost importance for our clients and their families.

Where Australians live and who they live with is of the utmost importance to occupational therapists in many clinical specialty areas. Whether working with children, the aged, people who are recovering from illness or injury, many occupational therapists may be working to assist a person to return home from a medical or rehabilitation setting, provide home based therapy services, or home modifications to enable access and occupational performance. Occupational therapists also assist children in educational settings and employees in their work environments.

The vast majority of Australians live with other people, although one quarter of Australians now live in single person households (ABS, 2017) and the majority continue to be women over the age of 60 (de Vaus & Qu, 2015). More Australians live alone for a shorter period of time due to factors such as partnership status, marriage separation, working arrangements and spousal death (de Vaus & Qu, 2015). Seventy-two per cent of Australians live in separate (free-standing) houses, a number that has reduced consistently over the last 40 years (ABS, 2017). The reduction in part is due to increased construction of high-rise units in urban areas. High-rise units (flats or apartments in four or more storey blocks) and townhouses or detached smaller dwellings now make up 26 per cent of Australian dwellings with higher density living increasing (ABS, 2017). High-rise living is more common for younger adults rather than older people or families with children (48 per cent of people living in high-rise units were aged 18 to 35 years, compared with 25 per cent in the general population). Older Australians continue to live in free-standing homes or residential care (ABS, 2012).

Occupational therapists work with people across the lifespan and therefore the statistics about the Australian population are important. The age distribution of Australians requires a closer look to further examine the role of occupational therapy across the lifespan (see Chapter 22) and to understand trends in relation to projected occupational therapy workforce needs. Ageing Australians are a major focus for occupational therapy—providing services within hospitals, rehabilitation, aged-care and community settings. Recently, the federal government has introduced navigation and information sites such as My Aged Care (see http://www.myagedcare.gov.au/), which have been set up to support older Australians and their families. Occupational therapists also work with the very young and adolescents, providing services in early intervention centres, schools, hospitals and community centres (see Chapter 23). Occupational therapists work with adults to enable occupational participation following the development of a mental health condition, disability or medical condition that requires facilitation of occupational performance, safety and participation in environments of importance to the person.

The median age (i.e., the age at which half the population is older and half is younger) of the Australian population is increasing and was 37 years in mid-2019 (ABS, 2019b). Over the next several decades, the population ageing is projected to have implications for Australia, including: health, size of the working-age population, housing and demand for skilled labour (ABS, 2019b). Australia's population is ageing as a result of several factors: sustained low fertility or reduction in chosen family size and increasing life expectancy for both men and women (ABS, 2019b). Consequently, compared to previous decades, Australia now has proportionally fewer children under 15 years of age in the population, and a proportionally larger increase in those aged 65 and over (ABS, 2019b). For example, over the last decade, the proportion of people aged over 65 years increased from nearly 12 to 15 per cent and the proportion of people aged 85 years and older doubled from 1 per cent to 2 per cent. In the past decade, the number of children under 15 years decreased from 22 per cent to 19 per cent; these age trends are expected to continue (ABS, 2019b).

The so-called working age population in Australia is aged 15 to 64 years and constitutes 66 per cent of the population (ABS, 2019c). One concern for the Australian health and care industries is that the non-working age group population (mainly people over 65) is growing faster than the working age population (people aged 15 to 64 years) (ABS, 2019c). This fact has direct implications for occupational therapists in that the profession will need to continue to build a sustainable workforce in order to appropriately service an ageing population who are likely to value independent and supported living in the community.

Where we live and work

Occupational therapists are specialists in modifying and facilitating a more enabling environment that will improve occupational participation for people of all ages, across different geographical and physical living environments. The diversity of living circumstances across Australia attests to the necessity for occupational therapists to be professionally adaptable and flexible to collaborate and work with different clients.

Occupational therapists may work with individuals, groups or communities in any area in Australia and may be exposed to technology to deliver health services (known as eHealth or telehealth) in areas that are regional or remote. The vast majority of Australians live in cities or regional inner or outer areas. The Australian Bureau of Statistics advises that the most populous states are New South Wales with 8 million people, Victoria with 6.6 million people and Queensland with 5 million residents (ABS, 2019d). Other states and territories have a substantially lower population, as Western Australia is the next populous with just 2.6 million. More than two-thirds of Australia's population live along the east coast, in a capital city and surrounding metropolitan area, or a major city or district, for example, the Gold Coast, Newcastle, Central Coast, Wollongong, Sunshine Coast, Townsville, Geelong and Cairns (ABS, 2015). The population of residents in Perth and Adelaide continues to grow and the trend is for these figures to continue to increase with migration. The population of Australia's large cities grew at double the rate of the rest of the country. Over recent years, the largest population declines were in Australia's regional areas (Australian Institute of Health and Welfare [AIHW], 2015). While major cities are experiencing a population boom, regional cities are experiencing slower growth and rural, remote and very remote areas in Australia are facing a decline in population.

Human beings value self-care, leisure, play and productive occupations. Cultures and geographical areas vary in their lifestyle opportunities and the daily occupations of people in the community. Australians value work (paid or unpaid), leisure, independence in self-care and care of significant others. Productive occupations are valued and a responsibility for the vast number of Australian adults of working age. Therefore, occupational therapists can expect to address return to work issues with their clients when health has deteriorated, when the client has been injured at work, or when the client acquires a condition of disability that changes their work capacity.

Australians are workers. There are nearly 12 million Australians in the workforce— over 8 million full-time workers and over 3.5 million part-time workers (ABS, 2019c). The Australian unemployment rate is approximately 4.7 per cent (ABS, 2020b). Currently, there are more people who consider themselves underemployed compared with previous decades, particularly people in casual work. Where people work and the types of occupations that people engage in have changed over the decades. One hundred years ago, being a farmer, labourer, tailor or tradesman was more common. Just a decade ago, the most common occupation in Australia was sales assistant, reflecting the large number of part-time sales assistants in the labour force (ABS, 2012). At that time, men were commonly in the occupations of truck driver, electrician and retail manager. For women, common occupations were office jobs and primary school teacher (ABS, 2012). By 2017, the most common occupations were: professionals (18.2 per cent), clerical and administrative workers (11.5 per cent) and managers (10.7 per cent). The most common industry for work is currently health care and social assistance (ABS, 2019c).

How we experience health and disability

Australia is a large agricultural country providing people with access to healthy eating, active and social lifestyles and easily accessible educational choices. Australian families most frequently have healthy lifestyles consuming fresh local foods. The Australian Institute of Health and Welfare (AIHW) is the premier government organisation that collects and reports information on a wide range of health and welfare issues affecting Australians. Every second year the AIHW presents a snapshot of the nation's health, providing occupational therapists with statistics about prevalence and incidence of health issues that affected men, women, children, young people, adults and older adults. Many of these trends will be evident in the way occupational therapy practice develops and responds to population issues. The reports provide a snapshot across a broad range of subjects—from hospitals, disease and injury, and mental health, to ageing, homelessness, disability autism and child protection—and may be found at the website https://www.aihw.gov.au/reports-data/health-welfare-overview.

In a country characterised by wide-open spaces and a vast coastline, it is no wonder Australians have a love of sport, high rates of leisure participation and many recreational opportunities. Many adults have work conditions that are favourable for occupation–leisure balance, with generous full-time work conditions: more than ten public holidays and recreational leave of four weeks for full-time workers. Two-thirds of Australians participate in physical recreation and sport (ABS, 2015). Australians engage in leisure at reasonably high rates with time use studies indicating that men participate in leisure more frequently than women and men have more free time than women (ABS, 2006). Yet, in 2014–2015, when surveyed about activity participation in the past week, just over half of the population had participated in sufficient physical activity to meet

Australian Heart Foundation guidelines, that is, less than half of Australian adults are active enough (Australian Government Department of Health, 2015).

It is important to acknowledge that families develop a health culture in relation to physical activity, food and exercise. Poverty or financial strain are associated with a family health culture, and therefore while children will benefit from a healthy family culture, they are also vulnerable to impoverished living conditions (Buddelmeyer & Lixin, 2009). Although Australians are living in a plentiful country with good quality fresh foods and in a culture that values time away from work and time engaged in sport and recreation, there may be a disparity with the necessary levels of participation needed to achieve optimum health.

Australians in general experience similar exposure to lifestyle determinants for ill health as people in other developed countries. As many as 30 per cent of Australian deaths are caused by modifiable risk factors that determine health: tobacco smoking, dietary behaviour, physical activity, alcohol consumption, sexual behaviours and vaccination behaviours (AIHW, 2018). Smoking rates sit at 15 per cent and are higher in regional and remote Australia. Sixty-four per cent of Australian adults and 28 per cent of school-aged children are overweight or obese (AIHW, 2018). Only 50 per cent of Australians meet the daily requirement for servings of fruit and only 7 per cent meet the guidelines for servings of vegetables (AIHW, 2014). Occupational therapists are wholly concerned with participation in occupations, lifestyle, productive time-use and health. Therefore, we need to know about current lifestyle habits and health sequelae. The next section discusses the major long-term health conditions in Australia and some prevalent disabilities.

Australians have long life expectancy—81 years for men and nearly 85 years for women (AIHW, 2018). Further, in 2018, cardiovascular disease was the leading cause of death for men and dementia was the leading cause of death for women. The most recent National Health Survey of 2014–2015 (ABS, 2016) identified the following prevalent conditions (percentage prevalence in the Australian community in brackets):

- mental health and behavioural conditions (more than 15 per cent);
- arthritis (15 per cent);
- asthma (11 per cent);
- hypertension (11 per cent);
- high cholesterol (7 per cent);
- heart disease (5 per cent); and
- diabetes mellitus type 2 (DMT2) (5 per cent).

The AIHW estimates that around 45 per cent of the population will experience a mental health condition in their lifetime (AIHW, 2018). It is well known that mental health conditions frequently co-occur with chronic health conditions including DMT2, Chronic Obstructive Pulmonary Disease and osteoporosis, as well as being overweight or obese (AIHW, 2014; 2015; 2018). One in four Australian children and teenagers will experience a mental health condition (AIHW, 2018). Mental health is a primary area of practice for occupational therapists and the need for health workers is expected to grow (AIHW, 2014). The history of the profession finds its roots in the mental health of people living in asylums over a century ago. The methods and context of delivery of services has changed dramatically, moving from segregated institutions to community based practice. However, the needs of the community remain strong—mental health is a major health concern in Australia.

While primary medical conditions, such as those listed, are of concern to occupational therapists, the potential secondary complications of these conditions almost always require contact with an occupational therapist. When people with one or more of these medical conditions experiences hospitalisation within a rehabilitation setting, they are very likely to receive the services of an occupational therapist. For example, cerebrovascular accidents (CVA) are a potential sequelae following hypertension and high cholesterol. Each year around 52,000 people have a CVA or stroke with about 440,000 Australians currently living following a CVA (National Stroke Foundation, 2014). There are many other groups of people within the estimated 4 million Australians who have a disability, 9 per cent of whom are children (Australian Government Productivity Commission, 2011). The most prevalent disability in Australia is autism with a prevalence rate of 1 in 150 persons (AIHW, 2017)

The AIHW released a report about disability in Australia in 2019 (AIHW, 2019). About one in five Australians has a disability, although people with disabilities have lower levels of employment, health and well-being and face discrimination at higher rates (AIHW, 2019). People with disabilities are known to be a vulnerable group with regards to physical, social and mental health outcomes (AIHW, 2019). The National Disability Insurance Scheme revolutionised the lives of people under 65 years living with disability in Australia. It is expected that 460,000 people will be supported by the scheme by 2021 (AIHW, 2019). Never before have people with disability experienced a scheme offering lifetime support for achievement of social and economic participation in their communities. As a consequence, health and disability services have been heavily influencing the roll-out of the scheme and occupational therapy is a part of the package of many participant schemes. Further, there are over 2.7 million unpaid family carers in Australia and carers frequently experience their own physical, mental health and occupation needs. The National Carer strategy is a federal government initiative set up to address the needs of carers and the Carer Gateway provides a publicly available navigation portal for carers to find services such as occupational therapists (see http:// www.carergateway.gov.au/).

Further, other groups of Australians have been identified as being more vulnerable to poor health outcomes than other Australians: Indigenous people are generally less healthy and have lower life expectancy; rural and remote residents have poorer health and access to services; people with a type of disability have poorer health outcomes; prisoners are known to have higher rates of disability and mental health issues; similar challenges are reported for refugees and socio-economically disadvantaged Australians (AIHW, 2015). Although such groups report better health, they are also likely to be higher users of health services and therefore occupational therapists are likely to provide services to people from these groups as well. Identifying vulnerable groups enables the occupational therapy profession to target and tailor services to the needs of communities.

3. Practice in Australia: Who are we as a profession?

Occupational therapy in Australia has evolved from being a nursing specialty known as occupation treatments in the 1920s (see Chapter 3) to being the diverse, registered (see Chapter 11), carefully governed (see Chapter 4), research-focused and evidence-based profession it is today (see Chapters 14 and 15). Occupational therapy became a registered profession nationwide in 2012.

In line with the distribution of Australia's population in the states and territories described above, there are over 22,000 practising registered occupational therapists working across the country with distribution approximately as follows: 28 per cent in New South Wales; 25 per cent in Victoria; 20 per cent in Queensland; 14 per cent in Western Australia; 8 per cent in South Australia; 2 per cent in the Australian Capital Territory; 1.5 per cent in Tasmania; and 1 per cent in the Northern Territory (Occupational Therapy Board of Australia, 2019). Further, 50 per cent of registered occupational therapists were under the age of 35 years and 91.5 per cent were female. The following were the most common areas of practice for professionals (percentage distribution in practice area): 20 per cent in rehabilitation; 17 per cent in paediatrics; 16 per cent in aged care; and 12 per cent in mental health (AIHW, 2013).

The job market for occupational therapists follows population needs and Australia's areas of need are clear. We already see emerging occupation-based practice areas to address newer practice areas related to refugee health and well-being, carer health, mental health and vulnerable populations. Technology has become a part of everyday practice within the practice, with moves towards telehealth evident in response to the COVID-19 pandemic of 2020. Technology and assistive devices are featured in Chapter 24. Occupational therapy students increasingly complete project fieldwork placements and fieldwork in non-traditional or emerging practice areas. Such valuable experiences create awareness of current needs and build creativity, thus equipping incoming occupational therapy professionals to respond to the ever-changing needs of the Australian population.

Conclusion

This book provides a detailed view of occupational therapy in Australia. As editors we aim to inspire, inform and encourage readers to embrace the complexities of the profession and commit to further growth so that all Australians, whether residing in major cities, regional or remote areas, will have access to occupational therapy services when they need it. We believe that occupational therapy is a profession with a strong track record of providing innovative and evidence-based practice. Embedded within our professional identity is a nascent potential to continue to expand on areas of practice aimed at being responsive to the needs of the Australian population and thereby improving people's lives.

Summary

- The book is a comprehensive text with three well-defined parts containing representational chapters.
- Australia has unique geography, population characteristics and distribution and occupational therapy practitioners are well placed to serve the country.
- The Australian population is growing, has an ageing element and many individuals with health conditions and disabilities who may select occupational therapy services across their lifespan.
- There are many sub-populations and areas of practice for occupational therapists to specialise in and provide evidence informed and responsive service now and as Australia progresses into the future.

Review questions

1. How large is Australia's population and describe the terms: working age population, third generation Australian and most populous states in relation to the current population trends?
2. What are the most prevalent health conditions in Australia and which sub-populations are at higher risk?
3. What is the most common health condition in Australia and what proportion of Australians seek health related services?
4. How many occupational therapists practice in Australia and what are the three most common areas of practice?

References

Australian Bureau of Statistics. (2006). *Time use on recreation and leisure activities, 2006*. Cat. no. 4173.0. https://www.ausstats.abs.gov.au/Ausstats/subscriber.nsf/0/91FB93C8E82F220C CA25771F0018AE29/$File/41730_2006.pdf

Australian Bureau of Statistics. (2012). *Australian social trends, April 2013*. Cat. no. 4102.0. https://www.abs.gov.au/AUSSTATS/abs@.nsf/Previousproducts/4102.0Main%20 Features1April%202013

Australian Bureau of Statistics. (2015). *Participation in sport and physical recreation, Australia, 2013–14*. Cat. no. 4177.0. https://www.abs.gov.au/ausstats/abs@.nsf/mf/4177.0

Australian Bureau of Statistics. (2016). *National health survey: First Results 2014–15*. Cat. no. 4364.0.55.001. https://www.abs.gov.au/AUSSTATS/abs@.nsf/DetailsPage/4364.0.55.0012014-15?OpenDocument

Australian Bureau of Statistics. (2017). *Census of population and housing: Australia revealed, 2016, Cultural diversity*. Cat. no. 2024.0. https://www.abs.gov.au/ausstats/abs@.nsf/mf/2024.0

Australian Bureau of Statistics. (2018). *Population projections, Australia, 2017 (base) to 2066*. Cat. no. 3222.0. https://www.abs.gov.au/ausstats/abs@.nsf/latestProducts/3222.0Media%20 Release12017%20(base)%20-%202066

Australian Bureau of Statistics. (2019a). *Estimates and projections, Aboriginal and Torres Strait Islander Australians, 2006 to 2031*. Cat. no. 3238.0. https://www.abs.gov.au/ausstats/abs@.nsf/ Products/C19A0C6E4794A3FACA257CC900143A3D?opendocument#:~:text=The%20 population%20of%20Aboriginal%20and,%25%20and%202.3%25%20per%20year

Australian Bureau of Statistics. (2019b). *Household and family projections, Australia, 2016 to 2041*. Cat. no. 3236. https://www.abs.gov.au/ausstats/abs@.nsf/mf/3236.0#:~:text=In%20 2041%2C%20there%20are%20projected,of%20all%20household%20in%202041

Australian Bureau of Statistics. (2019c). *Jobs in Australia, 2011–12 to 2016–17*. Cat. no. 6160.0. https://www.abs.gov.au/ausstats/abs@.nsf/mf/6160.0

Australian Bureau of Statistics. (2019d). *Australian demographic statistics, June 2019*. Cat. no. 3101. https://www.abs.gov.au/ausstats/abs@.nsf/mf/3101.0

Australian Bureau of Statistics. (2020a). *Population clock*. https://www.abs.gov.au/ausstats/abs@. nsf/0/1647509ef7e25faaca2568a900154b63

Australian Bureau of Statistics. (2020b). *Labour force, Australia, December 2019*. Cat. no. 6202.0. https://www.abs.gov.au/ausstats/abs@.nsf/mf/6202.0

Australian Government Department of Health. (2015). *Australia's physical activity and sedentary behaviour guidelines*. https://www1.health.gov.au/internet/main/publishing.nsf/content/F01F 92328EDADA5BCA257BF0001E720D/$File/brochure%20PA%20Guidelines_A5_18-64yrs.PDF

Australian Government Productivity Commission. (2011). *Disability care and support. Report no. 54: final inquiry report.* https://www.pc.gov.au/inquiries/completed/disability-support/report

Australian Institute of Health and Welfare. (2013). *Allied health workforce 2012.* http://www.aihw.gov.au/WorkArea/DownloadAsset.aspx?id=60129544590

Australian Institute of Health and Welfare. (2014). *Australia's health 2014.* Australia's health series no. 14. https://www.aihw.gov.au/reports/australias-health/australias-health-2014/contents/table-of-contents

Australian Institute of Health and Welfare. (2015). *Australia's welfare 2015—in brief.* Australia's welfare no. 12. https://www.aihw.gov.au/reports/australias-welfare/australias-welfare-2015/contents/table-of-contents

Australian Institute of Health and Welfare. (2017). *Autism in Australia.* Cat. no: WEB 187. https://www.aihw.gov.au/reports/disability/autism-in-australia/contents/autism

Australian Institute of Health and Welfare. (2018). *Australia's health 2018.* Cat. no: AUS 221. https://www.aihw.gov.au/reports/australias-health/australias-health-2018/contents/table-of-contents

Australian Institute of Health and Welfare. (2019). *People with disability in Australia.* Cat. no: DIS 72. https://www.aihw.gov.au/reports/disability/people-with-disability-in-australia/summary

Buddelmeyer, H., & Lixin, C. (2009, July 16–17). *Interrelated dynamics of health and poverty in Australia* [Paper presentation]. 2009 The Household Income Labour Dynamics in Australia (HILDA) Survey Research Conference, Melbourne, Vic., Australia. https://melbourneinstitute.unimelb.edu.au/assets/documents/hilda-bibliography/hilda-conference-papers/2009/Cai,-Lixin_paper.pdf

de Vaus, D., & Qu, L. (2015). *The nature of living alone in Australia (Australian Family Trends No. 9).* Australian Institute of Family Studies. https://aifs.gov.au/publications/nature-living-alone-australia

National Stroke Foundation. (2014). *Stroke in Australia: No postcode untouched.* National Stroke Foundation. https://strokefoundation.org.au/What-we-do/Research/Research-resources/No-postcode-untouched

Occupational Therapy Board of Australia. (2018). *Australian occupational therapy competency standards 2018.* https://www.occupationaltherapyboard.gov.au/Codes-Guidelines/Competencies.aspx

Occupational Therapy Board of Australia. (2019). *Occupational therapy registrant data.* http://www.occupationaltherapyboard.gov.au/About/Statistics.aspx

World Federation of Occupational Therapists. (2012). WFOT statement of occupational therapy. https://wfot.org/about-occupational-therapy

2   Australia's health and health care system

Stephen Isbel, Maggie Jamieson and Craig Greber

Chapter objectives

Upon completion of this chapter, the reader will be able to:

*   Provide an overview of the Australian health care system.
*   Describe major health challenges for Australians.
*   Describe how health care is funded in Australia.
*   Appreciate how the social determinants of health affect Australians.
*   Understand some of the areas where occupational therapists work.

Key terms

health policy; Australian Government; health funding; primary health care; secondary health care; Medicare; Aboriginal and Torres Strait Islander health; social determinants of health

Introduction

Australia's health care system is well regarded around the world with health outcomes, timely access to required services, facilities and funding comparing favourably to other Organisation for Economic Co-operation and Development (OECD) member countries (OECD, 2019). The system has different components including primary health care (community-based) and secondary health care (hospitals and specialist services), supported by a variety of regulatory, surveillance and professional organisations (Australian Institute of Health and Welfare [AIHW], 2018). The system is complex with different levels of government providing funding and oversight depending on the services being delivered. Some health care services are also delivered via a privately funded parallel system. Occupational therapists contribute to the health of Australians by providing services to all components of the system utilising all levels of government funding to a diverse range of individuals, groups and communities.

The Australian Government and health care

Australia has a federated system of government meaning that a central government (the Commonwealth) oversees the partially self-governing regions (States and Territories). This type of government requires each tier to cooperate in financing and delivering fundamental and essential services such as health (Duckett & Wilcox, 2015). Health care in Australia is funded in parts by most tiers of government and from private sources (such as private health insurance). The Commonwealth has the responsibility of administering the universal health insurance program (referred to as Medicare) and the Pharmaceutical Benefits Scheme. Hospital-based services are provided by the States and Territories with the Commonwealth contributing to the costs of running hospitals, primary health care and other recurrent costs. Private health care services, hospitals and aged care facilities are run by independent organisations but also receive some funding from the Commonwealth Government.

The Commonwealth contributes funds to the States and Territories for medical services and primary care, while the States are responsible for hospital service delivery and community health services such as mental health support and immunisation. Separation of responsibility and function makes the development of comprehensive, coordinated national policies and service provision difficult. This means that a government may make decisions about one part of the system without understanding the resultant implications for the other parts (National Health and Hospitals Reform Commission, 2009).

The health of Australians

Chapter 1 provided an overview of the health, living circumstances and some characteristics of Australians. This section provides an overview of life expectancy, health disparities and some of the social determinants of health as a precursor to describing and explaining the health care system. Australia is a diverse nation geographically, culturally, socially and regarding health status. Many communities live alongside each other and have a unique and often highly individualised sense of identity. It is important to recognise that Australia is diverse, the communities within Australia are diverse, and that diversity is acknowledged, celebrated and also accommodated within the health care system. In this chapter, the Aboriginal and Torres Strait Islander peoples provide an example of a unique community.

Life expectancy

Australia rates ninth for males (80.5 years) and ninth for females (84.6 years) in the member countries of the OECD (OECD, 2019). The most common causes of death in Australia are coronary heart disease, dementia and Alzheimer's disease, cerebrovascular disease, lung cancer and chronic respiratory diseases (Australian Bureau of Statistics [ABS], 2018a).

Aboriginal and Torres Strait Islander people

Aboriginal and Torres Strait Islander people are the indigenous peoples of Australia. Henceforth, Aboriginal and Torres Strait Islander people may also be described as Indigenous. Indigenous Australians are a diverse community and cannot be easily summed into a group with common characteristics, views, cultural beliefs and ways of living. Similarly, the health of Indigenous Australians including rates of chronic disease and the factors impacting health status cannot be summed in a few short paragraphs. Health statistics are documented according to the available data that tends to be reported in averages. Statistical averages do not capture the diversity within communities, cultural groups or people and nullify the diversity. In other words, diversity of peoples does not fit within the normal distribution of a bell curve. However, averages are how health and life factors are reported in government documents and some of these statistics will be presented here to illustrate some differences within the Australian community.

In 2016 there were approximately 798,000 people who identified as Aboriginal and Torres Strait Islander people (ABS, 2019a). Around 19 per cent of Aboriginal and Torres Strait Islander people live in remote and very remote areas, 44 per cent in regional areas and 37 per cent in major cities. Indigenous Australians have an overall younger profile than non-Indigenous Australians. For example, in 2016, 34 per cent of Aboriginal and Torres Strait Islander people were under the age of 15 compared to 18 per cent of non-Aboriginal and Torres Strait Islander people (AIHW, 2018). A further difference to non-Aboriginal and Torres Strait Islander people is the higher rates of co-habitation of multiple families, which was 5.1 per cent of Aboriginal and Torres Strait Islander people compared to 1.8 per cent of other families (ABS, 2017).

As described in Chapter 3, previous historical events, policies and approaches continue to influence the health and occupations of many Indigenous Australians. As health practitioners, it is important that occupational therapy students and practitioners resist imposing stereotypes or preconceptions on any person, group, community or organisation, remaining open and culturally sensitive to differences so that collaborations may be respectful and appropriate. Understanding historical factors may assist a deeper appreciation of the perspectives, viewpoints and health of many Aboriginal and Torres Strait Islander peoples.

Historical factors

The historical treatment of Aboriginal and Torres Strait Islander people explains some of the disparities seen in the demographic profile and health status when compared to non-Aboriginal and Torres Strait Islander people. Prior to European colonisation, Aboriginal and Torres Strait Islander people had been living in Australia for 50,000–120,000 years (Working with Indigenous Australian [WWIA], 2017). At the time of colonisation, it was estimated that about 500 Indigenous dialects existed and between 300,000 and 950,000 people existed in Australia (WWIA, 2017). However, due to disease, genocide and forced relocation, as much as 90 per cent of the Indigenous population died within ten years of European settlement (Harris, 2003). Aboriginal and Torres Strait Islander people had little representation in colonised Australia, only receiving the right to vote in elections in 1962. Compelled assimilation of Aboriginal and Torres Strait Islander people was the policy of the Australian Government up until 1962 meaning that many were forced from their traditional lands onto 'missions' (Australians Together, 2020). Another part of this policy was that many children from the Aboriginal and Torres Strait Islander community were taken away from their families under duress as a form of forced assimilation and integration (Australians Together, 2020). These are only some examples of historical events that continue to have long-term impacts that have resulted in social, economic, education and health inequalities for many people.

The health and well-being of Aboriginal and Torres Strait Islander people: Closing the gap

Generally speaking, compared to other Australians, Aboriginal and Torres Strait Islander people have poorer health and well-being on many indicators such as life expectancy, child mortality, incarceration, engagement in education and employment. Strong leadership from within the Aboriginal and Torres Strait Islander communities across Australia and advocacy by numerous experts from the medical, education, social, judicial and other sectors has resulted in policies and long-term strategies to enable both self-determination and ways to promote the health, lifestyle and cultural security and freedom of this population.

In response to the gap in health and well-being, the Commonwealth Government has set an agenda called 'Closing the Gap' (Commonwealth Government of Australia, 2020) which aims to achieved equality in a range of health, economic, education and social indicators within a generation. The key indicators in the strategy are: child mortality, early childhood education, school attendance, literacy and numeracy, year 12 attainment, employment and life expectancy. Results have been mixed with targets largely being met in early childhood education, partially met in year 12 or equivalent completions but unmet in school attendance, life expectancy, literacy and numeracy, and employment. Figure 2.1 shows that while the child mortality rate has been declining, there is still a significant gap between Indigenous and non-Indigenous Australians.

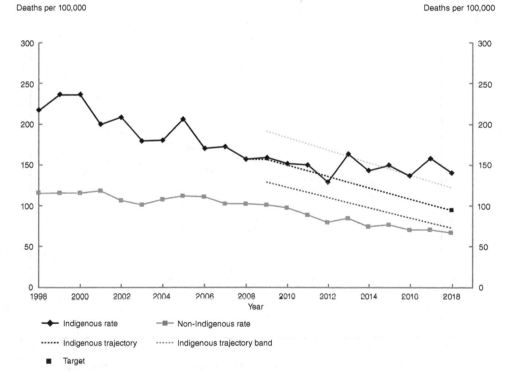

Figure 2.1 Child mortality rates, 0–4 years old, 1998–2018.
Source: Commonwealth Government of Australia, 2020

Figure 2.2 shows the upward trajectory of early childhood enrolment rates of Indigenous children. The target to have 95 percent of Indigenous four-year-olds in early childhood by 2025 is on track to be met.

The life expectancy for Indigenous males in 2015–2017 was 71.6 years and 75.6 years for Indigenous females compared to 80.2 years for non-Indigenous males and 83.4 years for non-Indigenous females (ABS, 2018b) (see Figure 2.3). The target to close the life expectancy gap is not on target. Mortality data is available each year (compared to life expectancy data which is available every five years). While the Indigenous mortality rates have improved, the gap has still not narrowed and the target in this area has not been met.

Strengths-based approach for engagement

Whilst the strengthening and sustained work within and outside Aboriginal and Torres Strait Islander organisations and communities show a gradual improvement in the health of Indigenous people, there is clearly more progress to be made. The ongoing health disparity and the slow progress in closing the gap has been a frustration for the Aboriginal and Torres Strait Islander community and successive governments. Strengths-based approaches that acknowledge the skills, experience, beliefs, values, wisdom and resilience of Aboriginal and Torres Strait Islander people are proposed to successfully

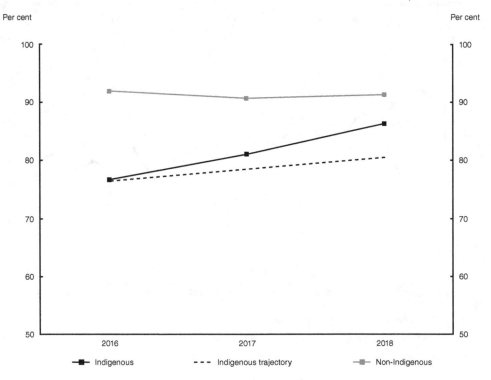

Figure 2.2 Early childhood education enrolment rates, 2016–2018.
Source: Commonwealth Government of Australia, 2020

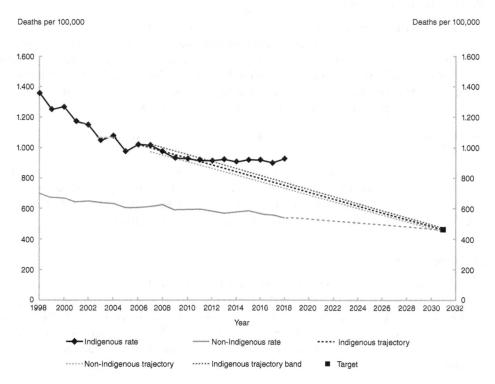

Figure 2.3 Age standardised mortality rates, trajectory to 2031 target.
Source: Commonwealth Government of Australia, 2020

engage communities with interventions aimed at closing the gap (Calma & Dick, 2007). Chapter 11 of this textbook proposes one way for occupational therapists to engage in a positive strength based approach with members of the Aboriginal and Torres Strait Islander community and how this may be implemented in practice to promote self-determination, cultural security and freedom, health, lifestyle and well-being. This approach is proposed by Indigenous Australians who are also expert occupational therapists.

Social determinants of health in Australia

The conditions in which people live and work or their social environment are related to health. The social determinants of health are shaped by factors such as employment, education, power and social support. The World Health Organization defines the social determinants of health as: 'The social determinants of health are the conditions in which people are born, grow, live, work and age. These circumstances are shaped by the distribution of money, power and resources at global, national and local levels." (World Health Organization, n.d.)

In Australia, the social determinants of health highlight some important differences that some groups experience. The following describes some key statistics examining some of the social determinants of health in Australia.

Socio-economic position

Socio-economic position is determined largely determined by level of education, income and occupation. In 2019, 68 per cent of Australians aged 20–64 had a non-school qualification and 33 per cent in this age group had a bachelor's degree (ABS, 2019b). Average household wealth in Australia passed 1 million dollars in 2017–2018 but with some clear disparity between groups, meaning the lowest 20 per cent of households controlled just 1 per cent of all household wealth (ABS, 2019c).

Early life

Conditions before birth and in the first years of life influence health and well-being into adult life. In Australia in 2015, 22 per cent of children starting primary school were assessed as being vulnerable in one or more developmental areas including language, cognition, communication and emotional maturity (AIHW, 2018).

Social exclusion

Social exclusion occurs when people are not able to equally access the resources, opportunity participation and skills (McLachlan et al., 2013) and this often results in poor health. About 4.3 million people in Australia experience some form of social exclusion including specific groups such as people over the age of 65, Aboriginal and Torres Strait Islander people and people with a disability (Brotherhood of St Laurence & Melbourne Institute, 2017).

Employment and work

Being employed is important not only for earning an income but for the self-identity and purpose that it brings and conversely being unemployed has a detrimental effect on health and well-being. In March 2020, 5.2 per cent of Australians were unemployed with 8.7 per cent of Australians reporting being underemployed (ABS, 2020).

Housing and homelessness

Having access to affordable, safe and uncrowded housing is an important social determinant of health. Being homeless is associated with poor physical and mental health and increases the risk of social exclusion (AIHW, 2018). The 2016 census recorded that 116,000 people in Australia were homeless (ABS, 2018c) and that 3.8 per cent of Australians lived in overcrowded houses and this was much higher (10 per cent) in Aboriginal and Torres Strait Islander communities (AIHW, 2018).

Chronic disease

Despite a relatively high life expectancy Australian's health is adversely affected by chronic diseases. In 2014–2015 a self-reported survey reported that 50 per cent of Australians had one or more of the following conditions: cardiovascular disease, back pain, chronic obstructive pulmonary disease, asthma, arthritis, cancer, diabetes or mental health conditions (ABS, 2016). Many of these diseases are caused by preventable factors such as tobacco use, obesity, dietary risks and high blood pressure (AIHW, 2019a) and continue to be a focus for all levels of government to address. There are numerous community-based programs in Australia that aim to address the preventable factors contributing to chronic disease. Occupational therapists have a key role in assisting people to engage in healthy lifestyles and occupations and these interventions can be accessed through health care plans managed by general practitioners and paid for through the Health Care Homes program (Australian Government, n.d.).

Primary health care

Primary health is usually the first point of service engagement and includes providers and services from across the public, private and non-government sectors (Standing Council on Health, 2014). A fundamental principle of primary health care is that collaboration is required at numerous levels between health care providers, including allied health, to meet individual health care requirements, with services being provided in multiple ways and venues including home environments. Primary health care, via general practitioners (GPs), is often the initial point of health care access but includes other professions, for example occupational therapy, physiotherapy, psychology, social work, speech therapy, nurses or dentists. Navigating the health system starts at access to primary care, yet an OECD report noted that the Australian health system is too complex for people (OECD, 2017). People are reliant on the professional providers having knowledge of the overall system which is becoming increasingly complex with calls of primary care to be strengthened, particularly around obtaining and measuring quality outcomes and establishing funding models that promote prevention and management of service provision as well as support of chronic health conditions (Calder et al., 2019).

Figure 2.4 describes the areas of primary health and how they relate to each other. Primary care acts as gatekeeper for hospital and specialist services with community-based services in supporting people and their families at home who have a health condition.

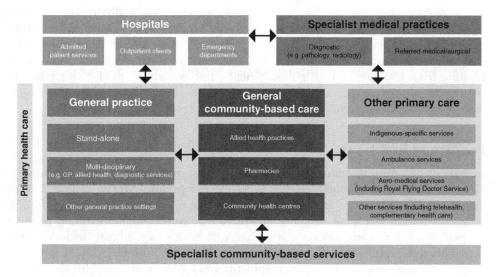

Figure 2.4 Primary health care.
Source: Australian Institute of Health and Welfare, 2014, p. 359

Secondary health care

In Australia, hospital services are provided by both public and private hospitals, accounting for 40 per cent of total health care expenditure. There are some 373,234 full-time equivalent staff employed in the hospital system. In the period 2017–2018, there were 1,350 hospitals in Australia (AIHW, 2019b) comprising: 693 public hospitals and 657 private hospitals. In 2017–2018, the 693 public hospitals in Australia provided 62,000 beds (about 2.5 beds per 1,000 people).

The numbers of hospital beds grew by 3.3 per cent per year in 2012–2013 and 2016–2017 (AIHW, 2019b). Public hospitals provide a wide range of services for those people admitted and not admitted into the hospital. There is considerable diversity in the hospital sector, from tertiary level services, in metropolitan areas to multi-purpose services in rural and remote locations. Major referral hospitals are found mainly in metropolitan areas and provided almost 38 per cent of all hospitalisations in the public system as well as 38 per cent of patient days (the number of days of admitted patient care provided) for public hospitals (AIHW, 2019b). The nature and experience of using the public hospitals have changed in the past 20 years, with increasing technology, changing surgical techniques and drives for efficiencies leading to shorter hospital lengths of stay.

In 2017–2018 there were 352,000 people who required emergency surgery with the bulk of the surgery (86 per cent) occurring in public hospitals, with the most common surgery being for appendicitis, hip fracture and heart attack (AIHW, 2019b). In the same time period there were 2.3 million admissions for elective surgery with 66 per cent of these occurring in the public hospitals commonly for addressing cataracts, malignant skin lesions and vision disorders (AIHW, 2019b).

Private hospitals

Australians who have private health insurance are able to choose to be treated in a private hospital with the doctor or specialist of their choice and for many procedures will not have to wait as long as those in the public system. Nationally, the private sector contributes a third of all hospital beds and is regulated by State Governments, through the granting of licences. The definition of public or private facility is not always clear-cut. In some instances, hospitals owned by charitable or religious organisations receive funding from the state to treat public patients, and as such are public hospitals, albeit with different governance arrangements from State-run facilities while also running their private services on the same site.

Funding of health care

In 2017–2018, Australia allocated 10 per cent of its gross domestic product (GDP) or $185 billion on health, which equates to $7,485 per person (AIHW, 2019c). The two main areas of expenditure in health are hospitals and primary health services. In 2017–2018, $74 billion was spent on public and private hospitals and $63.4 billion was spend on primary health care services. Other areas of health expenditure included capital expenditure to fund new hospitals and equipment ($9.3 billion) (AIHW, 2019c) and referred medical services that a general practitioner has recommended for their patients ($19.4 billion) (AIHW, 2019c). Figure 2.5 illustrates where funding is spent in the Australian health care system and which tier of government pays for each area. The tension

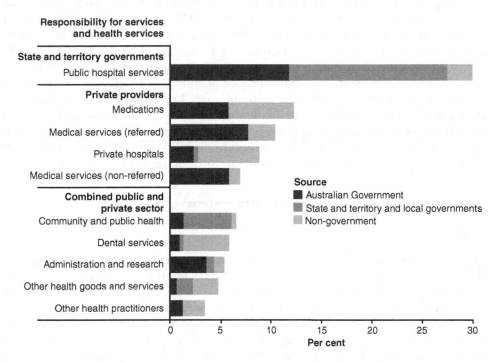

Figure 2.5 Health services—responsibility, funding sources and proportion of expenditure, 2015–2016.
Source: Australian Institute of Health and Welfare, 2018, p. 44

between health care funding and responsibility for delivering services can often lead to disagreement between the various levels of government.

Health policy in Australia

In the context of Federalism, the establishment of intergovernmental mechanisms, using State and Commonwealth agreements, has been progressed since 1992 following the establishment of the Council of Australian Governments (COAG). The COAG serves to bring together Commonwealth and State Governments to address topics in the national interest. In 2007, the COAG approved the establishment of the National Health and Hospitals Reform Commission. The reforms had at their core: i) funding changes whereby the federal government takes full public funding responsibility for primary health care and community-based care and 60 per cent of public hospital funding on an efficient activity basis; ii) governance through the establishment of Local Hospital Networks (LHNs), with a devolution of managerial accountability from State Governments; and iii) establishment of regional service coordination organisations now known as Primary Health Networks (PHNs) to better manage general practitioner (GP), specialist, hospital and community coordination as well as to work on preventive health provision. The COAG reforms also brought about a system that had policy focused on performance and accountability for efficient use of public funds to address need.

In August 2011, the National Health Reform Agreement (NHRA) (Council of Australian Governments, 2011) was signed by the COAG. The agreement detailed the shared intention of the Commonwealth, State and Territory Governments to work in partnership to improve health outcomes for all Australians and ensure the sustainability of the Australian health care system. Core elements of the agreement affirmed that other providers, both public and private providers, apart from Commonwealth and States, play a role in the delivery of health care. The NHRA established financial arrangements which aimed to improve access to services and improve public hospital efficiencies (Solomon, 2014). Medicare principles underpinned the agreement, and the agreement noted the interfaces between health, disability and aged care services. The addendum to the NHRA is currently under negotiation for the period 2020–2025.

Features of the Australian health care system

Medicare

Medicare is the universal health care scheme based upon the principle that all Australians should have equal access to health care. Medicare gives Australians access to free or subsidised health care from health professionals including doctors, optometrists and occupational therapists (Department of Human Services, 2019). For example, when consulting a general practitioner, rebates of up to 85 per cent of the scheduled Medicare fee are available, with the remaining 15 per cent the responsibility of the patient. If a doctor chooses to 'bulk bill', 85 per cent of the scheduled fee is charged to the government and the doctor receives this fee alone. However, if the doctor chooses to charge more, the patient will pay 'the gap' or the difference between the Medicare schedule and the actual consultation fee. Fee gaps can vary greatly between GP practices.

Occupational therapists can be reimbursed for their services through Medicare. For example, rebates are available for up to ten sessions provided by an allied mental health professional such as an occupational therapist, psychologist or social worker per calendar year to individuals with a mental illness (Department of Human Services, 2018). Patients need to be referred by a physician and have a detailed mental care plan in place to be able to access the rebates. Medicare-funded programs enable Australians with access to mental health programs or allied health sessions for people with chronic medical conditions. For populations such as Aboriginal and Torres Strait Islander peoples, such subsidies are doubled to address the wider health disparity that may be experienced by individuals in this population. Medicare is partially funded by an income tax levy of 2 per cent and a further 1.5 per cent for those people earning over a certain level of income per year (Australian Taxation Office, 2019).

Private health insurance

Australians eligible for Medicare are entitled to treatment as public patients in public hospitals, or they can choose to self-fund or use their private health insurance to be treated as private patients. In June 2017, 43.3 per cent of Australians had private health insurance (AIHW, 2017). In 2017, private patients (either patients using private health insurance or patients paying the full cost of their treatment directly) accounted for more than 13 per cent of all public hospital admissions with a total of 36 per cent of all admission to public and private hospitals combined (AIHW, 2017).

The National Disability Insurance Scheme

The National Disability Insurance Scheme or NDIS provides support for people with disabilities, their carers and families (Parliament of Australia, 2017). It was first trialled in 2013 and introduced across most of Australia in 2016 and is estimated to support 460,000 Australians by the end of 2020 (Parliament of Australia, 2017). The NDIS replaced the National Disability Agreement (NDA) which was described as ineffective, unfair and offered limited choice to many people with disabilities (Australian Government Productivity Commission, 2011). The premise behind the NDIS is to give people with a disability the choice and freedom to choose care and services that are reasonable and necessary. Recipients of the NDIS are able to self-manage funds that are allocated to them or they can elect to have someone manage their funds for them. For example, in many cases people with a disability require personal care assistance, transportation or equipment to be able to access their home and outside environment. Under the NDIS they can choose who provides these services as long as they are a registered provider of care. Many occupational therapists are registered providers of care which means they can charge recipients of the NDIS fees set by National Disability Insurance Agency (NDIA). Under the NDIS occupational therapists provide services such as aids and equipment, home modifications, transport assistance and mobility training (Occupational Therapy Australia, 2020).

Who delivers health care?

There are many medical, nursing allied health and support staff who deliver health care in Australia. Nurses and midwives are the largest group of registered health professionals in Australia (333,970) and are more than three times larger than the next group: medical practitioners (114,200) (Department of Health, 2018). In 2018, there were 18,447 registered occupational therapists in Australia (Department of Health, 2018). Occupational Therapists can work in public and private hospitals (secondary health care), in primary health and as private providers of non-referred medical services.

Occupational therapy in the health care system

The diverse domains of occupational therapy practice make it difficult to provide a definitive picture of how and where occupational therapists work in Australian health care. The experience of working as an occupational therapist varies by practice area, client group, employer, location, role and funding body. The diversity of roles and expanding scope of practice in occupational therapy provide opportunities for therapists to practise in both traditional and emerging domains. While traditional public sector secondary health services have long been a stronghold for occupational therapists, graduates can now expect to work in other organisations or as sole providers under the role of case managers, policy officers and rehabilitation consultants just to name a few (Broome & Gillen, 2014).

Another practice area where occupational therapists may find it challenging is working in generic, non-profession-specific mental health roles that could be filled by a nurse, psychologist, social worker or occupational therapist (Goh et al., 2019). Trying to maintain an occupational focus and professional identify can be challenging in these types of positions, particularly for new graduates. Many occupational therapists work with the growing number of ageing Australians and are remunerated through Commonwealth-funded schemes such as Medicare, My Aged Care the Department of Veterans Affairs, or directly by aged care providers. For Australians with disabilities, the National Disability Insurance Scheme (NDIS) can provide funds required to engage an occupational therapist. The NDIS is one of the most significant social policy changes in Australia in a generation and since the first trial of the NDIS in 2013, the opportunities for occupational therapists to provide services to people with disabilities has grown significantly.

Consider the experiences of two occupational therapists working differently in Australia in the following vignette highlighting some of the complexities involved with delivering occupational therapy services in Australia. In the vignette you will read about two occupational therapists who work across different areas that are administered by different levels of government. For example, the Department of Veteran's Affairs is a Commonwealth agency that sets fees for specific service which are then invoiced by the occupational therapists who provide services for veterans. The same is seen for the National Disability Insurance Scheme (NDIS) and My Aged Care (Commonwealth).

Box 2.1 Julie and Corina

Julie

Julie lives in the northern suburbs of Brisbane and works three days a week for Queensland Health. She is part of the Transition Care team that provides short-term care for older people following hospitalisation. She also works in a private practice owned by another therapist on Thursdays and Fridays, providing home-based services to clients who have DVA Gold Cards, as well as those funded through My Aged Care. Julie holds additional certification in driving assessment and also provides this service. She previously worked in acute hospital settings during her long career. She moved into Transition Care to build her skills in home modifications and adaptive equipment. Julie has attended numerous professional development events to build her skills and qualifications and is now an advanced skill occupational therapist in the area of community occupational therapy and driving assessment.

Corina

Corina runs her own private practice from a base location in Albany. She also employs two early career occupational therapists in her practice. From her base, Corina and her team provide outreach services to the Great Southern region of Western Australia. Corina uses the skills of her team to provide for a diverse range of children, adults and older people. Much of her own work is NDIS funded. This is because Corina has had 15 years' experience working with people with disabilities, having previously been employed by Disability Services and non-government organisations before the NDIS was rolled out locally. Corina did locums (temporary jobs) in mental health practice early in her career and has the skills to provide mental health OT services for clients on Medicare-funded

Mental Health Care Plans. Corina is a generalist occupational therapist who can work with a wide range of clients. She lacks experience in working with children so she addressed that shortfall when she recruited other staff. The other therapists have an interest in paediatrics and mostly work with children through NDIS funding, although occasionally the practice secures contracts with local schools to provide screening assessments and in-school services. Corina completed a small business training course when she first started her own practice and is currently enrolled in a Master of Business Administration.

Julie and Corina both enjoy their roles but are mindful of some of the challenges they face. Julie appreciates being able to work across both public and private sectors without the challenges of running her own practice. She has been able to focus on particular areas of occupational therapy and build a reputation. Her driving assessment skills are very much in demand. Managing to move between two part-time jobs is Julie's biggest challenge.

Corina enjoys the variety of her work and values the diverse skills and knowledge she holds. She relishes the autonomy of her private practice and working in rural and remote areas. Corina recognises the shortage of services for people in rural areas and understands the challenges of retaining her employees due to the amount of travel involved.

Conclusion

The Australian health care system is a complex mix of primary or community-based services, hospitals and specialist services. Funding is also complex, with various State, Territory and Commonwealth Government tiers taking responsibility for different aspects of health care delivery. Australia provides universal health care in the form of Medicare with private providers also playing a significant part in health care provision. Despite this complexity, Australians enjoy one of the best life expectancies in the OECD but there are significant health disparities between groups such as Aboriginal and Torres Strait Islander people. Challenges associated with increased health care costs, chronic diseases and the ageing population will continue to challenge the Australian health care system.

Summary

- Australia has a Federated system of government meaning cooperation at each level of government is required to fund and deliver health care.
- In general, Australians have a good health care system that compares favourably to other OECD countries.
- One of the features of the Australian health care system is Medicare, the universal health care model, allowing for affordable health care for all Australians.
- Australians have comparatively high life expectancy but challenges exist with chronic diseases and inequalities due to the social determinants of health.
- Aboriginal and Torres Strait Islander people have much poorer health compared to non-Aboriginal and Torres Strait Islanders.
- Occupational therapists have an important part to play across all parts of the health care system.

Review questions

1. Who funds the Australian health care system?
2. What are some factors that contribute to the poor health outcomes of Aboriginal and Torres Strait Islander people?
3. How do the social determinants of health relate to the health of Australians?
4. What is Medicare?
5. What is the NDIS?

References

Australian Bureau of Statistics. (2016). *National health survey: First results 2014–15*. Cat. no. 4364.0.55.001. https://www.abs.gov.au/AUSSTATS/abs@.nsf/DetailsPage/4364.0.55.0012014-15?OpenDocument

Australian Bureau of Statistics. (2017). *Census of population and housing: Reflecting Australia—stories from the Census, 2016*. Cat. no. 2071.0. https://www.abs.gov.au/ausstats/abs@.nsf/mf/2071.0

Australian Bureau of Statistics. (2018a). *Causes of death, Australia 2018*. Cat. no. 3303.0. https://www.abs.gov.au/ausstats/abs@.nsf/mf/3303.0

Australian Bureau of Statistics. (2018b). *Life tables for Aboriginal and Torres Strait Islander Australians, 2015–2017*. Cat. no. 3302.0.55.003. https://www.abs.gov.au/ausstats/abs@.nsf/mf/3302.0.55.003

Australian Bureau of Statistics. (2018c). *Census of population and housing: Estimating homelessness, 2016*. Cat. no. 2049.0. https://www.abs.gov.au/AUSSTATS/abs@.nsf/Lookup/2049.0Explanatory%20Notes12016?OpenDocument

Australian Bureau of Statistics. (2019a). *Estimates and projections, Aboriginal and Torres Strait Islander Australians, 2006 to 2031*. Cat. no. 3238.0. https://www.abs.gov.au/ausstats/abs@.nsf/Products/C19A0C6E4794A3FACA257CC900143A3D?opendocument#:~:text=The%20population%20of%20Aboriginal%20and,%25%20and%202.3%25%20per%20year

Australian Bureau of Statistics. (2019b). *Education and work, Australia, May 2019*. Cat. no. 6227.0. https://www.abs.gov.au/ausstats/abs@.nsf/mf/6227.0/#:~:text=Key%20statistics,-The%20Survey%20of&text=In%202019%3A,59%25%20or%20176%2C900%20people)

Australian Bureau of Statistics. (2019c). *Household income and wealth, Australia, 2017–2018*. Cat. no. 6523.0. https://www.abs.gov.au/ausstats/abs@.nsf/mf/6523.0

Australian Bureau of Statistics. (2020). *Labour force Australia*. Cat. no. 6202.0. https://www.abs.gov.au/ausstats/abs@.nsf/mf/6202.0

Australian Government. (n.d.). *Health care homes*. https://www.servicesaustralia.gov.au/organisations/health-professionals/subjects/health-care-homes

Australian Government Productivity Commission. (2011). *Disability and care support*. https://www.pc.gov.au/inquiries/completed/disability-support/report

Australian Institute of Health and Welfare. (2014). *Australia's health 2014*. Australia's health series no. 14. https://www.aihw.gov.au/reports/australias-health/australias-health-2014/contents/table-of-contents

Australian Institute of Health and Welfare. (2017). *Private health insurance use in Australian hospitals, 2006–07 to 2015–16: Australian hospital statistics*. Health services series no. 81. https://www.aihw.gov.au/reports/hospitals/private-health-insurance-use-hospitals/contents/table-of-contents

Australian Institute of Health and Welfare. (2018). *Australia's health 2018*. Australia's health series no. 16. https://www.aihw.gov.au/reports/australias-health/australias-health-2018/contents/table-of-contents

Australian Institute of Health and Welfare. (2019a). *Australian burden of disease study: Impact and causes of illness and death in Australia 2015*. Australian Burden of Disease series no. 19. https://www.aihw.gov.au/reports/burden-of-disease/burden-disease-study-illness-death-2015/contents/table-of-contents

Australian Institute of Health and Welfare. (2019b). *Hospital at a glance 2017–18*. https://www.aihw.gov.au/reports/hospitals/hospitals-at-a-glance-2017-18/contents/introduction

Australian Institute of Health and Welfare. (2019c). *Health expenditure Australia 2017–18*. Health and welfare expenditure series no.65. https://www.aihw.gov.au/getmedia/91e1dc31-b09a-41a2-bf9f-8deb2a3d7485/aihw-hwe-77-25092019.pdf.aspx

Australian Taxation Office. (2019). *Medicare levy*. https://www.ato.gov.au/individuals/medicare-levy/

Australians Together. (2020). *The stolen generations*. https://australianstogether.org.au/discover/australian-history/stolen-generations

Broome, K., & Gillen, A. (2014). Implications of occupational therapy job advertisement trends for occupational therapy education. *British Journal of Occupational Therapy*, 77(11), 574–581. https://doi.org/10.4276%2F030802214X14151078348558

Brotherhood of St Laurence & Melbourne Institute. (2017). Social exclusion monitor. https://www.bsl.org.au/research/social-exclusion-monitor/measuring-social-exclusion/

Calder, R., Dunkin R., Rochford C., & Nichols, T. (2019). *Australian health services: Too complex to navigate. A review of the national reviews of Australia's health service arrangements*. Australian Health Policy Collaboration, Policy Issues Paper No. 1 2019, AHPC.

Calma, T., & Dick, D. (2007). *Social determinants and the health of indigenous peoples in Australia: A human rights-based approach*. International Symposium on the Social Determinants of Indigenous Health, Adelaide. https://humanrights.gov.au/about/news/speeches/social-determinants-and-health-indigenous-peoples-australia-human-rights-based

Commonwealth Government of Australia. (2020). *Closing the Gap Report 2020*. Department of the Prime Minister and Cabinet. https://ctgreport.niaa.gov.au/

Council of Australian Governments. (2011). *National health reform agreement*. http://www.federalfinancialrelations.gov.au/content/npa/health/_archive/national-agreement.pdf

Department of Health. (2018). *Health workforce data*. https://hwd.health.gov.au/summary.html#part-1

Department of Human Services. (2018). *Better access initiative*. https://www1.health.gov.au/internet/main/publishing.nsf/Content/mental-ba

Department of Human Services. (2019). *About Medicare*. https://www.servicesaustralia.gov.au/individuals/subjects/whats-covered-medicare/about-medicare

Duckett, S., & Wilcox, S. (2015). *The Australian health care system*. Oxford University Press.

Goh, N. C. K., Hancock, N., Honey, A., & Scanlan, J. N. (2019). Thriving in an expanding service landscape: Experiences of occupational therapists working in generic mental health roles within non-government organisations in Australia. *Australian Occupational Therapy Journal*, 66(6), 753–762. https://doi.org/10.1111/1440-1630.12616

Harris, J. (2003). Hiding the bodies: The myth of the humane colonisation of Australia. *Journal of Aboriginal History*, 27, 79–104. https://doi.org/10.22459/AH.27.2011.07

McLachlan, R., Gilfillan, G., & Gordon, J. (2013). *Deep and persistent disadvantage in Australia*. Productivity Commission.

National Health and Hospitals Reform Commission. (2009). *A healthier future for all Australians – final report*. https://apo.org.au/node/17921

Occupational Therapy Australia. (2020). *What do occupational therapists do: Disability/NDIS*. https://aboutoccupationaltherapy.com.au/disabilityndis/

OECD. (2017). *Health at a glance 2017: OECD indicators*. OECD Publishing. https://doi.org/10.1787/health_glance-2017-en

OECD. (2019). *Health at a glance 2019: OECD indicators*. OECD Publishing. https://doi.org/10.1787/4dd50c09-en

Parliament of Australia. (2017). *The National Disability Insurance Scheme: A quick guide*. https://www.aph.gov.au/About_Parliament/Parliamentary_Departments/Parliamentary_Library/pubs/rp/rp1617/Quick_Guides/NDIS

Solomon, S. (2014). Health reform and activity-based funding. *Medical Journal of Australia*, 10, 564. https://doi.org/10.5694/mja14.00292

Standing Council on Health. (2014). *National primary health care strategic framework.* Common-wealth of Australia. https://www1.health.gov.au/internet/main/publishing.nsf/Content/nphc-strategic-framework

Working with Indigenous Australians. (2017). *History.* http://www.workingwithindigenous australians.info/content/History_2_60,000_years.html

World Health Organization. (n.d). *Social determinants of health. https://www.who.int/health-topics/social-determinants-of-health#tab=tab_1*

3 History of Australian occupational therapy

Anne Cusick and Rosalind Bye

Chapter objectives

Upon completion of this chapter, the reader will be able to:

- Trace key milestones in the professionalisation of occupational therapy in Australia.
- Identify events, politico-cultural trends and socio-economic challenges associated with the development of Australian occupational therapy.
- Consider ways the past might influence future trajectories of occupational therapy in Australia.

Key terms

sociology of professions; Australian history; occupational therapy; allied health

Introduction

The emergence of occupational therapy as a profession is a century-long, world-wide story of inspiration, ingenuity and incessant hard work. Australia was one of the first countries in the world to officially recognise occupational therapy as a health profession. Australia's unique social, cultural and political historical context shaped the scope, scale and style of occupational therapy in this country. Australian occupational therapy is similar to and different from the profession practised in other places around the world. As Barbara Anderson and Janet Bell (1988) noted in their landmark book *Occupational Therapy: Its place in Australia's history*, the history of occupational therapy in Australia is a 'fascinating story. It is one of which occupational therapists – indeed all Australians – can justifiably be proud.' (p. xii)

This chapter presents a chronology of ideas, events and developments that show how occupation treatments of the nineteenth century, turned into a new rehabilitation approach called 'occupational therapy' in the twentieth century. The chapter traces how occupational therapy today became a respected, regulated, research-based profession.

Australia before the British

Long before the British claimed Australia as their own, Aboriginal and Torres Strait Islander peoples lived in Australia. Archaeological evidence of artefacts shows community life for at least 65,000 years (Clarkson et al., 2017). Genetic evidence demonstrates continuity of Aboriginal peoples for 75,000 years (Malaspinas et al., 2016).

This evidence is important because it provides scientific validation of Aboriginal and Torres Strait Islander knowledge handed down over generations. It is important because the British justified their occupation and colonisation of Australia on the basis of *terrae nullius*, a Latin word meaning 'nobody's land', despite documentary evidence from European explorers and Asian traders that Aboriginal and Torres Strait Islander peoples had clearly lived in Australia for a very long time.

The British seizure of the Great Southern Land was and continues to be a source of injustice that engenders a sense of profound regret and shame for many non-Indigenous Australians. The seizure was compounded by enduring adverse impacts of colonisation on health and social participation of the First Australians (Ballyn, 2011). For Indigenous Australians, the health and well-being of individuals relied on the vigour and sustainability of community culture enacted through occupations of daily life in the context of 'Country' (Ganesharajah, 2009). Aboriginal and/or Torres Strait Islander communities, culture and connections to Country were decimated by British colonisation (Ballyn, 2011).

Many colonising practices implemented in Australia were unjust and inhumane (United Nations, 2007): dispossession, discrimination, dispersals, loss of self-determination, frontier violence, destruction of culture through forced assimilation and neglect. The strength and resilience of Aboriginal and Torres Strait Islander peoples to survive, flourish and today lead the way in decolonising practice is evident.

The indisputability of Aboriginal and Torres Strait Islander Peoples as First Australians is acknowledged here; as is the need for social justice, redress, reconciliation and collaboration to improve health outcomes (Australian Human Rights Commission, 2020). The history of occupational therapy from the perspective of Aboriginal and Torres Strait Islander Peoples is not presumed or assumed in this chapter. It is acknowledged with respect that this history is one that can only be told by them.

Western philosophical traditions

This history of occupational therapy thus starts with ideological roots based in Western philosophical traditions. The profession usually identifies philosophers in Ancient Greece as intellectual ancestors. Aristotle (384–322 BCE) is probably the most important because of his interest in practical wisdom, learning through doing and the need for purpose in everyday life (see 'Ancient Wisdom'). His ideas were used by philosophers, scientists and social reformers in the 1600s–1700s in Europe and Britain to improve and understand the human condition at a time called the 'Enlightenment'. According to Aristotle: 'For the things we have to learn before we can do, we learn by doing' (Aristotle, Book II, 1103.a33; cited in: Bynum & Porter (2006), *Oxford Dictionary of Scientific Quotations*, 21:9).

The Enlightenment movement proposed human beings could use reason (logic, mathematics, ethics, etc.) to solve problems, understand the world and improve society (Gottlieb, 2016). New concepts like human rights, progress, tolerance and freedom emerged in the Enlightenment, using concepts of the Ancient Greeks to describe and explain human experience. In the late 1700s reform of many social institutions was needed for Enlightenment concepts to become a reality. This was particularly so for prisons and asylums where inmates were incarcerated in barbaric conditions and their humanity was not respected. For Australia, and Australian occupational therapy over a century later, the Enlightenment prison reforms were of particular importance.

Enlightenment prison reforms

Australia was the transportation destination for British convicts when America was no longer available following the 1776 American Revolution. They were transported by boat in wave after wave of prison 'fleets'. Just before the First Fleet set sail in 1787, heroic efforts of enlightened prison reformers had effect and new prison laws were decreed (Howard, 1777; see 'Prisons in the eighteenth century'). The laws gave convicts basic rights to water, food, shelter, sunlight, clean air and daily occupations including exercise, work and sometimes schooling. These applied to all British prisons including Australian convict colonies and the prison ships they sailed in. Howard writes of prisons on the eighteenth century:

> There are very few [prisons] ... in which any work is done or can be done. The prisoners have neither tools, nor materials of any kinds; but spend their time in sloth ... [further] idiots and lunatics ... The insane, where they are not kept separate, disturb and terrify other prisoners. No care is taken of them although it is probably that by medicines, and proper regimen, some of them might be restored to their senses, and to usefulness in life.
>
> (John Howard, 1777)

Prison reformers like Howard (1777) identified that an absence of purposeful activity or daily routine (also called regimen) had terrible effects on the well-being of people incarcerated in prison (Howard, 1777). Consequently, occupation regimens were mandated in reforms and they formed a feature of well-run prisons. In prison ships sailing to Australia and in convict settlements, occupation regimens were thus implemented and used for a dual purpose – punishment and preparation for a new life in the colony (Foxhall, 2011). On the one hand, daily routines of forced labour with inadequate rations and little rest were so extreme and severe that many died (Davidson et al., 2003). On the other hand, some prisoners had occupation regimens set by enlightened doctors, governors or warders with their time served in custody a preparation, through occupation regimens, for new roles in the colony upon release (Foxhall, 2011). From 1788 to 1868, 168,000 mostly British convicts were transported to Australia. Naval and army personnel, traders, free settlers and local-born children of British decent steadily grew the migrant population. In the 1850s, Australia's gold rush heralded an explosion in the number and diversity of migrants coming to and staying in colonies of Australia. Increased prosperity enabled expansion in civic infrastructure including roads, hospitals, asylums and schools. In their design and operation many of these aimed to implement Enlightenment principles on a larger scale than previously possible. As former prison colonies, no institution better exemplified the scaling up of 'enlightened' care in institutions than the asylum.

Humane asylum reforms

Asylums were institutional settings where people were incarcerated not for crime, but because they had a condition that affected their mental function and behaviour. Most of the time this was a mental illness, but other times it could be a result of developmental disability, brain injury from trauma, or brain damage as a result of infectious disease, alcohol or drugs. In the 1700s through to the early twentieth century, people with these conditions were called 'insane', 'idiots', 'imbeciles', the 'inebriate' or 'incurable'. British and European asylums in the 1700s and early 1800s were almost worse than prisons because: people in them were not considered fully human; there was no end to their 'sentence'; and the basic rights awarded to convicts through prison reform laws in the late 1700s did not apply to asylums. Asylums only began to change when reformers showed that residents could improve when given the right conditions. One of those conditions was a daily routine of purposeful occupation.

An early asylum reformer in Britain was wealthy merchant William Tuke. In the 1790s, he provided funds for a new type of asylum to be developed in a town called York. With the help of like-minded people, he provided alternative residential care for people with mental illness. Instead of brutal physical treatment, people were treated humanely and were able to live in supervised, supported, comfortable living conditions. Participation in daily occupations, self-reflection and self-control were practices thought to bring order to the disordered mind. His 'humane treatment' showed that people with 'incurable conditions' could recover. The York asylum became famous and inspired people everywhere to lobby for humane treatment.

In France, people like Phillipe Pinel, Jean-Baptiste Pussin and Marguerite Pussin were also active in asylum reform. They used their positions as superintendents and staff at the Paris asylum to change the rules (Bewley, 2008). They removed physical restraints, gave adequate food, water, fresh air, and opportunities for people to move around and engage in activities. The Paris Asylum inspired many doctors to adopt scientific, case-based, humane treatment approaches in their asylum work.

Australia's first purpose-built asylum opened in 1838 in Sydney. It was built for 60 patients, and care was modelled on the York and Paris asylum approaches of humane treatment. Before psychiatric asylums, people in Australia with mental illness were cared for by families, housed in gaols, or taken to all-purpose asylums for the poor, blind, aged, destitute and infirm run by charities such as the Benevolent Society. The 1838 asylum was thus considered an advance in care but within a few years it was overcrowded, underfunded, with disturbing reports of abuse, patient and staff deaths and terrible living conditions. It was expanded in the years following the gold rush, with new buildings and humane treatment principles still in effect, but problems in living and working conditions, overcrowding, funding and staff capacity continued at this and other new asylums being built around the country.

Humane treatment in asylums

> Occupational treatment was the only curative measure of any value in restoring patients to sanity.
>
> Dr John O'Brien, 1888 Medical Superintendent Kew Asylums,
> Victoria (cited in Westmore & Monk, 2012)

Once inside asylums, most patients were rarely released. Their lives were a daily routine comprising self-care (meals, hygiene) and asylum care, including cleaning, laundry and sewing repairs for women, and manual labour, building maintenance, grounds maintenance, vegetable farming for asylum supplies for men (Garton, 1988). In well-funded asylums there were creative and productive occupations including crafts, music, gardening-for-pleasure, carpentry, games, picnics and sport (Royal Commission on Asylums for the Insane and Inebriate, 1886; Westmore, 2012; Westmore & Monk, 2012).

Asylum clerical, laundry and manual work was also routinely done by patients; this practice was so common that the term 'working patients' evolved (Westmore, 2012).

Federation Australia—the early 1900s

In 1901 Australian colonies agreed to become a Federation (Davidson et al., 2003). Australia became a nation. Nation-building was a common theme of debate and a theory promoted in Britain called 'eugenics' became popular amongst the elite in Australia. This theory proposed that population 'fitness' could be improved if people who were deemed 'defective' were separated from the rest of the community (Wyndham, 2003). Being 'defective' could arise from mental illness, developmental disability, brain damage, other medical conditions or sometimes just because a person's appearance, way of life or lifestyle was considered too different. They were put into institutions, often without consent. Incarceration was seen to be a way of removing individuals who could negatively affect 'population fitness' by their presence or by having children.

Forced incarceration in asylums was intended to be a humane way to protect the rest of the population: a mix of 'work, rest, food and sympathy' (Garton, 1988, p. 156; Monk, 2008). But the recession in the 1890s left asylums underfunded, overcrowded, without adequate resources, variable to poor oversight, little transparency and despite heroic efforts of some individuals, they became increasingly inhumane (Goggin & Newell, 2005).

Occupation and therapy in the United States of America

While things stagnated in Australia during the Federation years, the United States of America (USA) saw four precursors to the development of the occupational therapy profession:

(a) The linking of 'occupation' to 'therapy' by Julia Lathrop in the so called 'mental hygiene movement' (Crowley-Cyr, 2005; Metaxas, 2000);

(b) The work of Susan Tracy to promote occupation as therapy for nursing the infirm (Metaxas, 2000; Tracy, 1910);

(c) The use of a bio-psycho-social model of treatment for mental illness by psychiatrist Dr Adolf Meyer and social worker Mary Brooks Meyer, at Johns Hopkins Hospital which featured the healing use of occupation (Lamb, 2014; Meyer, 1977); and

(d) The appointment of Eleanor Clarke Slagle as first Director of Occupational Therapy at Johns Hopkins Hospital in 1912 and the establishment of an influential medical coalition to advocate for 'occupation therapy' to be more widely adopted and developed into an independent profession.

World War One—1914–1918

In 1914 Britain became involved in war and 40 per cent of all Australian men aged between 18 and 44 enlisted; 61,527 died and 80 per cent of survivors were disabled or had permanent injuries (Noonan, 2014). On top of this tragedy, the 1918 influenza epidemic in Europe was conveyed home by returning soldiers and over 12,000 Australians were killed. Tens of thousands became infected. The task of caring for sick and war-injured people was a national challenge.

During the war Australia had an ad-hoc approach to returned soldiers—many were left unsupported. But in the final year of the war, in 1917 when America entered as an ally, Australia observed new and better models of repatriation, rehabilitation and resettlement of military personnel. Instead of bed rest, institutional convalescence and withdrawal from society, their model was centralised, coordinated and directed to-wards: active rehabilitation (called reconstruction); accelerated recovery; and community resettlement. This model suited Australia, a nation with few economic resources following war, and with so many returned service personnel and thousands of people affected by the pandemic. The new recovery-orientated rehabilitation approach was better and cheaper than long-term custodial care. It has also been shown to work in a range of settings—tuberculosis sanatoriums in Scotland, army field hospitals in Europe and hospitals in the USA.

Under the new approach, the Australian Government had to deliver treatments on a large scale to enable recovery. In the USA, the military had recruited and deployed 'reconstruction aides' to provide physical and occupational rehabilitation (Gavin, 1997; Lowe, 1992; McDaniel, 1968). Reconstruction aides were the precursors of occupational therapists (see occupation treatments). They received specialised training over-seen by Dr William Rush Dunton (Dunton, 1918; 1919), president of the newly formed American Society for the Promotion of Occupational Therapy (1917, later to be called the American Occupational Therapy Association). While the value of reconstruction aides was clear, the cost of training both physical and occupational therapists was too much so only one of these roles was selected for formal training—physical therapy. The assumption was that occupation therapy could be delivered by nurses or volunteers. It was an opportunity lost. It took 30 years and another war before dedicated occupational therapy training was implemented and dedicated positions were established.

> Occupation treatments existed long before the term 'occupational therapy' was first used. George Edward Barton described services at his Philadelphia USA facility as 'occupational therapy' designed to 'retrain or adjust' people for 'gainful living': Occupational therapy was 'not the making of an object but the making of a man'.
>
> (Barton, 1919)

Post-war Australia and the pioneer occupational therapists—1920s and 1930s

Australia, already burdened with post-war reconstruction and lingering social and eco-nomic impacts of the pandemic, faced new problems with a poliomyelitis epidemic emerging in the late 1920s and exploding in the 1930s. Polio was an infectious disease that could not be prevented or treated. Traditionally rest and immobilisation of affected limbs was prescribed, but the active rehabilitation approach in post-war USA promoted new physical therapy techniques including massage, exercise and use of technologies such as prosthetic braces and negative pressure ventilators ('iron lungs'). This active approach also used graded occupations to increase functional capacity and maintain psychological well-being.

An effective treatment:

> is a satisfactory method of hastening recovery in both mental and physical cases. Occupational Therapy is a definite and proven therapeutic measure having as its

advocates a great many members of the medical and surgical professions and practically all mental specialists.

(Howland, 1933, p. 4)

The polio epidemic provided momentum to formalise and extend physical therapy training in Australia. Despite success of occupational therapy interventions (see An effective treatment) and the proliferation of training courses in the United Kingdom, Canada and the USA, occupational therapy training in Australia remained informal. Training was provided by people who had previously 'practised' occupation treatments giving classes to nurses and volunteers including tradesmen, teachers and artists (Oppenheimer, 2019). 'Hospital Auxiliaries' (small charities attached to individual hospitals or asylums) often organised these courses. Auxiliary members, such as Stella Pines in South Australia, were great advocates of occupational therapy.

Unsurprisingly then, the first dedicated 'occupational therapist' job in Australia was funded by the Mental Hospital Auxiliary at Mont Park Hospital Victoria in 1934. It was taken by nurse Lucy Syme who had previously trained 'on the job' in nurse-administered occupational therapy at Broughton Hall Psychiatric Hospital in Sydney. Three years later, the first overseas trained diploma qualified occupational therapists started practice in Australia (see Table 3.1). Their practice was informed by biomedical, scientific and vocational approaches of American occupational therapy augmented by treatment modalities favoured by the United Kingdom occupational therapy courses influenced by the Arts and Crafts Movement (Schemm, 1994).

By the end of the 1930s the pioneers had introduced occupational therapy to the following specialisations (Anderson & Bell, 1988): physical rehabilitation, paediatric,

Table 3.1 Australian occupational therapy pioneers

- 1933: Ethel May Francis attends the Philadelphia School of Occupational Therapy USA graduating with a Diploma. After further training at the first School of Occupational Therapy in the UK, Dorset House, she returns to Victoria, Australia working in mental health. In 1937 she goes to Sydney. As the first occupational therapist there she says she needs to 'practise and prove occupational therapy to the medical profession'. She joins the first multidisciplinary allied health service in Australia a 'child guidance' clinic at Rachel Forster Hospital. She leads the establishment of occupational therapy adult and paediatric services and departments in the 1940s and 1950s.
- 1934: Nurse Lucy Syme is employed in the first 'occupational therapist' advertised position in Australia at Mont Park Hospital, Victoria after training 'on the job' at the Broughton Hall psychiatric service in Sydney.
- 1934 Sylvia Docker from Sydney attends the London School of Occupational Therapy, the second school established in the UK. Already qualified as a physiotherapist, her focus is on occupational therapy with people who have physical conditions. She returns to Australia in 1938, working in Melbourne at 'Crippled Children's' Services and the Austin Hospital until 1941. She plays an active role in Australia's response to the poliomyelitis epidemic and in 1941 is appointed Director of Occupational Therapy in the Sydney Training School, the first specialised facility to offer occupational therapy Diplomas in Australia.
- 1937: Joyce Keam from Tasmania trains at the Maudsley Psychiatric Hospital, with further study at Dorset House, returning in 1939 to Victoria to work as a private practitioner in mental health at Alencon Private Mental Hospital. In 1941 she established an occupational therapy department at the 2,000-bed military hospital at Heidelberg, Victoria, was appointed the first occupational therapy advisor in the Australian Army and achieved the rank of Major.

psychiatric and acute general medical services. They also put Australian occupational therapy on the international map by maintaining letter contact with professional colleagues overseas, receiving and sending occupational therapy professional association journals and bulletins.

World War II and the birth of Australian occupational therapy—1940s

Occupational therapy employment opportunities expanded across the globe in World War II. Tens of thousands of people suffered adverse consequences of combat, prisoner of war experiences, civilian deprivation or attack (Beaumont, 2001). Army reconstruction aides from the USA were re-invigorated as part of special medical services and this time the full range of professional titles were used under the banner of allied health (Vogel, 1968). Occupational therapists, physical therapists and dietitians were employed.

After the ad-hoc approach following World War I, Australia wanted to support its military personnel better this time (Bearup, 1996). The USA rehabilitation and repatriation system was seen as best practice and Australia adopted a similar planned approach. As part of this, dedicated occupational therapy positions were included (Walker, 1961). In a milestone for occupational therapy in Australia, the army decided to appoint only qualified occupational therapists, same as the USA. But there were only three in all of Australia—Francis, Docker and Keam. With the needs of the Australian Army front and centre, in 1940 Francis successfully applied to the Hospital Commission to start an occupational therapy course. It was led by Professor Dawson, Psychiatrist at the University of Sydney, with Francis teaching occupational therapy subjects. It was then coordinated by the Australian Physiotherapy Association (APA) from 1941 and later transferred to the Australian Association of Occupational Therapists. The first graduate of this occupational therapy diploma program was Gwendoline Sims in 1941. Twenty-five years later in 1966, she gave the first Sylvia Docker Memorial Lecture, a prestigious biennial award given by the occupational therapy professional association. The lecture was established to acknowledge Sylvia Docker who was appointed by the APA as Occupational Therapy Director in 1942 (Docker, 1959). Docker oversaw the development of a new facility called the Sydney Training Centre (STC). Her first intake into the new diploma program (implemented after Gwendoline Sims graduated), was 27 students.

In those first years, the standard course was 18 months (Docker, 1959). Most of these early occupational therapy graduates were already in, or they had volunteered for, the Australian Army as commissioned lieutenants. They could be deployed anywhere to provide services to accelerate soldiers' recovery enabling return to action, repatriation or medical discharge (Neuhaus & Mascall-Dare, 2014). Some graduates went overseas to staging hospitals; others went to repatriation hospitals interstate. Some of these were vast tent-cities where over 2,000 troops and workers were housed (Anderson & Bell, 1988). These were often the first occupational therapists ever encountered by patients, doctors and nurses. They not only had to establish their department facilities and programs, but also had to carve out a professional role and reputation, earning respect in places with a strong biomedical and military hierarchy (Walker, 1961).

After the war, Australia adopted a coordinated and controlled demobilisation, repatriation and reconstruction plan (Macintyre, 2015). By 1947 most military hospitals had become Repatriation Hospitals and most females, including occupational therapists, were discharged from the army and encouraged to return to home duties (Walker, 1961). Many did not and occupational therapists continued to work in Repatriation Hospitals.

The post-war rehabilitation and 'baby-boom' offered new employment opportunities which kept the STC, now with 54 graduates, busy training occupational therapists. These services included: Commonwealth Rehabilitation Centres for non-combat conditions, tuberculosis sanatoriums, mental hospitals for returned service personnel, civilian mental asylums, new paediatric and adult services in special and general civil ian medical hospitals and new community health clinics (Anderson & Bell, 1988). The STC could not meet graduate demand and a second training course opened in 1948 in Victoria (Cameron, 1977). In concert with the development of occupational therapy education, occupational therapists formed associations to promote the profession and encourage high quality practice through continuing professional learning, research and supervision (see Historical milestones of the OT association).

Historical milestones of the OT Association*

- 1944—The Occupational Therapists' Club formed in Sydney.
- 1945—The *OT Bulletin* is published.
- 1945—First group meeting of occupational therapists held in Queensland.
- 1945—The Occupational Therapists' Club in Sydney is renamed the Australian Association of Occupational Therapists (AAOT).
- 1946—AAOT Constitution is approved.
- 1947—Victorian Division is established
- 1948—Queensland Division is established
- 1948—New South Wales Division is established.
- 1949—Western Australia establishes an OT Club.
- 1951—AAOT is identified as a federal (national) association distinct from the state divisions.
- 1951—AAOT becomes a foundation member of the World Federation of Occupational Therapists.
- 1952—*The OT Bulletin* becomes the *Australian Occupational Therapy Journal*.
- 1953—Western Australian Division is established.
- 1953—First meeting of the Federal Council of AAOT.
- 1953—World Federation of Occupational Therapists Course Accreditation Standards applied in Australia for the first time.
- 1961—All state divisions become members of the federal association.
- 1963—South Australian Division is established.
- 1971—Tasmanian Division is established.
- 1979—Australian Capital Territory Division is established.
- 1986—Northern Territory Division is established.
- 2010—All divisions consolidated within the AAOT, now Occupational Therapy Australia Ltd, also known as OT AUSTRALIA (OTA).

Source: Adamson et al., 2017; Anderson & Bell, 1988; https://www.otaus.com.au/about/about-ota

Australian nation-building and building of the profession—1950s to 1960s

For most of the 1950s and 1960s Australia had a single conservative government (Knott, 2016). It used a combination of managed markets, social safety nets and private businesses to create an Australia that charted what was called a 'middle way' between market and welfare states (Bolton, 1990). There was centralised regulation and management of financial markets, capital infrastructure and social policies, but an expectation that individuals, families and communities would help themselves. The conservative 'middle way' required: high levels of citizen conformity; a culture of self-reliance; assimilation and integration of post-war migrants; and a safety-net approach to education, health and social services (Bolton, 1990). The safety net provided limited government assistance for some defined groups (returned-service personnel, the so-called 'certifiably insane', or the demonstrably poor); everyone else paid or relied on charity which involved dramatic expansion of volunteering in Australia (Oppenheimer, 2005).

This 'middle way' provided steady and growing employment for occupational therapists in Commonwealth repatriation and rehabilitation services, state civilian hospitals, and in a vast array of small and large specialty services developed by charities (Macintyre, 2015; Oppenheimer, 2005). This diversified occupational therapy employment specialties, salaries, conditions, career opportunities and increased demand for training.

The 1950s–1960s refocused attention on asylums as the national emergencies of war and reconstruction subsided. They had continued in much the same way as the Federation years. Post-war reforms identified that many asylums had chronically poor conditions including serious understaffing and overwork, inadequate staff training, overcrowding, inadequate residential/sanitation facilities, compromised patient and staff safety, ill treatment of patients by staff and of staff by patients, and a system that was 'unscientific, obsolete and inhuman … [which treated patients as] convicts and animals' (*The Sunday Herald*, 1949). Occupational therapy provided by qualified occupational therapists was one of many reforms introduced to change the culture and conditions inside residential care institutions in the late 1950s and 1960s. As agents of change, some occupational therapists in institutions experienced difficult and sometimes dangerous working conditions (Anderson & Bell, 1988).

As workforce needs expanded in Australia across a range of sectors, graduates were in high demand. There were never enough (see 'In high demand'). At that time, most women who got married or became pregnant were forced to resign their jobs because of employment law, organisation policies and social convention. As women were paid only part of a male wage, salaries were poor, women were cheaper to hire and few men were attracted to the profession. Further, there were restrictions on recognition of overseas qualifications, so the pool of qualified migrant therapists was limited. There was thus an urgent need to expand training.

By 1961 there were four courses in Australia—all at diploma level: New South Wales, Victoria, Queensland (originally a combined degree with physiotherapy but later a discipline specific diploma) and Western Australia. All courses included: biomedical and behavioural sciences; training in assessment, planning and implementation of treatment for a variety of physical and mental conditions; how to understand and use research in practice; practical training in arts, crafts and trades; and fieldwork in hospitals or other services. All courses used teacher expertise, information from *The Bulletin* (the precursor of the *Australian Occupational Therapy Journal*) and published sources primarily from the United States where textbooks had been available since 1911.

In high demand:

> the career of Occupational Therapist. Perhaps this is the one for you. Candidates to be at least 18 years old and to have Matriculation or an equivalent examination. A well adjusted personality, interested manner, sense of responsibility, good health, understanding, resourcefulness, ingenuity and manual dexterity. Training: Three year course at Occupational Therapy School. Students do 40 weeks in hospitals. [...] Tremendous demand for qualified personnel. Graduates wishing to travel have no difficulty obtaining positions overseas.
>
> (*The Herald*, January 1952)

Training was provided in a variety of private–semi-private institutions often in affiliation with the professional association. A government review in 1964 showed that health professional training was fragmented, inefficient and insufficient for projected population growth. The Australian Government changed legislation and funding to ensure health professional training took place in government accredited institutions—colleges or universities—with approved courses. At that time terms such as 'paramedic', 'allied health' or 'auxiliary health professions' were used to describe non-nursing and non-medicine courses. Nowadays 'allied health' is the most common term and it comes from this 1960s period.

As more courses emerged across the country, ways to assure public safety and practitioner quality were sought. Practitioner registration had occurred for medicine and nursing for a long time. Registration restricts the right to practise by limiting the use of professional titles and identifying entry criteria and scope of practice. Western Australia was the first state to register occupational therapists for practice (1960). Other states and territories followed in later decades with nationwide registration occurring in 2012 (see Registration milestones).

Registration milestones:

- 1960 Registration for occupational therapists in Western Australia
- 1974 Registration for occupational therapists in South Australia
- 1981 Registration available to occupational therapists in Queensland
- 1986 Registration for occupational therapists in Northern Territory
- 1986 The inaugural conference of Australian Occupational Therapy Registration Boards held to discuss common issues. State associations where there was no registration were invited (Tasmania, New South Wales, Victoria, Australian Capital Territory)
- 2012 National registration for all occupational therapists in all states and territories through the Commonwealth of Australia Government body, the Australian Health Practitioner Regulation Agency Occupational Therapy Registration Board

(https://www.ahpra.gov.au/)

Another mark of quality in training was the World Federation of Occupational Therapists (WFOT) education standards, set in place soon after the Federation's establishment in 1952. Australia played an active role in establishing WFOT, so not surprisingly, Australia was one of the first countries to adopt WFOT course standards.

From managed to market economies—1970s to 1990s

In the 1970s to 1990s a number of policy changes created a very different environment for occupational therapy education and practice. A series of governments shifted Australia from a managed to market economy, from regulated to deregulated employment and services, and from conservative to liberal social perspectives. The changes were dramatic and for some the changes were traumatic (Smyth & Cass, 1998). In education, higher qualification levels were introduced to prepare graduates for increasingly complex roles. Instead of diplomas, most courses in the late 1970s were bachelor's degrees and occupational therapists holding diplomas studied to 'upgrade' their qualifications.

These were tense times for the profession. Some therapists saw the introduction of degrees as unnecessary credential-creep. They saw it as a threat to 'hands-on' experience that had earned occupational therapy a 'can-do' reputation for success. Other therapists saw that bachelor's degrees were essential in a sector that was becoming increasingly specialised and research-based. Vigorous debates happened in education and in practice and some of this can be seen in journal publications from the time which explored: occupational therapy's role; identity and foundations; occupational therapy 'art' versus 'science', 'practice' versus 'theory', 'experience' versus 'qualifications', 'caring' versus 'career', 'technical' versus 'professional', and 'expertise' versus 'evidence'.

These 1970s debates were well timed. Colleges had funding arrangements that permitted both practice and theory to have equal investment. Courses had high contact hours, technical instruction in a range of hands-on modalities and some had paid student internships. The college years thus provided a period of transition from the relatively autonomous practice-oriented courses of the 1950s–1960s to multidisciplinary streamed-academic-practice approaches of the 1970s–1980s. The transition in the 1970s also gave Australian occupational therapy a chance to clarify and consolidate professional definitions, assumptions, roles and scope of practice.

These events proved to be fortuitous because the 1980s began with a severe recession that increased unemployment, led to government expenditure cuts to many social services including health, and provided a platform for extensive restructuring of labour and employment laws and conditions. This directly affected occupational therapy which, until then, had most graduates employed in public sector positions. The introduction of market-driven approaches to health and human services led to reductions in the number of government occupational therapy positions, increased competition for the few public sector jobs that were available, and more graduates seeking employment opportunities in 'non-traditional', 'emerging role' or 'generic' occupational therapy and allied health positions.

The increasingly competitive health sector led the occupational therapy association to accelerate efforts to promote research capacity building in the profession. There was an urgent need for research evidence to show occupational therapists were effective, efficient and essential. During the 1980s the association sponsored research and quality improvement workshops, research prizes and awards, included research as an essential competency in course accreditation guidelines, promoted research in conference programs, and looked to universities and occupational therapy managers to lead efforts to develop researchers and build the occupational therapy knowledge base (see Table 3.2).

By the 1990s, when the next economic recession hit Australia, occupational therapy had successfully adapted and was embedded across health, education, human services and industry sectors with a growing evidence base to support practice. Changes in

Table 3.2 Important milestones within the profession of occupational therapy during the 1990s

Status of the profession	Important progress and milestones
Professional standing	Agreed professional definitions.
	An official Australian history of profession from 1940s to the 1960s, released in association with Australian Bicentenary of British settlement (Anderson & Bell, 1988).
	A professional association actively engaged in advisory, accreditation and advocacy activities.
	Australian leadership roles in the World Federation of Occupational Therapists.
	Consistent standards applied for recognition of overseas qualifications.
	Minimum competency standards for graduating occupational therapists.
	Registration in some states.
	Association awards to recognise contributions in service, research and leadership.
Professional education	Nationally consistent professional course accreditation standards.
	Undergraduate and postgraduate university courses in all jurisdictions except Tasmania, Northern Territory and Australian Capital Territory.
	Accreditation requirements including continuing professional development.
	Occupational therapy submissions to government inquiries.
Professional scholarship and research training	A dozen or so occupational therapists have studied for or attained a doctorate.
	Doctoral courses available in occupational therapy.
	Increases in the number of articles, issues, submissions, readers and status of the *Australian Occupational Therapy Journal.*
	Increases in the number of research submissions, international and scholarly speakers, specialty streams, and participants in national and state conferences.
	Appointment of an Occupational Therapy Professorial Chair to a university.
Professional employment	Occupational therapists and occupational therapy in national and state government workforce planning.
	Employment opportunities extended from clinical roles to community development, public health, policy, education and research.
	Expansion of employment in private enterprise and industry;
	Diversification of fields of practice to all sectors of the Australian economy, all national health priority areas and all regions of the country.
	Increased multidisciplinary team and sole-therapist roles.

migration, employment and corporate regulation in the 1990s saw Australia shift from a closed Euro-centric culture to one strategically engaged with the Asia-Pacific in a market-driven globalised world (Galligan et al., 2001). This engagement was increasingly reflected in the occupational therapy profession. Despite the recession, graduates from the dozen or so education programs in Australia obtained employment and prospective domestic and international student demand for courses was high. About this time occupational therapy courses across the country were relocated from colleges to universities as part of a nationwide restructure of post-school education (previously only Queensland was university-level).

Global and local—2000–2020

At the beginning of the new millennium Australia was a more diverse country. The immensely successful 2000 Paralympic Summer Games held in Sydney was an iconic event for Australia and the world. It was the first time that Paralympic athletes were assured of the same experience, support and conditions as other Olympic athletes. As an indication of public engagement, over 1,000,000 tickets were sold for Paralympic events – more than ever before. The high profile of the event, visibility of competitors and mass participation of Australians as volunteers and spectators was a turning point in Australia's history. It was a positive and exciting time for occupational therapists and disability/health community stakeholders and consumers.

In 2001 the World Health Organization published a new model of functioning, disability and health (ICF) that embraced a bio–psycho–social approach and recognised social models of disability and social determinants of health (WHO, 2001). This model explicitly identified, defined and operationalised concepts of activity and participation. This brought fresh, interdisciplinary attention to constructs that had been occupational therapy's 'core business' for decades. But it was only the beginning of a journey to articulate and attain human rights for all people regardless of disability or diagnosis to achieve greater participation as respected, safe and responsible citizens.

Practical consequences of an increased focus on human rights were felt in Australia in years that followed. There was legislation reflecting Australia's commitment to international conventions (for example, Australian Government Department of Foreign Affairs and Trade, 2020). Government enquiries into policy and practices in institutions were held (for example, Royal Commissions [https://www.royalcommission.gov.au/], or Productivity Commission Enquiries [https://www.pc.gov.au/]). New consumer-directed service models were introduced and provider arrangements were restructured (for example, the Australian Government My Aged Care [https://www.myagedcare.gov.au/] or the National Disability Insurance Scheme [https://www.ndis.gov.au/]). Occupational therapy played an important role in contributing to these changes through submissions by OT Australia and individual therapists, and implementing change through service consultation and provision and advocacy engagement with consumers.

In *research* there is more occupational therapy scholarship in conferences and journals about human rights, experience of the dispossessed, displaced and disadvantaged particularly in relation to occupational deprivation, maintenance of meaningful daily occupations in times of trauma and change, and adaptation through occupation to new socio-economic environments. Increasingly, collaborative and co-constructed approaches to research are being applied. For 20 years, occupational therapy contemporary research and practice has been framed by biopsychosocial models of health and well-being and social models of disability (WHO, 2001), understanding of public health practice and principles, and implementation of evidence-based practice approaches (Cusick, 2001).

In *practice*, human rights approaches are influencing the uptake of more collaborative, power-sharing, equal models of care, including shared care, family and person-centred practice, consumer directed care and recovery-oriented care. Occupational therapists, many of whom continue to work in biomedical specialties, are agents of cultural change introducing these rights-based approaches in provider-orientated contexts.

In *education*, deregulation of higher education in the 2000s meant any university could offer an occupational therapy course—government control of type, location and size of courses was lifted. Places in occupational therapy courses were in high demand, so many universities embraced the opportunity. From five courses in 1971 there are now over 20—most of them being launched after 2000 (see: Approved Occupational Therapy Programs—https://www.ahpra.gov.au/education/approved-programs-of-study.aspx?ref=occupational%20therapist). The increase in number and type of courses, together with targeted government funding, has helped diversify the student body to include more 'first-in-family' candidates, mature age students, people from low socio-economic or culturally and linguistically diverse backgrounds.

In *employment*, law reforms have reduced formal discrimination of people from different backgrounds or with non-normative identities. Informal discrimination, institutional racism and institutional discrimination still occur, but for occupational therapists and the people they work with, there are legislative and policy frameworks now available that can be used to identify discrimination where it occurs and engage stakeholders to change practice and shift attitudes. Employment opportunities have also diversified: from public institutions to small-to-medium enterprises; from occupational therapy-specific positions to inter-professional roles where occupational therapy skills and knowledge are applied; and from the health care and social assistance sector to one where occupational therapists now work across a range of industry sectors including education and training, public administration and safety, and professional, scientific and technical services.

In *policy*, occupational therapy finds itself at the heart of local, national and global reforms as the implications of human rights-based approaches to understanding health and disability are worked through (WHO, 2001). Links between the person, environment, activity, participation and health well known to occupational therapists are now of concern to everyone in human services, health and disability policy, planning, practice and research.

Twenty-first century challenges: 2021 and beyond

Eighty years ago, in 1941, there were four qualified occupational therapists in Australia. In the space of one lifetime occupational therapy has grown in scope, scale and esteem to be a driving force in health and human services in Australia. The profession starts the third decade of this century with more than 23,000 registered occupational therapists in Australia (Occupational Therapy Board of Australia, 2019).

While the future is unknown, it is clear the world is changing at a rapid pace, with technology, infectious diseases, environmental catastrophe, economic and employment upheaval, and conflict continuing to be major disruptors in the way people live their lives and engage in occupations across the lifespan. There are advances in technology and health, and social, political and cultural change will accelerate—but despite this change, people will still need and want to engage in occupations in everyday life situations. Occupational therapy enables this engagement.

Conclusion

Australia is the driest inhabited continent on earth (Geoscience Australia, 2020). For something to grow in Australia it needs to be tough, adaptable and resilient. It needs deep roots to survive fires, droughts and storms. It needs strong branches to shelter saplings from harsh conditions for which they are not yet ready. It needs seeds able to ride the winds and cover vast distances to find new fields.

This chapter shows that occupational therapy has grown, indeed flourished, in Australia. It is tough, adaptable and resilient. Australian occupational therapy has roots reaching deep into colonial history. It has branches all over the country, economy and society which spread the benefits of occupational therapy and protect new and emerging therapists and therapies. It has seeded enterprises in new fields across policy, practice, research and education.

As Australian occupational therapy faces the inevitable socio-economic and politico-cultural fires, droughts and storms of the twenty-first century, there is no doubt it will continue to grow. It will be the profession's roots that give it strength and sustenance. This is why Australian occupational therapists need to know and be inspired by their own history. It will be the profession's branches that protect and extend the terrain already covered. As Rachel Norris, Chief Executive Officer of OT Australia (2012–2018) and one of the leaders of Australia's more recent occupational therapy history, noted in 2018, 'there are many more chapters to be written' for our profession (Norris, 2018). The profession's remarkable history will ensure it can ride the winds of change and write new history chapters into the future.

Summary

- Principles of the Enlightenment informed the use of occupation-based regimens in Australian colonial institutions.
- Challenging events including war, epidemics, recession and deregulation were catalysts for the uptake and growth of occupation as therapy in the early twentieth century and the formation of the occupational therapy profession over the last 80 years.
- The pace of politico-cultural, socio-economic, environmental and technological change in the twenty-first century is accelerating. Australian occupational therapy's history indicates an agile capacity for adaptation and action.

Review questions

1. Plot a timeline of events and trends relevant to the development of occupational therapy in Australia.
2. What similarities and differences do you see in past and present contexts that are relevant to the development of occupational therapy in Australia?
3. Ask an older person about their recollections of events or trends they consider to be 'historic'. How might these events or trends have affected the growth of occupational therapy in Australia?
4. Think about occupational therapists you have met or read about—who are the 'history makers' of today and why?

References

Adamson, L., Norris, R., Russell, M., & Zakrzewski, L. (2017). The role of occupational therapy professional associations and regulatory bodies in Australia. In T. Brown, H. Bourke-Taylor, S. Isbel, & R. Cordier (Eds.), *Occupational therapy in Australia: Professional and practice issues* (pp. 49–61). Allen & Unwin.

Anderson B., & Bell J. (1988). *Occupational therapy: Its place in Australia's history.* Australian Association of Occupational Therapists.

Australian Government Department of Foreign Affairs and Trade. (2020). *International Relations—United Nations*. https://www.dfat.gov.au/international-relations/international-organisations/un/Pages/united-nations-un.aspx

Australian Human Rights Commission. (2020). *Aboriginal and Torres Strait Islander Social Justice: Close the gap indigenous health campaign*. https://www.humanrights.gov.au/our-work/aboriginal-and-torres-strait-islander-social-justice

Ballyn, S. (2011). The British invasion of Australia convicts: Exile and dislocation. In M. Renes (Ed.). *Lives in migration: Rupture and continuity; Essays on migration* (pp. 16–29). Observatori Centre d'Estudis Australians, Universitat de Barcelona. http://www.ub.edu/dpfilsa/ebook1contents.html

Barton, G. E. (1919). *Teaching the sick: A manual of occupational therapy and re-education*. W. B. Saunders Co. Digitised by Harvard University, 2007.

Bearup, C. (1996). *Occupational therapists in wartime*. Australian Association of Occupational Therapists.

Beaumont, J. (2001). *Australian defence: Sources and statistics in the Australian centenary history of defence volume VI*. Oxford University Press. https://trove.nla.gov.au/version/42710949

Bewley, T. (2008). *Madness to mental illness: A history of the Royal College of Psychiatrists*. Royal College of Psychiatrists Archive. https://catalogues.rcpsych.ac.uk/

Bolton, G. C. (1990). *1945–1966 the Middle Way. The Oxford history of Australia, volume 5, 1942–1988*. Oxford University Press.

Bynum, W. F., & Porter, R. (2006). *Oxford dictionary of scientific quotations*. Oxford University Press. https://10.1093/acref/9780198614432.001.0001

Cameron, B. S. (1977). *The work of our hands: A history of the occupational therapy school of Victoria*. Lincoln Institute.

Clarkson, C., Jacobs, Z., Marwick, B., Fullagar, R., Wallis, L., Smith, M., Roberts, R. G., Hayes, E., Lowe, K., Carah, X., Florin, S. A., McNeil, J., Cox, D., Arnold, L. J., Hua, Q., Huntley, J., Brand, H. E. A., Manne, T., Fairbairn, A., … Pardoe, C. (2017). Human occupation of northern Australia by 65,000 years ago. *Nature, 547*, 306–310. https://doi.org/10.1038/nature22968

Crowley-Cyr, L. (2005). The incarceration archipelago of lunacy 'reform' enterprises: An epochal overview. *James Cook University Law Review, 3*(12), 33–64. http://www.austlii.edu.au/au/journals/JCULawRw/2005/3.html

Cusick, A. (2001). OZ OT EBP 21C: Australian occupational therapy, evidence-based practice and the 21st century. *Australian Occupational Therapy Journal, 48*(3), 102–117. https://doi.org/10.1046/j.0045-0766.2001.00281.x

Davidson, G., Hirst, J., & Mcintyre, S. (2003). *The Oxford companion to Australian history*. Oxford University Press.

Docker, S. (1959). Development of occupational therapy in Australia, *Australian Journal of Occupational Therapy, 6* (3), 2–8, https://doi.org/10.1111/j.1440-1630.1959.tb00824.x

Dunton, W. R. (1918). *Occupation therapy: A manual for nurses*. W. B. Saunders Co, Classic Reprint Series, Forgotten Books, 2013. http://www.forgottenbooks.com/

Dunton, W. R. (1919). *Reconstruction therapy*. W. B. Saunders Co., Classic Reprint Series, Forgotten Books, 2013. http://www.forgottenbooks.com/

Foxhall, K. (2011). From convicts to colonists: The health of prisoners and the voyage to Australia, 1823–1853. *Journal of Imperial and Commonwealth History, 39* (1), 1–19. https://doi.org/10.1080/03086534.2011.543793

Galligan, B., Roberts, W., & Trifiletti, G. (2001). *Australians and globalisation: The experience of two centuries*. Cambridge University Press.

Ganesharajah, C. (2009). *Indigenous health and wellbeing: The importance of country*. Australian Institute of Aboriginal and Torres Strait Islander Studies. https://aiatsis.gov.au/sites/default/files/products/report_research_outputs/ganesharajah-2009-indigenous-health-wellbeing-importance-country.pdf

Garton, S. (1988). *Medicine and madness: A social history of insanity in New South Wales 1880–1940*. University of New South Wales Press.

Gavin, L. (1997). Reconstruction aides. In *American women in World War I: They also served* (Chapter 5). University Press of Colorado.

Geoscience Australia. (2020). Deserts. Geoscience Australia. https://www.ga.gov.au/scientific-topics/national-location-information/landforms/deserts

Goggin, G., & Newell, C. (2005). *Disability in Australia: Exposing a social apartheid.* University of New South Wales Press.

Gottlieb, A. (2016). *The dream of enlightenment: The rise of modern philosophy.* Penguin.

Howard, J. (1777). *The state of the prisons in England and Wales with preliminary observations, and an account of some foreign prisons.* Classic Reprint Series, Forgotten Books, 2013. http://www.forgottenbooks.com/

Howland, G. (1933). Editorial. *Canadian Journal of Occupational Therapy, September* (1), 4–5. https://journals.sagepub.com/doi/pdf/10.1177/000841743300100101

Knott, J. (2016). *Australian's Prime Ministers: Robert Menzies—In Office.* National Archives of Australia. http://primeministers.naa.gov.au/primeministers/menzies/

Lamb, S. D. (2014). *The pathologist of the mind: Adolf Meyer and the origins of American psychiatry.* Johns Hopkins University Press.

Lowe, J. F. (1992). The reconstruction aides. *American Journal of Occupational Therapy, 46*(1), 38–43. https://doi.org/10.5014/ajot.46.1.38

Macintyre, S. F. (2015). *Australia's boldest experiment: War and reconstruction in the 1940s.* University of New South Wales Press.

McDaniel, M. L. (1968). *Professional activities and problems 1947–1961. Occupational Therapy Educational and Training Programs, Part IV.* United States Army. https://history.amedd.army.mil/corps/medical_spec/publication.html

Malaspinas, A., Westaway, M. C., Muller, C., Sousa, V. C., Lao, O., Alves, I., Bergstrom, A., Athanasiadis, G., Cheng, J. Y., Crawford, J. E., Heupink, T. H., Macholdt, E., Peischl, S., Rasmussen, S., Schiffels, S., Subramanian, S., Wright, J. L., Albrechtsen, A., Barbieri, C. ... Willerslev, E. (2016). A genomic history of Aboriginal Australia. *Nature, 538,* 207–213. https://doi.org/10.1038/nature18299

Metaxas, V. A. (2000). Eleanor Clarke Slagle and Susan E Tracy: Personal and professional identity and the development of occupational therapy in progressive era America. *Nursing History Review, 8,* 39–70.

Meyer, A. (1977). The philosophy of occupation therapy. Reprinted from the Archives of Occupational Therapy, Volume 1, pp. 1–10, 1922. *American Journal of Occupational Therapy, 31*(10), 639–642.

Monk, L. A. (2008). *Attending madness at work in the Australian colonial asylum.* Rodopi.

Neuhaus, S. J., & Mascall-Dare, S. (2014). Betwixt and between: Allied health care and the struggle for recognition. In S. J. Neuhaus & S. Mascall-Dare (Eds.), *Not for glory: A century of service by medical women to the Australian Army and its allies* (pp. 109–150). Boolarong Press.

Noonan, D. (2014). *Those we forget: Recounting Australian casualties of the First World War.* Melbourne University Press.

Norris, R. (2018). Occupational Therapy Australia, CEO's report. *Connections, June,* 4–6.

Occupational Therapy Board of Australia. (2019). *Registrant data: Reporting period: 01 October 2019 to 31 December 2019.* https://www.occupationaltherapyboard.gov.au/About/Statistics.aspx

Oppenheimer, M. (2005). Voluntary action and welfare in post-1945 Australia: Preliminary perspectives. *History Australia, 2* (3) 2:3, 82.1–82.16. https://doi.org/10.2104/ha050082

Oppenheimer, M. (2019). The professionalisation of nursing through the 1920s and 1930s: The impact of war and voluntarism. In K. Darian-Smith & J. Waghorne (Eds.), *The First World War, the universities and the professions in Australia, 1914–1939* (pp. 213–252). Melbourne University Publishing.

Royal Commission on Asylums for the Insane and Inebriate, Victoria. (1886). *Report of the Royal Commission, Minutes of Evidence, Q.5541. Victorian Parliamentary Papers, 2,* 224.

Schemm, R. L. (1994). Bridging conflicting ideologies: The origins of American and British occupational therapy. *American Journal of Occupational Therapy, 48*(11), 1082–1088. https://doi.org/10.5014/ajot.48.11.1082

Smyth, P., & Cass, B. (1998). *Contesting the Australian way: States, markets and civil society.* Cambridge University Press.

The Sunday Herald. (1949, 15 May). p. 6.

Tracy, S. E. (1910). *Studies in invalid occupations: A manual for nurses and attendants.* Whitcomb and Barrows, Classic Reprint Series, Forgotten Books, 2013. http://www.forgottenbooks.com/

United Nations. (2007). *United Nations Declaration on the Rights of Indigenous Peoples.* General Assembly Resolution 61/295. https://www.un.org/development/desa/indigenouspeoples/declaration-on-the-rights-of-indigenous-peoples.html#:~:text=The%20United%20Nations%20Declaration%20on%20the%20Rights%20of,Bangladesh%2C%20Bhutan%2C%20Burundi%2C%20Colombia%2C%20Georgia%2C%20Kenya%2C%20Nigeria%2C%20

Vogel, E. (1968). *Medical training in World War II: Dietitians, physical and occupational therapists*, p. 163. United States Army Medical Department. http://history.amedd.army.mil/corps/medical_spec/chaptervi.html#c

Walker, A. S. (1961). *Medical services of the Royal Australian Navy and Royal Australian Air Force with a section on women in the Army Medical Services. Australia in the War of 1939–1945. Series 5—Medical.* Australian War Memorial. https://www.awm.gov.au/collection/C1417327

Westmore, A. (2012). *Occupational therapy & art therapy in Victorian mental health institutions.* Museum Victoria Collections. http://collections.museumvictoria.com.au/articles/11540

Westmore, A., & Monk, L. (2012). *Confinement & seclusion in Victorian mental health institutions.* Museum Victoria Collections. http://collections.museumvictoria.com.au/articles/11532

World Health Organization (WHO). (2001). *International Classification of Functioning, Disability and Health.* WHO. https://www.who.int/classifications/icf/en/

Wyndham, D. (2003). *Eugenics in Australia: Striving for national fitness.* Galton Institute.

4 The role of occupational therapy professional associations and regulatory bodies in Australia

Lynne Adamson, Rebecca Allen, Julie Brayshaw, Samantha Hunter, Adam Lo, Carol McKinstry and Anita Volkert

Chapter objectives

Upon completion of this chapter, the reader will be able to:

- Describe the role of professional associations at national and international levels, particularly that of Occupational Therapy Australia (OTA) and the World Federation of Occupational Therapists (WFOT) and their relationship with each other.
- Discuss the registration of occupational therapy practitioners in Australia and the bodies that participate in the process of registration.
- Describe the accreditation of occupational therapy education programs and assessment of internationally qualified occupational therapists.
- Demonstrate the importance of professional and regulatory bodies to occupational therapists and the interrelationship between these organisations and practitioners.

Key terms

professional association; accreditation; regulation; standards of practice

Introduction

This chapter describes four independent yet interrelated organisations which support the practice of occupational therapy in Australia. The organisations in focus are Occupational Therapy Australia (OTA), the national professional association, the World Federation of Occupational Therapists (WFOT), the international professional association, the Occupational Therapy Board of Australia (OTBA), the profession's registration board, and the Occupational Therapy Council of Australia Ltd (OTC), the body responsible for the accreditation of occupational therapy education programs in Australia and assessment of internationally qualified practitioners. While each operate and are structured independently, there are effective working relationships which enhance the role of the individual entities as well as the contributions each brings to the profession and practice of occupational therapy in Australia. The role and relationship of these organisations are explored.

Introducing the four organisations

Occupational Therapy Australia (OTA)

Occupational Therapy Australia (OTA) is the peak national professional association for occupational therapists in Australia. Professional associations are membership-based organisations, which have their genesis in medieval England when trade guilds were formed as collectives for craftsmen who sought to develop and guarantee standards of craftsmanship, ensure a fair price for goods and develop collective solutions to mutual areas of concern (Ernstthal, 2001; Rusaw, 1995). While professional associations as we know them in the twenty-first century have evolved significantly, the issues of leading a profession, guiding standards of practice and knowledge dissemination remain core to the mission and objectives of these organisations (Stokes, 2016). The role of professional organisations, such as OTA, is underpinned by a defined mission with objectives which may include raising the standards of education and practice, promoting the profession to key stakeholders and developing competencies which underpin practice.

Prior to 2010, occupational therapists in Australia were represented by state and territory based organisations. In 2010, the Australian state and territory occupational therapy associations amalgamated into one single entity called Occupational Therapy Australia. State and territories have divisional managers and councils that oversee the provision of local services with most services being developed and coordinated at the national level. OTA has a Chief Executive Officer (CEO) who works closely with a board of directors to oversee the leadership and management of the organisation. The majority of board of directors are elected by members while some are co-opted for specific skills.

As a member-based organisation, OTA exists to provide a range of services to its members and especially welcomes membership from students across all years and new graduates. OTA provides a variety of supports for early career therapists and some of these are highlighted in this chapter. The profession and its association in Australia do not exist in a national or international vacuum. The growth of the profession and its influence occur through participation and relationship with other organisations—the Occupational Therapy Australia Research Foundation, the World Federation of Occupational Therapists, the Occupational Therapy Board of Australia, and the Occupational Therapy Council of Australia Ltd. OTA also networks with other national occupational therapy professional associations both in Australia and internationally. Nationally, OTA has strong links with other professional organisations, including Indigenous Allied Health Australia, Allied Health Professions Australia, Speech Pathology Australia, the Australian Physiotherapy Association, the Australian Hand Therapy Association, and the Australian Rehabilitation and Assistive Technology Association.

World Federation of Occupational Therapists (WFOT)

The international organisation for occupational therapists commenced in 1951 with ten members, including Australia, and today comprises links with 101 member organisations around the world. At the first meeting a constitution was written with objectives focused on:

- the promotion of occupational therapy;
- the advancement of the practice and standards of occupational therapy;
- the promotion of education and training of therapists; and
- organising international congresses.

These objectives are still relevant today, as the WFOT continues with its mission to promote occupational therapy as an art and science internationally. The WFOT supports the development, use and practice of occupational therapy worldwide, demonstrating its relevance and contribution to society. The WFOT provides position papers on issues relevant to occupational therapists globally and also sets the minimum education standards for entry-level occupational therapy programs worldwide. The WFOT contributes to many international initiatives through links with the World Health Organization (WHO).

In the same way OTA is the professional association for occupational therapists in Australia, the WFOT is the professional association for occupational therapists worldwide who seek to belong to an international professional body for occupational therapists. In Australia, members of OTA automatically belong to the WFOT, as OTA pays an annual organisation membership fee. The WFOT is managed by an executive management team, comprising a president, vice presidents, executive director and program coordinators who meet annually. A council consisting of a delegate from each member country meets every second year. The WFOT organises an international occupational therapy congress that is held every four years since the inaugural Congress in 1954 at Edinburgh, United Kingdom. Congresses are truly international events, hosted by member countries across all five continents, including Sweden, 2002; Australia, 2006; Chile, 2010; Japan, 2014; South Africa, 2018; and France, 2022.

Occupational Therapy Board of Australia (OTBA)

In Australia, professional registration is an important mechanism for upholding standards of practice for health professionals and to ensure the protection of the public in accessing health services. Occupational therapy is one of 16 health professions regulated by nationally consistent legislation under the National Registration and Accreditation Scheme (NRAS). Practitioners are required to comply with the Health Practitioner Regulation National Law Act 2009 (the National Law), so understanding registration is an important part of education in these professions.

There is a legal requirement that anyone who uses the title or practises as an 'occupational therapist' must be registered by the Occupational Therapy Board of Australia. The functions of the Board include:

- registering occupational therapy practitioners and students;
- deciding the requirements for registration;
- developing standards, codes and guidelines for the profession;
- approving accreditation standards and accredited programs of study;
- overseeing the assessment of overseas trained practitioners who apply for occupational therapy registration; and
- considering and making decisions on notifications (complaints) made against registered practitioners.

The Board is made up of six practitioner members who are occupational therapists and three community members, all of whom are appointed by the Ministerial Council. To fulfil its responsibilities, the Board works closely with the Australian Health Practitioner Regulation Agency (AHPRA) which oversees the regulation of all registered health professions in Australia.

Under the National Law, all students enrolled in an approved occupational therapy program of study must be registered with the Occupational Therapy Board of Australia. There are no fees for student registration and students do not need to apply for registration. Twice a year, each university provides details of all new and existing occupational therapy students to AHPRA who manage student registration on behalf of the Board. After completing their studies, graduates must make an application to the Board for registration as an occupational therapist before they commence practice.

As noted in the list above, other roles of the regulator include overseeing the assessment process for overseas qualified practitioners who apply to register in Australia and approving programs of study as meeting the standards required for students to graduate with the knowledge, skills and professional attributes to practice the profession. To fulfil these responsibilities, the Board has assigned the Occupational Therapy Council of Australia Ltd (OTC) to undertake these roles.

Occupational Therapy Council of Australia Ltd (OTC)

The OTC is an independent, not-for-profit organisation, established as a public company limited by guarantee. Its operation is overseen by a board of directors, comprising experienced occupational therapists as well as independent and community representatives. The OTC's role is set out in the National Law, with two core functions. Firstly, the OTC develops and reviews accreditation standards for occupational therapy education. These standards outline what is expected of the education providers (universities) that deliver occupational therapy education and are regularly reviewed through extensive consultations to ensure they reflect contemporary practice. Accreditation standards are particularly relevant to students of occupational therapy as they are the mechanism to confirm that entry-level programs of study in occupational therapy meet the expectations of the profession and the public so that graduates will be competent and safe to practise. The OTC regularly assesses programs against the standards by reviewing performance of a program and seeking the views of students, practitioners, employers, practice education supervisors and educators. The second core role of the OTC is to conduct assessments of internationally qualified practitioners to ensure they meet competencies relevant to practise as an occupational therapist in Australia.

Exploring the roles and contributions of the organisations to professional practice

The occupational therapy organisations described in this chapter have both unique and collaborative roles related to professional practice. These roles can be summarised as being facilitators of:

* knowledge: sharing and professional learning;
* professional practice: standards and research; and
* change: lobbying and advocacy.

Facilitators of knowledge sharing and professional learning

All four organisations contribute in diverse ways. Professional associations have been described as knowledge agents (Karseth & Nerland, 2007), and organisations that facilitate knowledge development and knowledge transfer.

Continuing professional development

Provision of continuing professional development (CPD) is core to the mission of professional associations. The OTBA, through registration standards, requires practitioners to engage in ongoing professional development activities through their careers to ensure they maintain their competence and provide safe and effective health services. The OTC, through accreditation standards, requires graduates to be prepared for life-long learning via CPD. OTA has become a key stakeholder in the delivery of formal CPD programs including a biennial national scientific conference, practice-oriented events and an extensive range of workshops, webinars and other development activities such as journal clubs. CPD programs are targeted at qualified occupational therapists and many of the offerings are highly useful and relevant for new graduates/early career therapists. OTA also shares knowledge and information with student members by providing each member with access to the journal and magazine, regular updates via online e-news and access to the member-only section of the website where professional resources can be obtained. Other member services include a mentoring program for qualified occupational therapists, access to professional and educational resources on the OTA website; networking and learning opportunities via special interest and regional groups, career forums relevant to students and new graduates, local professional news and informal support; discounted rates for CPD; and access to specific online communities of practice to provide support in key practice areas.

OTA has provided a mentoring program for its members for many years, where the mentee is linked with a more experienced therapist in the same area of practice or for a specific career or professional need (Doyle et al., 2019). The program assists both new graduates as well as established therapists providing opportunities to seek mentoring from experienced therapists in the field or their sector of practice. Mentoring and supervision are key aspects of support to new graduates as they develop professional knowledge. Supervision is a management strategy to direct work and ensure efficient and effective use of resources, and typically occurs in the workplace. In contrast, mentoring concentrates on professional and career development and can occur separate to workplace activities (Braveman, 2016; Doyle et al., 2019).

The WFOT promotes professional knowledge through collaborative international activities to develop competency standards, position papers and international congresses. Online educational opportunities reflect the international nature of the profession and create wide possibilities for sharing knowledge and cross-cultural learning across the widely dispersed profession. The *World Federation of Occupational Therapists (WFOT) Bulletin* is the official publication of the WFOT and is published biannually in April and October. Its aim is to promote awareness and understanding of the WFOT and its activities and services. This includes the development of the occupational therapy profession worldwide, promotion of cross-cultural awareness and understanding, the international exchange of professional knowledge and experience, as well as being a platform for constructive engagement in dialogue and debate. Articles are published in the official languages of WFOT: English, Spanish, French and German.

The registration standards developed by the OTBA require practitioners to plan, record and reflect on their professional development activities. Practitioners are also expected to participate in interactive learning with others. Through this mechanism, the OTBA maintains a key role in ensuring ongoing development and sharing of professional knowledge. The OTC accreditation standards require universities to develop graduates' commitment to life-long learning and capacity for self-reflection.

Facilitators of professional practice—standards and research

All four organisations have significant, albeit different, roles to play in the development of professional standards. Bringing their unique perspectives and roles together, all agree that it is vital for standards to be in line with the diversity of occupational therapy practice and updated as practice changes, addressing emerging health care needs, technological advances and public expectations.

Registration standards

A key function of the OTBA is to establish registration standards which a therapist must meet to be eligible to register as an occupational therapist. The National Law requires the Board to establish standards for:

- professional indemnity insurance which must be maintained by occupational therapists;
- how it will consider any criminal history when deciding if it is relevant to professional practice;
- continuing professional development;
- English language skills for people applying for registration; and
- recency of practice which determines eligibility for practice.

The initial application and annual renewal processes require practitioners to make declarations about whether or not they meet the mandatory registration standards. AHPRA and the OTBA audit a proportion of occupational therapists each year, asking them to provide evidence that they have met the registration standards. Audits are important to provide an assurance of public protection by ensuring that occupational therapists are meeting the registration standards. In addition to registration standards, the OTBA has developed codes and guidelines to guide the profession. These include a Code of Conduct, a social media policy, guidelines for mandatory notifications, and guidelines for advertising regulated health services.

Competency standards

The OTBA has developed the current professional competencies which describe the standards expected for competent practice by occupational therapists for registration and for regulation of the profession by the Board. These competency standards (OTBA, 2018) replace the previous Australian competency standards for new graduate occupational therapists that were developed by Occupational Therapy Australia. The standards focus on four conceptual areas of occupational therapy practice, namely: professionalism; knowledge and learning; occupational therapy process and practice; and communication. Each of the four competency standards is further described by a number of practice behaviours. The practice behaviours communicate to an occupational therapist and the public the expected behaviours an occupational therapist should demonstrate under each competency standard.

All competency standards are developed within a cultural and social timeframe in Australia. The current standards specifically acknowledge the need for occupational therapists to enhance their cultural responsiveness and capabilities for practice with Aboriginal and Torres Strait Islander Peoples. The need for respectful, collaborative, safe and culturally responsive practice is supported in the competency standards, where occupational therapists recognise that historical, political, cultural, societal, environmental and economic factors influence clients' health, well-being and occupational participation. The competency standards apply to all occupational therapists, including those working in research, education, management or other roles not involving direct contact with clients. They have been designed for regulatory use and are the benchmark for the standard of practice deemed suitable by the profession.

OTA is responsible for assessing occupational therapists as Better Access to Mental Health endorsed occupational therapists within the Medicare Benefits Scheme. This Scheme provides people with mental health disorders access to a defined number of low cost or free allied health services. Criteria are set by the Australian Department of Health and OTA membership is one of these criteria, in addition to being registered with the OTBA, having a minimum of two years of supervised experience in mental health—specifically the delivery of Focused Psychological Strategies—and ongoing supervision and development plans. Applicants submit a portfolio which is assessed by a panel of experienced occupational therapists.

The OTC is responsible for conducting assessments of occupational therapists who hold an international qualification not approved by the OTBA. Occupational therapists wishing to work in Australia are required to have their qualifications assessed and are required to undertake a period of supervised practice before gaining general registration status. The OTC is also appointed by the Federal Department of Home Affairs to assess occupational therapy qualifications for skilled migration. This process assists practitioners to understand Australian health care settings and ensures Australian competency standards are met.

Education standards

In Australia, the Health Practitioner Regulation National Law 2009 (National Law) mandates that for each registered profession there will be standards of education which determine the requirements for an educational program to ensure its graduates are provided with the knowledge, skills and professional attributes to practise that profession in Australia. The National Law requires that education programs are accredited by an independent process, which for occupational therapy is carried out by the OTC. As part of its international commitment, OTA assesses Australian accredited education programs against the WFOT standards. OTA contributes to program accreditation through regular liaison with education programs, students, graduates and other professional organisations.

Developing accreditation standards for occupational therapy education programs is an important responsibility. Not only will the public be reassured that graduating therapists are appropriately qualified, but they will also know that during an education program, there will have been an adequate amount of clinical practice to ensure necessary skills and knowledge have been tested in supervised situations.

Setting, reviewing and monitoring standards are important professional activities, requiring liaison between the regulatory bodies, professional associations, education providers, practitioners and community members. Consultation processes are always set in place when standards are reviewed, when changes might be determined as necessary or as part of ongoing quality improvement. Students are considered an important part of consultation processes. Reflection and reporting on learning experiences provide valuable input to any review process. Educators and accreditors will seek participation of students in both ongoing program review and the formal reaccreditation process.

Standards to enhance practice

A role of professional associations, which have government regulated professionals as members, is to develop standards to enhance practice. OTA contributes to this function through the development of guides to good practice, position statements and guidelines in key domains of practice, as well as provision of CPD to support the requirement for mandated requirements of CPD for ongoing registration.

Like OTA, the WFOT develops position statements. Both organisations have leadership roles in the profession and strong relationships with organisations relevant to the profession. Position papers present the official stance of organisations and are developed in response to an issue, concern or need of members. They can be a useful resource to guide practice and to advise the public and other stakeholders about the profession's view on important issues. As a result, these resources are useful for students to facilitate understanding of professional issues and to assist in understanding what the profession regards as good practice. Consequently, these can assist in supporting assignments, clinical and other practice education experiences. A recent example is the WFOT Position Statement on Occupational Therapy and Human Rights (2019). This paper outlines the importance of occupation to people, the impact of occupational injustice and the 'right for all people to engage in the occupations they need to survive, define as meaningful, and that contribute positively to their own well-being and the wellbeing of their communities' (WFOT, 2019).

Supporting research

Research is integral to a profession's development and is imperative to improve the quality of services provided by the profession. The OTBA and the OTC have a role in research as both organisations use evidence and best practice to support their standards. OTA actively supports research development and research dissemination in the profession. It has a well-established journal, the *Australian Occupational Therapy Journal* (AOTJ), which is internationally recognised as a provider of high quality, peer-reviewed information. The journal has an editorial board of skilled and internationally renowned researchers, educators and clinical experts.

Both OTA and WFOT conferences include the latest research and evidence-based practice studies. These occur every two years for OTA and every four years for the WFOT. Students are encouraged to attend and often participate as volunteers. Students and new graduates have presented findings from their honours thesis and other projects at these events. In 2013, the Occupational Therapy Australia Research Foundation was launched to support and build research capacity in the profession in Australia through providing research grants and awards. The WFOT recently developed a program area devoted to research. The program team focuses its activities on the priority areas for research that are determined from the international occupational therapy community. In 2017, OTA also established the Occupational Therapy Australia Research Academy to recognise outstanding scholarship and enhance research capacity building in the occupational therapy profession. As of 2020, there have been a total of 21 Fellows inducted into the Academy.

Facilitators of change

The standards set by the four organisations can be an important facilitator of change. Professional associations such as the OTA and WFOT can take a direct role in lobbying, advocating for change and promoting the profile of the profession. The focus of the OTBA and OTC differs. However, the standards they set facilitate action in areas identified for change. For example, the OTBA (2018) competency standards specifically require all occupational therapists to enhance their cultural responsiveness and capabilities for practice with Aboriginal and Torres Strait Islander Peoples and the OTC accreditation standards for education providers support this expectation as one of the ways occupational therapy can contribute to the National Scheme's Aboriginal and Torres Strait Islander Health and Cultural Safety Strategy 2020–2025 (AHPRA, 2020).

Increasing the profile of the profession—lobbying and advocacy

Lobbying and advocacy have been recognised as core to professional association functions. Andrews et al. (2013) identified the role associations have in influencing and developing policy and practice. Advocacy is described as actions which support policy recommendation or a cause (Shaw, 2014). Lobbying is the practice of influencing an agenda, often of a legislative nature pertaining to concerns of a profession (Matthews, 2012).

Occupational therapists practise in a range of areas influenced by government policy and have been part of many significant changes since emerging as a profession. OTA regards lobbying and advocacy as a collective responsibility and actively supports this key work by contributing to submissions, senate hearings and initiating meetings with politicians and government department representatives to discuss topics of concern both federally and at state and territory level.

The WFOT is actively involved with lobbying and advocating for the occupational therapy profession at the international level. This is a key area of responsibility for members of the executive with each having a regional responsibility. Other relationships include those with the UN, WHO, Rehabilitation International, World Bank and other NGOs. Some of the areas of advocacy at the international level include human rights, mental health, and disaster preparedness and response.

Increasing the profile of the profession—promotion and communications

Promotion of the profession occurs in many ways such as through lobbying and advocacy activities but also through direct promotional campaigns. OTA celebrates the profession during OT Week, which is the third week of October each year. A theme is chosen to assist national and local campaigns to promote events and the profession, and occupational therapists across the country find ways of celebrating and promoting the profession at this time. World Occupational Therapy Day is the opportunity to heighten the visibility of the profession's development work and to promote the activities of WFOT locally, nationally and internationally. It is held on 27 October each year. Celebrations are held around the world and on social media to celebrate World Occupational Therapy Day. OT Week and World Occupational Therapy Day are important in the occupational therapy calendar to promote and celebrate the profession and many students in OT have participated in OT Week activities at their universities to both celebrate and promote the profession.

Conclusion

In this chapter, the four chief organisations that represent different sectors of the occupational therapy profession were profiled. OTA is the peak body that represents the occupational therapy discipline in Australia while the WFOT advocates for the profession at the international level. OTC accredits the occupational therapy education programs in Australia and reviews all international applicants seeking a review of their occupational therapy education for parity purposes with the Australian education of occupational therapists. OTBA is the national registration body for all occupational therapists who wish to practise in Australia and is designed to ensure competent and safe practice to protect the public. It is important for occupational therapy students to be familiar with the roles and responsibilities of these four organisations. Participation in relevant student activities will enhance educational experiences and prepare graduates to be active within the occupational therapy profession.

Summary

- As students in occupational therapy it is important to understand some of the key external organisations which contribute to shaping and supporting the profession.
- There are four key organisations which shape the practice of occupational therapy in Australia which become increasingly relevant as students progress to graduation.
- The organisations are: i) Occupational Therapy Australia (OTA), the professional association; ii) the World Federation of Occupational Therapists (WFOT), the international professional association for occupational therapists; iii) the Occupational Therapy Board of Australia (OTBA), the profession's registration board; and iv) the Occupational Therapy Council of Australia Ltd (OTC), the body responsible for the accreditation of occupational therapy programs in Australia and assessment of internationally qualified occupational therapists.
- Each of these organisations has a role in facilitating knowledge sharing and professional learning, facilitating professional practice standards and research, and facilitating change through lobbying and advocacy.
- While these organisations intersect, their roles are unique and contribute to a diverse range of functions to support the profession, raise its profile and enhance occupational therapy practice.

Review questions

1. Summarise the key distinctions between OTA, OTBA and OTC.
2. Why do OTA, OTBA and OTC each have distinct roles?
3. What are the benefits of belonging to OTA?
4. Why is registration of a profession important? How do the four separate organisations contribute directly or indirectly to supporting registration?
5. What benefits does being part of WFOT bring to a national professional group, and to an individual practitioner?

Websites for the four organisations

- Occupational Therapy Australia: www.otaus.com.au
- Occupational Therapy Board of Australia: www.occupationaltherapyboard.gov.au
- Occupational Therapy Council of Australia Ltd: www.otcouncil.com.au
- World Federation of Occupational Therapists: www.wfot.org

References

Andrews, H., Perron, L., Plaetse, B. V., & Taylor, D. J. (2013) Strengthening the organizational capacity of health professional associations: The FIGO LOGIC Toolkit. *International Journal of Gynaecology and Obstetrics, 122*(3), 190–191. https://doi.org/10.1016/j.ijgo.2013.06.002

Australian Health Practitioner Regulation Agency. (2020). *National Scheme's Aboriginal and Torres Strait Islander health and cultural safety strategy, 2020–2025.* https://www.ahpra.gov.au/About-AHPRA/Aboriginal-and-Torres-Strait-Islander-Health-Strategy.aspx

Braveman, B. (2016). *Leading and managing occupational therapy services: An evidence-based approach.* F. A. Davis Co.

Doyle, N. W., Gafni Lachter, L., & Jacobs, K. (2019). Scoping review of mentoring research in the occupational therapy literature, 2002–2018. *Australian Occupational Therapy Journal, 66*(5), 541–551. https://doi.org/10.1111/1440-1630.12579

Ernstthal, H. (2001). *Principles of association management* (4th ed.). American Society of Association Executives.

Health Practitioner Regulation National Law Act 2009. https://www.ahpra.gov.au/About-AHPRA/What-We-Do/Legislation.aspx

Karseth, B., & Nerland, M. (2007). Building professionalism in a knowledge society: Examining discourses of knowledge in four professional associations. *Journal of Education and Work, 20*(4), 335–355. http://dx.doi.org/10.1080/13639080701650172

Matthews, J. H. (2012). Role of professional organisations in advocating for the nursing profession. *Online Journal of Issues in Nursing, 17*(1), Manuscript 3. http://ojin.nursingworld.org/MainMenuCategories/ANAMarketplace/ANAPeriodicals/OJIN/TableofContents/Vol-17-2012/No1-Jan-2012/Professional-Organizations-and-Advocating.html

Occupational Therapy Board of Australia. (2018). *Australian Occupational Therapy Competency Standards.* https://www.occupationaltherapyboard.gov.au/Codes-Guidelines/Competencies.aspx

Rusaw, C. (1995). Learning by association: Professional associations as learning agents. *Human Resource Development Quarterly, 6*(2), 215–226. https://doi.org/10.1002/hrdq.3920060209

Shaw, D. (2014) Advocacy: The role of health professional associations. *International Journal of Gynaecology and Obstetrics, 127*(Supplement 1), S43–S48. http://www.sciencedirect.com/science/article/pii/S0020729214004251

Stokes, G. (2016). Relevance and professional associations in 2026: Towards a new role for thought leadership. In J. Guthrie, E. Evans, & R. Burritt (Eds.). *Relevance and professional associations in 2026* (pp. 44–47). RMIT University & Chartered Accountants, Australia & New Zealand. https://www.psc.gov.au/sites/default/files/Relevance%20and%20Prof%20Associations%20in%202026.pdf

World Federation of Occupational Therapists. (2019). *Position statement: Occupational Therapy and Human Rights (revised).* https://www.wfot.org/resources/occupational-therapy-and-human-rights

5 The scope of practice of occupational therapists in Australia

Roles, responsibilities and relationships

Kieran Broome and Ann Kennedy-Behr

Chapter objectives

Upon completion of this chapter, the reader will be able to:

* Know the personal, legislative, professional and role-specific limitations on scope of practice.
* Be familiar with the opportunities for occupational therapists to undertake a broad range of activities and responsibilities.
* Know avenues to advance and extend their scope of practice.

Key terms

scope of practice; roles; responsibilities

Introduction

Most students ask the question 'what do occupational therapists do?' Scope of practice describes what occupational therapists are able to do; in other words, the activities that they are competent to undertake, who they work with and where they work. Scope of practice can change as the profession and the needs of society evolve; however, the core scope of practice for occupational therapy is retained. Scope of practice in Australia is influenced by a number of different factors (Occupational Therapy Australia, 2017) (see Table 5.1).

General factors

* the minimum or threshold competency standards that your university training is accredited against by the registration board, the Occupational Therapy Board of Australia (OTBA) and the accrediting body, the Occupational Therapy Council of Australia Ltd (OTC);
* the general consensus of the profession, usually represented by the professional association Occupational Therapy Australia (OTA);
* federal and state laws such as the *Health Practitioner Regulation National Law Act 2009*; and
* the health care context, such as professional boundaries.

There are international differences in scope of practice. For example, dysphagia (swallowing problem) management is a specialised part of occupational therapy education and practice in the United States, but is not undertaken by occupational therapists in Australia. In Australia, dysphagia is central to the scope of practice of speech pathologists.

Table 5.1 Factors that impact occupational therapy's scope of practice

Factor	Example
Education and training you receive at university	Laurie is an occupational therapist. When she was a student, one of her lecturers taught the basics of how to use switches for people with severe disabilities to control their environment (e.g., lights, TV). On graduation, Laurie felt confident that 'recommending switches' was within her scope of practice. For some more complex cases, she sought extra support, supervision and training to improve and refresh her skills.
Competency standards	Peter is an occupational therapist. He designs home modifications (e.g., grab rails and ramps) on a regular basis. He received introductory education and training in home modification at university, in line with the occupational therapy competency standards. He keeps his skills current by reflecting on his practice and engaging in continuing professional development.
The registration board	Martha was interested in doing acupuncture as an occupational therapist. After visiting the websites and communicating with the Occupational Therapy Board of Australia (the registration board) she decided that acupuncture was a 'significant departure from accepted standards of practice' for occupational therapists, so she could not do acupuncture as an occupational therapist. She decided to do another degree as a Traditional Chinese Medicine (TCM) practitioner, but was clear with her clients and in her advertising about when she was working as an occupational therapist or a TCM practitioner.
The professional association	Max is an occupational therapist working in workplace rehabilitation. With support from his team, he began doing home modifications in his work. He joined the relevant professional association interest group to make sure that he developed and maintained competence in home modification, and to help align his work with the principles of occupational therapy.
Federal and state laws	Marie is an occupational therapist. She saw her podiatrist colleagues had done additional training to prescribe antibiotics. She thought this could be useful for her clients. After talking to her supervisor, she found out that there are laws that limit the prescribing of medication, with only specific professions with specific training allowed. Therefore, under the current laws, she could not prescribe medication as an occupational therapist.
Specific circumstances	Harvey is an occupational therapist working as a private practitioner in mental health. One of his clients had a hand injury from self-harming. Although Harvey had previous experience in hand therapy, he was out of practice. Also, the Medicare funding that the client was receiving to see Harvey only covered psychological therapies. Harvey decided to refer the client to another occupational therapist.
What your employer expects	Ashley works as an occupational therapist for an aged care assessment team. Although Ashley has many skills in providing interventions such as home modifications and equipment, her current role only includes assessment and deciding on levels of care required. In her current role, she is not able to provide intervention.

Individual factors

*   the accredited education and training you receive at university;
*   your ongoing learning as an occupational therapist, including appropriate continuing professional development;

- specific circumstances such as the job that you are in or how your work is funded; and
- relevant experience.

What do occupational therapists do?

Central to occupational therapy is the aim of enabling people to be involved in meaningful occupation, and engaging in occupations. All occupational therapists should be able to assess how well a person is functioning in daily activities, and how engaged they are. An occupational therapist will find out what is meaningful to the client. They should be able to identify factors that can support or hinder engagement in occupation, including personal components (e.g., vision, thoughts), occupation components (how people do things) and environment components (e.g., ergonomics, stressful environments). Because occupation is central to the scope of occupational therapy, occupational therapists should be able to identify and support engagement in occupations that promote health and wellness such as independent living, employment, education, play, leisure, socialising, rest and sleep. Due to complexity, some areas of practice such as driving assessment and rehabilitation may require further training.

Occupational therapists may assess and provide intervention for specific aspects of the person, occupation and environment. The Canadian Model of Client-Centred Enablement describes a range of different skills that occupational therapists might use to promote occupational performance and engagement including: adapt, advocate, coach, collaborate, consult, coordinate, design/build, educate, engage and specialise (Townsend & Polatajko, 2007). This model is broadly applicable in the Australian context. Examples of activities that occupational therapists do in Australia include:

- building a strong therapeutic relationship with the client, centred around the client's needs;
- facilitating the development of clients' goals;
- using occupation in a therapeutic way (e.g., engaging adolescents with eating disorders in adventure activities to build their self-esteem);
- working with parents or caregivers to support the client (e.g., problem-solving toileting issues);
- establishing or rehabilitating skills required for everyday living (e.g., dressing, social skills);
- educating clients and carers on different ways of doing things (e.g., how to manage stress during a job interview);
- using talking therapies such as coaching, motivational interviewing or micro-counselling;
- recommending and supporting people to use equipment and devices (e.g., wheelchairs);
- fabricating devices and orthotics to promote occupational performance (e.g., making a hand splint);
- designing modifications to the environment (e.g., lift into a pool, ergonomic seating in a workplace, training personal care workers in how to help people with dementia with daily tasks);
- educating people on their health and the impact of occupations on their health;
- coordinating care by planning and referring to relevant health professionals and support services; and
- advocating for the needs of clients at individual, group, community and societal levels.

Occupational therapists may also develop specific skills that draw upon and build on their foundational training in occupational therapy. These often require further training, consolidation of skills or extended experience. Examples include:

- coaching (e.g., occupational performance coaching; Graham et al., 2009);
- focused psychological strategies (e.g., acceptance commitment therapy; Hayes et al., 2006);
- rehabilitation of specific skills and abilities (e.g., cognitive rehabilitation);
- manual therapy for musculoskeletal injuries;
- management of specific conditions (e.g., injury management, wound management, or oedema management);
- specific therapeutic modalities such as functional electrical stimulation (Howlett et al., 2015); and
- being an expert witness in a legal case.

While some of these activities may overlap with other professions or seem out of place, there are often historical, philosophical, economic or competency reasons why they may fall into the scope of occupational therapy. For example, oedema management often involves the use of compression garments, which can be difficult to get on and off and require adjustments to positioning and physical activity that draw upon the broader skills of occupational therapists. In addition, an occupational therapist may be the member of the treating team who has advanced training in compression garment prescription; they are an occupational therapist first and an oedema practitioner second.

To identify whether an activity is within your scope of practice you should ask yourself the following questions:

- Is it clearly linked to enabling occupational performance and engagement in occupations?
- Am I knowledgeable and skilled in this activity?
- Do I need advice/support from my supervisor or someone more experienced?
- Is it supported by my workplace, profession and the health care context?
- Would it be better provided by another health professional?

Occupational therapists will also complete a range of activities that are common across the health professions, including:

- communicating effectively with others;
- following workplace procedures such as documentation, handover of clients and safe home visiting;
- managing a health service (e.g., prioritising workloads, being a team leader);
- quality improvement, which involves continually monitoring and improving your practice;
- using research to improve practice;
- conducting and supporting new research;
- working as part of a team;
- contributing to education of others (e.g., supervising other occupational therapists, occupational therapy students); and
- risk management.

Who do occupational therapists work with?

In Australia, occupational therapists work with people across the lifespan. Some occupational therapists work with newborn children, for example helping parents and children to improve feeding and to undertake activities that help promote positive attachment between the child and the caregiver. At the other end of the spectrum, occupational therapists work with people who are dying, helping people to remain independent as long as possible and to continue to engage in meaningful occupation for as long as they wish/are able.

Occupational therapists also work with individuals, groups, communities and broader society (Craik et al., 2007; OTA, 2017). Including the family and a person's community is an important part of working with individuals. At times it can be challenging to balance the needs of the individual with the needs of the family and caregivers. Examples of working with individuals, groups, communities or society include:

- Individual: Working with a child with autism and their family to develop skills for forming friendships.
- Group: Facilitating a group for people with intellectual disability to learn to live independently in the community.
- Community: Working with a council to make sure that facilities such as children's play areas and walkways are accessible for people with disabilities.
- Society: Advocating for efficient and effective support services to help people with severe mental illness to find and maintain employment.

Who we work with is often influenced by funding. Occupational therapists may be paid directly by the person or their insurer. They may work for the public service (e.g., a public hospital). They may receive funding through a government scheme such as the National Disability Insurance Scheme, My Aged Care, Medicare or Department of Veterans Affairs. We might also be contracted by organisations such as councils, workplaces or lawyers to provide specific services. Regardless of the funding source OTs must always ensure they are working within their scope of practice.

Where do occupational therapists work?

Because people live their lives in many different places, occupational therapists work in many different settings. Occupational therapists commonly work in places such as community-based services (visiting people in their homes or running clinics), hospitals, schools, aged care facilities, workplaces and prisons. Occupational therapists work across sectors, for example private practice, public services (such as housing services) and non-governmental or charitable organisations. Some may work in education, research, policy or development roles. Occupational therapists can work in highly specialised services such as a large metropolitan hospital or may work remotely such as flying in to a mine site or visiting remote communities. Not all people with occupational therapy degrees will work in roles with the title of occupational therapist. Some occupational therapists may take on roles with titles such as case manager, occupational rehabilitation consultant, manager, policy advisor or professional development officer (Broome & Gillen, 2014). Below is a case study of an occupational therapist who works in a multi-faceted community role.

Case study: A day in the life of a community occupational therapist

In the morning, Shaun the occupational therapist checks and responds to his emails and phone messages. He then checks new referrals to the occupational therapy service, prioritises which need to be seen sooner, and sends letters to referrers and clients to let them know they are on a wait-list.

Then Shaun visits two clients at home. At the first visit he reviews the client's progress with their stroke rehabilitation plan. The client has made some progress in their ability to cook independently but has found it difficult to find the motivation to practise regularly. The therapist explores with the client ways to remain motivated, and updates the rehabilitation plan.

At the second visit, a client with motor neurone disease has lost a significant amount of strength. Shaun identifies that the client may soon need a power-driven wheelchair and some other devices and strategies. He measures the client, talks through the options, client needs and potential funding sources, and assesses the house for modifications that may need to happen. Shaun helps her to identify new ways to be meaningfully occupied in life, as she feels depressed after stopping playing golf. Shaun also notices that she has been losing weight and offers a referral to the dietitian.

After lunch, Shaun runs an education group alongside the physiotherapist for the local pain management program. He focuses on different ways to manage the physical and emotional aspects of pain so that people are able to be as active and independent as possible.

Later in the afternoon, he documents his sessions, designs home modifications, organises a trial of a power-driven wheelchair with an equipment supplier, liaises with and refers to the dietitian and plans his activities for upcoming days including booking home visits with the most urgent clients. He also does some research on equipment that might help one of his clients, and does some work updating an education booklet for his pain program clients with the latest research findings.

What do occupational therapists *not* do as part of their scope of practice?

In Australia, the following activities are not part of occupational therapy practice by law (Health Practitioner Regulation National Law Act 2009):

- *Invasive procedures* such as surgery or injections (although we may, for example, help someone with diabetes and a hand tremor to find ways to inject themselves with insulin).
- *Manipulation of spinal or peripheral joints.*
- *-Prescribe or administer medications* (although we may, for example, help someone with memory problems find ways to get in to a regular medication routine or open their medications).

Occupational therapists should not undertake assessments or interventions that require a *high degree of specific skill and knowledge* that are typically *central to another profession*, X-rays for radiographers, or prosthetics for prosthetists (although we may, for example, help

---

Case study: A day in the life of a paediatric occupational therapist

Lynne works in a large outer-regional town in Queensland at the community health centre based in the middle of town. Her role is to provide occupational therapy services to children both in the town and in the surrounding area. One of the things Lynne enjoys about her role is that no two days are alike. Today, Lynne is assessing a three-year-old boy, Thomas. His parents have had concerns about his development and their GP referred them to Lynne to assess his play skills and gross and fine motor skills. Lynne spends time talking to Thomas's parents, asks them about his daily routines, his self-care skills, and his likes and dislikes. Lynne carefully observes the way Thomas interacts with his parents, how he explores the play items that are in the room and how he responds to her conversation with him. Following the assessment session, Lynne prepares a detailed report which is to be shared with the GP and with Thomas's parents.

Lynne then drives to the local primary school to observe three children in their classrooms and provide advice to their teachers on how to support these children. One of the children, Michael, is five and has been referred for handwriting difficulties. Lynne observes that Michael sits at a desk that is too high for him, that his feet do not touch the floor, and that he is often distracted by the two children that sit either side of him. He hunches his shoulders while he is writing and grips his pencil very tightly. Lynne suggests to the teacher that Michael be placed at a smaller desk and that he only have one child next to him if possible. She also gives Michael some handwriting tips in a fun, child-friendly way. Lynne then visits two other classrooms, and provides support to both the children and the teachers. The remainder of the day is spent on documentation and preparing for a talk that she is giving tomorrow at a new mums group, talking about the importance of 'tummy time' and supporting infant play.

---

someone with a new prosthetic to learn how to use it during home and community activities). Some interventions, such as *physical agent modalities* (e.g., therapeutic ultrasound, electrical stimulation, shortwave diathermy [electromagnetic energy], light therapy, electrical stimulation, iontophoresis, superficial and deep heating agents, and cryotherapy, dry needling, etc) should not be used routinely, although these may be used on occasion to support other occupational therapy interventions.

How do I broaden my scope of practice?

There are many ways to move beyond the skills and knowledge that you establish in your pre-registration university degree. Experience in your workplace, under appropriate supervision and support, will allow you to reflect on your practice and be self-directed in your research and development. Occupational therapists use other strategies to extend their knowledge such as attending special interest groups, workshops and conferences, regular reading of the literature, peer support and work-shadowing, pursuing specific extra qualifications such as accreditation in a specific skill or postgraduate university study. For example, if you were working with children you might choose to attend a workshop on the Cognitive Orientation to Daily Occupational Performance

(CO–OP) Approach (Polatajko & Mandich, 2004). You would then need to continue implementing and reflecting on this in your practice and updating skills as required. Occupational therapists may also conduct their own research to advance their own personal knowledge base and the knowledge of the profession.

Other concepts related to scope of practice

What has been described so far can broadly be considered the general scope of practice of occupational therapists. Other concepts around scope of practice include:

- Advanced scope of practice: Practice which is significantly more advanced when compared with new graduate competency and involves a greater depth or breadth of skills, knowledge and attitudes.
- Extended scope of practice: Undertaking activities that are outside of the traditional scope of a profession, and which may require further training, oversight and relevant legislation changes if applicable (e.g., occupational therapists ordering X-ray investigations).
- Delegated scope of practice: Considered and appropriate delegation of selected tasks to supporting health professionals (e.g., therapy assistants) and students. Attention should be paid to providing sufficient training, oversight and supervision, the selection of appropriate tasks, and ensuring that the supervising occupational therapist retains responsibility for higher level professional tasks such as clinical decision-making and treatment planning.

Legal requirements to work in Australia as an occupational therapist

As per Chapters 4 and 7 it is your legal responsibility to:

- work within the scope of practice that you are competent in performing;
- maintain your registration as an occupational therapist;
- maintain appropriate insurance for your activities;
- complete relevant and appropriate continuing professional development to maintain and develop your competency; and
- act with integrity.

Conclusion

Scope of practice describes the tasks, activities, roles and responsibilities that occupational therapists undertake. Your scope of practice will be influenced by a range of personal, legislative, professional and role-specific factors. Occupational therapists work with individuals, groups and communities, across the lifespan. While the goal of occupational therapy remains the same across different roles, there is a range of different activities that are specific to each role and client. For example, one occupational therapist might make a splint in a hospital for a client to improve his/her hand function, while another might assess a professional fisherman's ability to perform tasks safely on a boat. Occupational therapists will identify what is important and meaningful for the client, but may use diverse techniques such as ergonomics, play, relaxation, dressing training or driving assessment to help achieve the client's goals. While as a new graduate you will hold basic competency in a broad range of generic occupational therapy skills, you will need to continue to develop, hone and expand your scope of practice across your career.

Summary

- This chapter describes the tasks, activities, roles and responsibilities that occupational therapists undertake.
- Scope of practice is influenced by a range of personal, legislative, professional and role-specific factors.
- While the goal of occupational therapy remains the same across different roles, there is a range of different activities that are specific to each role and client.
- Occupational therapists continue to develop, advance and expand their scope of practice throughout their career.

Review questions

1. What professional association might influence your scope of practice as an occupational therapist?
2. Margie is a new graduate occupation therapist. She has been working with some psychologists who are specially trained psychotherapists. Margie would like to start doing this in her practice. Is this in her scope of practice?
3. If you were an occupational therapist working with children, describe a range of activities that you might do in a normal day.

References

Broome, K., & Gillen, A. (2014). Implications of occupational therapy job advertisement trends for occupational therapy education. *British Journal of Occupational Therapy*, 77(11), 574–581. https://doi.org/10.4276/030802214X14151078348558

Craik, J., Davis, J., & Polatajko, H. J. (2007). Introducing the Canadian Practice Process Framework (CPPF): Amplifying the context. In E. A. Townsend & H. J. Polatajko (Eds.), *Enabling occupation II: Advancing an occupational therapy vision for health, well-being, and justice through occupations* (pp. 229–246). CAOT Publications ACE.

Graham, F., Rodger, S., & Ziviani, J. (2009). Coaching parents to enable children's participation: An approach for working with parents and their children. *Australian Occupational Therapy Journal*, 56, 16–23. https://doi.org/10.1111/j.1440-1630.2008.00736.x

Hayes, S. C., Luoma, J. B., Bond, F. W., Masuda, A., & Lillis, J. (2006). Acceptance and commitment therapy: Model, processes and outcomes. *Behaviour Research and Therapy*, 44, 1–25. https://doi.org/10.1016/j.brat.2005.06.006

Health Practitioner Regulation National Law Act 2009 (Qld) (Austl.). https://www.legislation.qld.gov.au/view/html/inforce/current/act-2009-045

Howlett, O. A., Lannin, N. A., Ada, L., & McKinstry, C. (2015). Functional electrical stimulation improves activity after stroke: A systematic review with meta-analysis. *Archives of Physical Medicine and Rehabilitation*, 96, 934–943. https://doi.org/10.1016/j.apmr.2015.01.013

Occupational Therapy Australia (OTA). (2017). *Occupational therapy scope of practice framework*. Occupational Therapy Australia.

Polatajko, H. J., & Mandich, A. (2004). *Enabling occupation in children: The Cognitive Orientation to daily Occupational Performance (CO-OP) approach*. CAOT Publications ACE.

Townsend, E. A., & Polatajko, H. J. (2007). *Enabling occupation II: Advancing an occupational therapy vision for health, well-being, and justice through occupations*. CAOT Publications ACE.

6 Values and philosophy of occupational therapy

Alison Wicks

Chapter objectives

Upon completion of this chapter, the reader will be able to:

- Reflect on their personal values.
- Appreciate the difference between values and philosophy.
- Contemplate the values and the unique philosophy of occupational therapy.
- Acknowledge that values and philosophy shape practice.

Keywords

ethics; occupation; health; personal values; philosophy; professional values

Overview

The values and philosophy of occupational therapy are significant as they underpin practice. Values are ideals to which people are committed and relate to what they consider to be important. As such, values influence how occupational therapy services are provided, how individual occupational therapists practise and inform the design of occupational therapy education programs. The profession's values are embodied in the Occupational Therapy Australia Code of Ethics and Code of Conduct and shape the Australian Occupational Therapy Competency Standards. The profession's philosophy is the basic framework that explains why occupational therapists do what they do. The unique philosophy of occupational therapy consisting of assumptions about humans and occupation is what distinguishes occupational therapy from other health professions. Occupational therapy's philosophy clarifies why occupational therapists use occupation as a therapeutic medium in practice and why they work with clients to enable them to participate in their occupations of choice.

The key message of this chapter is that it is important for students, as future occupational therapy professionals, to be aware of their own values, and those of the occupational therapy profession. Moreover, the chapter emphasises that it is also essential that students understand the philosophy that is at the core of occupational therapy. Collectively, values and philosophical principles shape occupational therapy practice.

Introduction

This chapter discusses how values and philosophy shape occupational therapy practice in Australia. In the chapter values refer to the fundamental beliefs that guide how occupational therapists practise. Philosophy refers to a framework of assumptions and principles that clarifies why occupational therapists use occupation to enable participation in occupations.

Whilst all members of a profession have their personal set of values, they are expected to take on the values held by their profession. It is important to note that other professionals may have personal values that are similar to those of occupational therapists. Perhaps other professions have values comparable to those of the occupational therapy profession. However, the philosophy of occupational therapy is unique. In fact, its philosophy is what makes occupational therapy practice and its contribution to the health and well-being of individuals, communities and populations so distinctive.

Values

Values are the various views people hold about what is important, worthwhile, and of merit, but they are not necessarily held as truths. The values people hold relate to what they judge to be important in life and to standards by which they live. Consequently, values guide behaviour and the choices people make. Some examples of personal values may include beliefs about: being honest; having integrity; respecting others; being there for family and friends; caring for the environment or making a difference in the world.

The degree to which certain values have priority at any given time varies, influenced by specific circumstances and contexts. Values are not necessarily static since they can change in response to new experiences, new learning or critical events. In addition, values do not exist in isolation from each other. People tend to have clusters of values and these clusters are integrated into their value system.

Personal values are developed over time. They are moulded by social, cultural and political contexts and life experiences. Families are particularly influential in the development of values early in life. When young, people generally adopt the values of parents and those closest to them, such as grandparents and friends. As individuals grow and develop, education, exposure to diverse groups of people outside the family, and new experiences in different social settings may result in modification of these values or taking on additional values. Sometimes people may even discard original, family-based values. Furthermore, when personal values and those of family members or one's peers are no longer aligned, tensions may arise within these relationships. Besides the family and peers, the workplace, religion, culture, social media and major historical events also influence which values people adopt.

When individuals join a profession such as occupational therapy they bring their personal values with them. The diverse personal values of occupational therapists who work in Australia have been shaped by their culture and their way of life. Additionally, their personal values are moulded by their occupational therapy education program. For example, during practice education, students integrate the knowledge they have acquired, start to make sense of what they are doing, model the behaviour of their supervisors and begin to act as therapists, demonstrating the values and attitudes of their new profession. In fact, it is likely some students will experience a transformation of personal values in the process of becoming a professional. Ideally, there is alignment between personal and professional values.

Professional values of occupational therapists

Professional values guide the behaviour of members of an occupational group. They are deliberately selected by the occupational group as those values that shape the group's identity, principles and beliefs and are generally defined within their code of ethics (Frankel, 1989). To some extent perhaps, values held by today's Australian occupational therapists are shaped by values of previous occupational therapists who developed both the training and practice in our country. The first occupational therapists to work in Australia in the 1940s were Ethel Francis, Sylvia Docker and Joyce Keam. These three women would have held values espoused at the time by their respective education centres in the United States and United Kingdom. Whilst their personal values are unknown, it is highly likely that each possessed the characteristics that were considered requisite for an occupational therapist in the early days of the profession in Australia. Docker described these characteristics as: being able to mix well with all types of people; being patient; possessing a natural understanding of others; and having a fundamental wish to do her [sic] part in the world (Anderson & Bell, 1988, p. 5).

Interestingly, a study conducted seven decades after the founding of the Australian profession of occupational therapy revealed somewhat similar values. The exploration of the professional values of Australian occupational therapists working in the twenty-first century revealed three main categories: values related to the client and client-therapist relationship, such as honouring the client's priorities and goals and understanding the client; values related to occupational therapy knowledge, skills and practice such as using and updating knowledge, problem solving and working with a team; and selfless values—for example, warmth, empathy, humility, fairness and honesty (Aguilar et al., 2012).

As there is little additional research on professional values of Australian occupational therapists, it is necessary to review recent studies on the values of other health professionals. In New Zealand, research on doctors', nurses' and allied health professionals' personal and professional values identified that the values considered most relevant to health care practitioners were altruism, equality and capability (Moyo et al., 2016). Another Australian study which conducted an inter-professional analysis of common values among seven health professions proposed a model of two core values incorporating all identified themes: the rights of the client and the capacity of a particular profession to serve the health care needs of clients (Grace et al., 2017, p. 325).

In 2013, when the Australian Government's Department of Health developed its National Practice Standards for mental health workers, it outlined the values and attitudes that underpin how mental health practitioners apply their knowledge and skills when working with people, carers, families and communities. These values are: respect; advocacy; working in partnership; and excellence. In addition, the attitudes of mental health workers, that is the interaction of their values, beliefs and feelings, are expected to be: respectful; compassionate, caring and empathic; ethical, professional and responsible; positive, encouraging and hopeful; open-minded; self-aware; culturally aware; and collaborative (Department of Health, 2013).

Values of the profession

Each profession usually has its own set of values. The values of a profession guide how its members work and set the standards for the profession. Professional values guide reasoning and inform ethical decisions (Purtilo & Doherty, 2011). As with personal values, professional values are shaped and influenced by social, institutional, cultural and political contexts (Aguilar et al., 2012). They may also have an historical basis, in that they have been developed from the values of the founding organisation. For instance, the values of the profession of occupational therapy in Australia are largely influenced by the values of the World Federation of Occupational Therapists (WFOT), established in 1952 to promote the art and science of occupational therapy internationally. In 2019, WFOT had 101 member organisations around the world (WFOT, 2019a). Occupational Therapy Australia (OTA) is one of its founding members.

The WFOT has produced an overarching guide to ethical practice, framed by the values it upholds, to support occupational therapists in performing their professional role. The WFOT Code of Ethics is based on tasks of the profession and the responsibilities towards recipients of occupational therapy, other professions and employees, and towards society on a local and global level (WFOT, 2019b).

Each member organisation is expected to develop its own Code of Ethics that incorporates values particular to the professional context in its own country, in relation to: personal attributes; responsibility to clients; conduct in collaborative practice; developing professional knowledge; promotion; and development. The Occupational Therapy Australia (OTA) Code of Ethics is founded on the bio-ethical principles of beneficence, non-maleficence, honesty, veracity, confidentiality, justice, respect and autonomy. This Code embodies the ethos, that is, the set of common values, of the Australian occupational therapy profession. Essentially, it requires its members to discharge their duties and responsibilities, at all times, in a manner which professionally, ethically, and morally compromises no individual with whom they have professional contact, irrespective of that person's position, situation or condition in society (OTA, 2014). The OTA Code of Ethics describes appropriate conduct for occupational therapists in any professional circumstance and serves as a guide for practitioners in the following broad domains: relationships with, and responsibilities to patients and clients; professional integrity; professional relationships; and responsibilities and standards.

Some examples of statements in the OTA Code of Ethics 2014 are:

- Confidentiality: Beyond the necessary sharing of information with professional colleagues, occupational therapists are to safeguard confidential information relating to patients and clients (p. 4).
- Discrimination: Occupational therapists shall not discriminate in their professional practice, on the basis of ethnicity, culture, impairment, language, age, gender, sexual preference, religion, political beliefs or status in society (p. 6).
- Loyalty: Occupational therapists shall be loyal to their professional organisation and their fellow members of the profession and shall respect and uphold their dignity (p. 8).

In addition to the Code of Ethics, Australian practitioners are required to adhere to the Australian Occupational Therapy Competency Standards 2018 (OTBA, 2018) and the

Code of Conduct (OTBA, 2014). Collectively these codes and the standards have been developed to ensure both practice and public safety in Australia (OTCA, 2019, p. 12).

It is important to note that there is wide-ranging consultation with key stakeholders when the Australian occupational therapy codes are reviewed, ensuring alignment with and relevance to changing social values and regulatory environments. Any changes will consequently impact the competency standards. For example, the competency standards which were launched in February 2018 and came into effect in January 2019 reflect evolving cultural and social attitudes, especially in regard to Aboriginal and Torres Strait Islander peoples. 'These competency standards recognise that Aboriginal and Torres Strait Islander peoples are the Traditional Custodians of this country and hold many cultural values and beliefs which are diverse, complex and evolving' (OTBA, 2018). The revised Standard 2.4—*understands and responds to Aboriginal and Torres Strait islander health philosophies, leadership, research and practices*—illustrates how change in attitudes are reflected in the standards.

It is presumed students will be informed of these standards and codes early in their studies as they should adhere to them during their practice education. Students are also expected to have developed detailed knowledge of these standards and codes at program completion (OTCA, 2019, p. 12). It goes without saying that all registered occupational therapists should be conversant with them at all times. In addition, the practice of students and registered occupational therapists needs to be guided by the profession's philosophy.

Philosophy

The term philosophy can be confusing. It can refer to a specific academic discipline that studies the fundamental nature of knowledge, reality and existence. Likewise, it can refer to a framework of assumptions that explain thinking and behaviour. Assumptions are ideas or principles that are taken for granted as the basis for argument and action (Hooper, 2008 cited in Hooper & Wood, 2014). The latter description of philosophy is adopted for this chapter.

As for all professions, occupational therapy needs a philosophy. Indeed, it is considered the basic element of practice. It is the foundation upholding all that practitioners do, and provides the basis on which to make professional decisions. A profession needs a philosophy that is sufficiently general to accommodate contextual variations and changes as ideas, research, practice and experience demand (Wilcock, 2000). A profession's philosophy helps practitioners: develop a professional identity; hone a practice that is unique; and explain the complexity of the profession to themselves and to others (Hooper & Wood, 2014). An occupational therapy philosophy is required to enable occupational therapists to understand and to articulate to others the boundaries of occupational therapy practice and enable practitioners to concentrate efforts within a distinctive domain of concern—adding or discarding services according to philosophy, rather than fashion or self-consciousness (Wilcock, 1999).

The philosophy of occupational therapy has evolved and will continue to evolve as the profession influences, and is influenced by other professions, disciplines and movements. The assumptions that currently form its framework focus on the human–occupation relationship.

Adolf Meyer (1922), an American psychiatrist, was credited with providing the profession of occupational therapy with its philosophical footing. Through his work in psychiatric institutions at the beginning of the twentieth century, he recognised the health-promoting power of occupation and stated that the 'proper use of time in some helpful and gratifying activity' (p. 1) was important in the treatment of the people with neuropsychiatric conditions. However, it was Edmund Barton in 1914 who coined the term occupational therapy (Anderson & Bell, 1988). By embedding the word occupation in the profession's name, occupation became the domain of a new health profession that used occupation as its primary therapeutic medium. And so the first assumption in the philosophical framework of occupational therapy is that 'Humans have an innate need for occupation for health and well-being'.

No other health profession focuses on occupation to the same extent as occupational therapy, nor appreciates its complexity and relationship to health and well-being (Whiteford, 2007). During their education, occupational therapy students learn about occupation and come to understand that occupations are active, meaningful, purposeful and contextualised, and impact health (Molineux, 2010). Moreover, they learn to appreciate that occupations give structure to daily life through the establishment of rhythm and routine, and that participation in occupations provides a sense of accomplishment and promotes self-identity (Christiansen & Townsend, 2010). In fact, students come to realise that for many people, occupations are their reasons for living.

Meyer (1922) was also influential in embedding humanistic values within the profession's philosophy. According to Yerxa (1991), Meyer perceived patients with mental illness as persons who had problems with daily living and who required normalisation of their activities and environments. The view held by occupational therapists that 'persons have the potential to be capable, competent and productive citizens while living with a disability or chronic condition' (Yerxa, 1991) was fostered by Meyer and strengthened by the emergence of humanistic psychology in the mid-twentieth century. Key elements in humanistic psychology are: understanding of the person as a whole; the role of intentionality in human existence; and the importance of the end goal of life for the healthy person (Buhler, 1971). The second assumption in the current philosophical framework of our profession is 'Humans are unique, with unique capacities to realise their potential, to grow and self-actualise'.

The establishment of the discipline of occupational science in 1989 to generate knowledge of occupation and its relationship to health has provided critical evidence to further support the philosophy of occupational therapy (Yerxa et al., 1990). The research undertaken by occupational scientists is generating new understandings about occupation. A case in point is the work of Cutchin and Dickie (2013). They have adopted a transactional perspective of occupation highlighting the interconnectedness between occupation and the environments in which it takes place. Similarly, Whiteford and Wright-St Clair (2005) have shown that 'no communication, no interaction, no intervention that takes places between a practitioner and client is context free'. Hence a third assumption in occupational therapy's philosophical framework is 'Humans are complex, multileveled systems who act on and interact with their environments'.

These three assumptions are incorporated in the following statement: 'Ever changing occupational humans, interconnected with ever changing environments occupy time with ever changing occupations and thereby transform and are transformed by their actions, environments and states of health' (Hooper & Wood, 2014).

A fourth assumption currently completes the profession's philosophical framework: 'All humans have a right to occupation'. Undoubtedly influenced by the social justice movement, WFOT has published a new position statement on Human Rights (WFOT,

2019c). Position statements are used by large organisations to make public their official philosophy. The WFOT, in its capacity as the international organisation for the promotion of *occupational therapy,* uses position statements as a platform for projecting the profession's philosophy, values and stance on particular issues that are relevant to the profession of occupational therapy and civil society.

The first principle of the Human Rights position statement, as stated below, clearly emphasises why occupational therapists enable people to engage in the occupations they need, want and are expected to do.

Occupational therapists are concerned with human rights in pursuing occupational justice for all. Occupational justice requires universal rights to occupation, broadly defined and recognising differences related to the cultural, social, political (current and historic) and geographical context. Occupational justice is the fulfilment of the right for all people to engage in the occupations they need to survive, define as meaningful, and that contribute positively to their own well-being and the well-being of their communities.

So the philosophical framework underpinning occupational therapy, forged by the founders of the profession and shaped by the world in which we are living, is quite profound. As occupational scientists continue to discover the diverse functions and meanings of occupations (Reed et al., 2013) and the various contextual factors that influence occupation (Galvaan, 2015), additional assumptions will be added to the framework. The current philosophy is based upon the premise that all people, regardless of age, context and capacity, have a need, indeed a right, to participate in personally meaningful occupations for their health and survival (Wilcock & Hocking, 2015).

Conclusion

Shared values and a common philosophy are important elements in any profession. In occupational therapy, they are interrelated and shape occupational therapy practice, as shown in Figure 6.1.

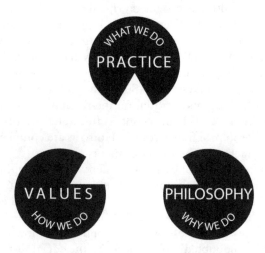

Figure 6.1 The relationship between values, philosophy and practice in occupational therapy.

For the profession of occupational therapy in Australia, it is important that all members of the profession be committed to a set of common values and an agreed philosophy. Shared values and an agreed philosophy empower the profession and, in addition, build trust among its members. Mutual commitment to a set of beliefs and a central principle that governs practice also builds trust in the profession of occupational therapy among stakeholders and clarify expectations of clients.

Strong congruence of personal values and philosophy with those of the occupational therapy profession can catalyse meaningful, satisfying and sustaining work over the course of an entire career (Hooper & Wood, 2014). Hence, students need to reflect upon their own values, know the values embedded within the Australian occupational therapy profession and understand the unique philosophy that provides a foundation to occupational therapy. Such reflection and understanding are critical as students are the future members of the occupational therapy profession.

Summary

- The values of a profession guide how its members work and set the standards for the profession.
- Occupational therapy's values are beliefs and ideals that guide how occupational therapists practise. They are embodied in the Occupational Therapy Australia Code of Ethics and Code of Conduct.
- Some important occupational therapy professional values are:
  - *showing respect*
  - *having integrity*
  - *being culturally aware*, and
  - *being collaborative.*
- The philosophy of a profession is the foundation upholding all that practitioners do, and provides the basis on which to make professional decisions.
- Occupational therapy's philosophy, consisting of assumptions about humans and occupation, explains why occupational therapists use occupation to enable participation in occupation.
- The assumptions that currently make up occupational therapy's philosophical framework are:
  - *Humans have an innate need for occupation for health and well-being.*
  - *Humans are unique, with unique capacities to realise their potential, to grow and self-actualise.*
  - *Humans are complex, multileveled systems who act on and interact with their environments.*
  - *All humans have a right to occupation.*
- Together, values and philosophy shape occupational therapy practice.

Review questions

1. What are some of the values you hold personally?
2. Who or what shaped your personal values?
3. Why does our profession need to hold values and have a foundational philosophy?
4. Is the philosophy of occupational therapy what you expected?
5. Do you foresee any challenges in maintaining the professional philosophy?
6. Do you think some of the profession's values will remain constant?
7. How might the profession's values and philosophy change in the future?

References

Aguilar, A., Stupans, I., Scutter, S., & King, S. (2012). Exploring professionalism: The professional values of Australian occupational therapists. *Australian Occupational Therapy Journal, 59*(3), 209–217. https://doi.org/10.1111/j.1440-1630.2012.00996.x

Anderson, B., & Bell, J. (1988). *Occupational therapy. Its place in Australia's history*. Australian Association of Occupational Therapists.

Buhler, C. (1971). Basic theoretical concepts of humanistic psychology. *American Psychologist, 26(4)*, 378–386. https://doi.org/10.1037/h0032049

Christiansen, C., & Townsend, E. (2010). *Introduction to occupation: The art and science of living* (4th edn). Prentice Hall.

Cutchin, M., & Dickie, V. (2013). *Transactional perspectives on occupation*. Springer.

Department of Health. (2013). *National practice standards for mental health workforce 2013. Part 2. Values and attitudes*. https://www1.health.gov.au/internet/publications/publishing.nsf/Content/mental-pubs-n-wkstd13-toc~mental-pubs-n-wkstd13-2

Frankel, M. S. (1989). Professional codes: Why, how, and with what impact? *Journal of Business Ethics, 8*, 109–115. https://doi.org/10.1007/BF00382575

Galvaan, R. (2015). The contextually situated nature of occupational choice: Marginalised young adolescents' experience in South Africa. *Journal of Occupational Science, 22*(1), 39–53. https://doi.org/10.1080/14427591.2014.912124

Grace, S., Innes, E., Joffe, B., East, L., Coutts, R., & Nancarrow, S. (2017). Identifying common values among seven health professions: An interprofessional analysis. *Journal of Interprofessional Care, 31*(3), 325–334. https://doi.org/10.1080/13561820.2017.1288091

Hooper, B., & Wood, W. (2014). The philosophy of occupational therapy: A framework for practice. In B. Schell, G. Gillen, M. Scaffa, & E. Cohn (Eds.), *Willard & Spackman's occupational therapy* (12th edn, pp. 35–46). Lippincott, Williams & Wilkins.

Meyer, A. (1922). The philosophy of occupation therapy. *Archives of Occupational Therapy, 1*(1), 1–10.

Molineux, M. (2010). The nature of occupation. In M. Curtin, M. Molineux, & J. Supyk-Mellson (Eds.), *Occupational therapy and physical dysfunction* (pp. 17–26). Churchill Livingstone.

Moyo, M., Goodyear-Smith, F., Wellerm, J., Robb, G., & Shulruf, B. (2016). Healthcare practitioners' personal and professional values. *Advances in Health Science Education, 21*(2), 257–286. https://doi.org/10.1007/s10459-015-9626-9

Occupational Therapy Australia. (2014). *Code of ethics*. https://otaus.com.au/publicassets/f3bceaea-49ff-e811-a2c2-b75c2fd918c5/OTA%20Code%20of%20Ethics%202014.pdf

Occupational Therapy Board of Australia. (2014). *Code of conduct*. https://www.occupationaltherapyboard.gov.au/Codes-Guidelines/Code-of-conduct.aspx

Occupational Therapy Board of Australia. (2018). *Australian occupational therapy competency standards*. https://www.occupationaltherapyboard.gov.au/Codes-Guidelines/Competencies.aspx

Occupational Therapy Council of Australia. (2019). *Guidelines and evidence guide for the accreditation of Australian entry level occupational therapy education programs*. https://www.otcouncil.com.au/wp-content/uploads/OTCAccStdsEvidence-Guide-September-2019-v1-1.pdf

Purtilo, R., & Doherty, R. (2011). *Ethical dimensions in the health professions* (5th edn). Elsevier/Saunders.

Reed, K., Smythe, L., & Hocking, C. (2013). The meaning of occupation: A hermeneutic (re)view of historical understandings. *Journal of Occupational Science, 20*(3), 253–261. https://doi.org/10.1080/14427591.2012.729487

WFOT. (2019a). *Member organisations*. https://www.wfot.org/membership/member-organisations

WFOT. (2019b). *Code of ethics*. https://www.wfot.org/resources/code-of-ethics

WFOT. (2019c). *Position statements: Occupational therapy and human rights—revised*. https://www.wfot.org/resources/occupational-therapy-and-human-rights

Whiteford, G., & Wright-St Clair, V. (2005). *Occupation and practice in context*. Elsevier.

Whiteford, G. (2007). The Koru unfurls: The emergence of diversity in occupational therapy thought and action. *New Zealand Journal of Occupational Therapy, 54*(1), 21–25. https://search.informit.com.au/documentSummary;dn=304618481933208;res=IELHEA

Wilcock, A. (1999). The Doris Sym Memorial Lecture: Developing a philosophy of occupation for health. *British Journal of Occupational Therapy, 62*(5), 192–198. https://doi.org/10.1177/030802269906200503

Wilcock, A. (2000). Development of a personal, professional and educational occupational philosophy: An Australian perspective. *Occupational Therapy International, 7*(2), 76–86. https://doi.org/10.1002/oti.108

Wilcock, A., & Hocking, C. (2015). *Occupational perspective of health* (3rd edn). SLACK Inc.

Yerxa, E. J. (1991). Seeking a relevant, ethical and realistic way of knowing for occupational therapy. *American Journal of Occupational Therapy, 45*(3), 199–204. https://doi.org/10.5014/ajot.45.3.199

Yerxa, E. J., Clark, F., Frank, G., Jackson, J., Parham, D., Pierce, D., Stein, C., & Zemke, R. (1990). An introduction to occupational science: A foundation for occupational therapy in the 21st century. *Occupational Therapy in Health Care, 6*(4), 1–17. https://doi.org/10.1080/J003v06n04_04

7 Ethical and legal responsibilities of occupational therapy practice

Angus Buchanan, Dave Parsons and Ben Milbourn

Chapter objectives

Upon completion of this chapter, the reader will be able to:

* Provide details of the general ethical responsibilities of health care professionals including occupational therapists.
* Explain the legal responsibilities of being a health care practitioner.
* Provide an overview of the regulatory authorities relevant to Australian occupational therapy practice.
* Identify key legislative acts that impact on Australian occupational therapy practice.

Key terms

ethics; ethical practice; legislation; professional practice

Introduction

This chapter introduces ethical principles, the code of conduct and some relevant legislation that governs the practice of occupational therapy in Australia. Ethics, the code of conduct and relevant legislation provide all health professionals with a guiding framework for their practice. Broadly speaking, ethics provide a general set of principles that guide and influence an occupational therapist's judgement in their practice, while the code of conduct is more focused, providing targeted guidance for how occupational therapists should act in specific situations related to occupational therapy practice. Legislation refers to laws that have been enacted, are legally binding and must be followed. Breaches in ethical principles, the code of conduct and legislation can have a considerable impact on an occupational therpist's career; thus they must be understood and adhered to by all registered occupational therapists. Understanding ethical principles, the code of conduct and relevant laws is also critical to the practice of occupational therapy students who are required to demonstrate the highest levels of behaviours in their classes, assessments, fieldwork practice and personal life.

On completion of tertiary studies, students register with the Occupational Therapy Board of Australia (OTBA) and must conduct their duties and responsibilities in a manner which is professional, ethical and legal. There are severe penalties that may be imposed by the OTBA, employer and/or the legal system if an occupational therapist (or occupational therapy student) is found to be knowingly or unknowingly engaging in unethical or illegal behaviours. While not a breach of professional ethics per se, occupational therapy students may face severe penalties for breaches in university policies, for example, academic misconduct or the student charter.

It can be difficult to define exactly what an ethical issue is. Every occupational therapy student must be able to articulate an ethical framework that guides their thinking and reasoning when considering the range of potential issues that will be encountered. Students place themselves at significant risk of investigation of their professional conduct if they are unable to identify situations that might be unethical and even illegal in all aspects of their lives. Clients and their families may also be placed in considerable jeopardy if students who work with them engage in unethical activities, particularly where clients may be in vulnerable situations.

There are two core documents that guide the ethical and legal practice of Australian occupational therapists: the Code of Ethics (OTA, 2014) and the Code of Conduct (AHPRA, 2014a). The principles outlined in the codes are designed to guide occupational therapists' professional reasoning, ethical and legal decision-making. The principles also support the establishment of effective ongoing working relationships with clients and their families. All occupational therapy students and practitioners should be using the codes as a foundation for ethically appropriate professional practice as well as their clinical reasoning and decision-making.

Overview of ethics

Ethics is a broad area of philosophy too expansive to fully address in this chapter; however, there are specific facets that are essential for a practising occupational therapist to understand and engage with. The principles of normative ethics, and more specifically *bioethics*, are the most relevant for the practice of occupational therapy. Bioethics can be defined as the study of moral problems that impact human well-being (Freegard, 2012). Before examining the nature of ethics, it is important to understand why it is relevant to occupational therapy practice.

Occupational therapists have a fiduciary obligation to clients. A fiduciary obligation is where a professional has: i) special duties due to trust and confidence placed in them by their client; ii) the ability to dominate and influence the client due to their status in the relationship; and iii) a duty to serve their clients' welfare without abusing their special status in the relationship (Kutchins, 1991; Lohman & Brown, 1997). This special ethical obligation to clients is in addition to the everyday morality that members of society must exhibit.

The fiduciary obligation is often greater for health professionals than for other types of workers. For example, if an occupational therapist was completing a home visit and their client disclosed that they were experiencing mental health issues, the occupational therapist has the professional obligation to encourage their client to seek the appropriate help and support. If the client shares the same information with a tradesperson working at their home, the tradesperson has no such fiduciary obligation.

The most common and widely recognised practical implementation of the bioethical principles is the Four Principle Approach as described by Beauchamp and Childress (1994). This approach provides a set of four core principles that all health professionals including occupational therapists should follow throughout their practice. The four principles are outlined below:

Autonomy

Health professionals should espouse the principle of autonomy: 'To respect an autonomous agent is, at a minimum, to acknowledge that person's right to hold views, to make choices and to take actions based on personal values and beliefs' (Beauchamp & Childress, 1994, p. 125).

Clients have the right to their personal values, views and beliefs and these come before the values, views and beliefs of the therapist in regard to decisions made about the client's care or as a result of the interaction with the occupational therapist. As part of this process it is critical the occupational therapist be aware of their own values, views and beliefs and have an understanding of how these may influence their own decision-making and behaviour. The occupational therapist must recognise their own influence in the context of providing a service to their clients.

Non-maleficence

The principle of non-maleficence is an obligation of the health practitioner to not inflict harm intentionally and is closely aligned by the maxim in medical ethics: 'Above all do no harm' (Beauchamp & Childress, 1994). While simple in definition, in practice this principle can be quite complex, with numerous ambiguities in the definitions of harm and injury (Beauchamp & Childress, 1994). Occupational therapists might also cause harm or injury to their clients without intent; due to a duty of care, they might breach this ethical principle (Beauchamp & Childress, 1994). Occupational therapists must be mindful of the consequences of their actions and their behaviour, and any potential harm or injury to their client, regardless of their original intent.

Beneficence

The principle of beneficence is an active process by which occupational therapists must take positive steps for the benefit of their clients. This principle outlines that occupational therapists are not only obligated to respect their client's autonomy and cause no harm or injury, but must contribute to their welfare (Beauchamp & Childress, 1994). Beneficence also encompasses the kindness and empathy that occupational therapists should have for their clients. Occupational therapists must do all in their power to actively engage with often vulnerable populations, to enhance client health and well-being throughout the therapeutic process.

Justice

The principle of justice can be broadly described as the 'fair, equitable, and appropriate treatment in light of what is due or owed to persons' (Beauchamp & Childress, 1994, p. 327). This principle is complex and can be understood on a number of levels. Freegard (2012) identifies four ways to determine the equitable and fair distribution and allocation of scarce resources in the health sector: i) justice as fairness—those with equal needs should be served equally without discrimination or prejudice; ii) comparative justice—those with the greatest needs should receive more of the available resources without discrimination or prejudice; iii) distributive justice—resources should be allocated based on a set of societal norms that are pre-determined; and iv) compensatory justice—those who experience discrimination or prejudice should receive more resources to address this imbalance.

The most notable characteristic of the Four Principle Approach is that each principle should not conflict with another. If conflict does arise, practitioners need to consider the reasoning that may elevate one principle over another. No principle is inherently superior to another and all are interrelated (Freegard, 2012). The framework then acts as a guide to decision-making with consideration of each particular principle, acknowledging that every ethical situation is unique and there is no one formula or hierarchy that can be applied that will work in all instances.

The principles outlined in this section are not all-encompassing and there are other principles that occupational therapists must consider. These include:

- confidentiality;
- procedural justice;
- duty;
- veracity; and
- fidelity.

These principles form part of a code of ethics that occupational therapists and other health professionals are obliged to implement within their practice.

The Code of Ethics for occupational therapists

A code of ethics is a transparent disclosure that provides guidance of how a profession or organisation is expected to behave and function, and is intended to be a reference for users in their decision-making. A code of ethics can also be used as a framework to facilitate discussions about ethics and to improve management of dilemmas that might be encountered by an occupational therapist. Any code of ethics and conduct should always complement relevant laws, standards, policies and rules.

In Australia, a code of ethics for occupational therapists has been developed by Occupational Therapy Australia (2014). The introduction in the code states:

> The ethos of the occupational therapy profession and its practice requires its members to discharge their duties and responsibilities, at all times, in a manner which professionally, ethically, and morally compromises no individual with whom they have professional contact, irrespective of that person's position, situation or condition in society.
>
> (OTA, 2014, p. 2)

The Code of Ethics is consistent with the bioethical principles of beneficence, non-maleficence, honesty, veracity, confidentially, justice, respect and autonomy.

The Code of Ethics addresses four core aspects of ethical practice. Firstly, it highlights the critical importance of an occupational therapist's understanding *Relationships with, and Responsibilities to, Patients and Clients*. This includes issues such as client confidentially, engaging in personal relationships, respecting the rights of your client and withdrawal of services for patients and clients. Secondly, the importance of *Professional Integrity* is articulated, covering aspects including advertising, discriminatory practices and personal conduct related to the use of alcohol and drugs. *Professional Relationships and Responsibilities* is identified as the third aspect of the Code of Ethics. This includes loyalty to the profession, public comment representing the profession, understanding working relationships, engaging in ongoing professional development and the conduct of ethical research. Lastly, all occupational therapists must ensure they maintain *Professional Standards* which addresses the boundaries of competence, including keeping clear and concise records of occupational therapy services for the information of patients, clients and records (OTA, 2014).

All occupational therapists (and occupational therapy students) must be aware of the Code of Ethics and have a working understanding of how the code applies to their own specific practice context. Implementation of the Code of Ethics in practice is dynamic, and may at times raise ethical issues that should always be explored and resolved if possible. For example, one practice context may provide short one-off interventions and have limited opportunity to form deep relationships with clients. In another setting a family and their child may be seen for an extended period. Over time, it is possible to get to know the family well and become very friendly with them. As an occupational therapist it would be important to consider the ethical implications of forming a personal relationship with the family. Would this impact on the outcomes of the client, the establishment and maintenance of professional trust?

Occupational Therapy Board of Australia Code of Conduct

To work legally as an occupational therapist in Australia, practitioners must be registered with the Occupational Therapy Board of Australia (OTBA). The role and function of the board is outlined in the OTBA Code of Conduct (AHPRA, 2014a, p. 2). The code of conduct states that the OTBA is:

> Responsible for the registration of practitioners and students, setting the standards that practitioners must meet, and managing notifications (complaints) about the health, conduct or performance of practitioners.

The Australian Health Professional Regulatory Agency (AHPRA) works in partnership with the National Boards to implement the National Registration and Accreditation Scheme, under the Health Practitioner Regulation National Law.

The core role of the National Boards and AHPRA is to protect the public. The final statement is of great importance. It is imperative practitioners understand the key role of the OTBA is to protect the public, not to uphold the individual needs of registered occupational therapists.

The OTBA Code of Conduct released by the OTBA aims to enable occupational therapy practitioners to deliver effective regulated health services. It achieves this by providing practitioners with guidelines in a variety of practical and applied areas of professional behaviour. These include:

• providing good care;
• working with patients or clients;
• working with other practitioners;
• working within the health care system;
• minimising risk;

- maintaining professional performance;
- maintaining professional behaviour;
- ensuring practitioner health;
- teaching, supervising, assessing; and
- undertaking research.

Legal responsibilities of being a health care practitioner

Under the *Health Practitioner Regulation National Law Act 2009*, occupational therapists in each state of Australia must meet nationally consistent registration standards to be able to practise occupational therapy. The OTBA has mandatory standards which include:

- continuing professional development (CPD);
- criminal history disclosure;
- English language skill competency;
- professional indemnity insurance; and
- recency of practice (AHPRA, 2014a).

The OTBA (AHPRA, 2014b) provides the following guidance for registered occupational therapists and occupational therapy students transitioning into practitioners:

1. Occupational therapists must complete a minimum of 30 hours of CPD per year directed towards maintaining and improving their competence in occupational therapy practice.
2. Occupational therapists must disclose their complete criminal history when applying for occupational therapy registration.
3. Occupational therapists must be able to provide evidence of English language skills that meet the OTBA English language skills registration standard.
4. Registered occupational therapists must not practise their profession unless they have appropriate private indemnity insurance.
5. Occupational therapists must work at least six months full-time equivalent in any five-year period.
6. Occupational therapists must be aware of their responsibility under the National Law to notify the Boards in relation to certain impairments.

Occupational therapists also have a legal obligation to make a mandatory notification if they have formed a reasonable belief that a health practitioner has behaved in an unethical or illegal manner. This constitutes notifiable conduct in relation to the practice of their profession. Notifiable conduct as defined by Occupational Therapy Registration (AHPRA 2014c) includes:

- practising while intoxicated by alcohol or drugs;
- sexual misconduct in the practice of the profession;
- placing the public at risk of substantial harm because of an impairment (health issue); or
- placing the public at risk because of a significant departure from accepted professional standards.

These guidelines have been developed under Section 39 of the *Health Practitioner Regulation National Law Act 2009*. The aim of the mandatory notification requirements is to prevent the public from being placed at risk of harm. AHPRA should be notified if a health professional believes that an occupational therapy student or practitioner has behaved in a way which presents a serious risk to the public. In Australia, an occupational therapist may be suspended and possibly struck off the professional register for failing to recognise and manage risks within their caseload, breaching professional boundaries and for failing to act within the scope of practice as an occupational therapist.

Occupational therapy students are automatically registered with the OTBA by OTBA receiving occupational therapy enrolment details from tertiary institutions for student registration. AHPRA can be notified for student breaches of the same ethical and conduct standards expected of qualified practitioners. This includes if the education provider reasonably believes, 'a student enrolled with the provider has an impairment that, in the course of the student undertaking clinical training, may place the public at substantial risk of harm' (AHPRA, 2014b, p. 11).

Another example of legislation in Australia that may impact on how an occupational therapist performs their professional role in the workplace includes the Commonwealth *Freedom of Information Act 1982*. All clients have the right to request access to their medical notes. Occupational therapists should always strive to be professional, clear and objective in what is recorded. The *Disability Discrimination Act 1992* is another example of legislation which influences professional practice. Disability discrimination may happen when people with a disability are treated less fairly then people without a disability. Occupational therapists need to be aware how their occupational therapy practice impacts on the lives of the people they work with who may have a disability.

Occupational therapists working in different Australian states and territories must become familiar with relevant laws at all three levels of government and how these may impact on the care provided to clients. For example, each jurisdiction will have its own Mental Health Act outlining specific criteria for providing treatment, care, support and protection for people who experience a mental illness as well as providing protection of legal rights.

Case study: Jessica

Jessica is a third-year occupational therapy student and currently on a four-week placement at a private in-patient community facility for young adults with acute mental health conditions. Her occupational therapy practice education supervisor is Megan. At the admissions meeting, a new client called Sally is discussed. Sally has been diagnosed with depression and an anxiety disorder. Jessica recognises the name as someone she knew at school. They were good friends but have drifted apart. Jessica has not seen her in about two years but is still friends with her on social media and sees what she is doing. As her real friendship is over, Jessica does not consider that her previous friendship with Sally is important. Jessica chooses not to say anything about her previous friendship with Sally at the meeting or to Megan later on. The Consultant Psychiatrist would like Sally to be included in a number of occupational therapy groups in the coming week. Megan asks Jessica to meet Sally and conduct an initial interview and set some goals with Sally. Jessica meets with Sally who is very surprised and embarrassed to meet someone who knows her. Sally is reluctant to share information with Jessica and is not very responsive to the questions during the initial assessment. Jessica realises that she probably already knows quite a lot about Sally so thinks it will easier to terminate the session and set goals based on what she already knows about Sally. Jessica feels pleased with herself that she has been kind to Sally and saved her needing to spend time to set her goals as she already has the necessary information. Jessica lets Megan know that she has done the interview and documents in the client notes what she has found out including what she says are Sally's goals.

Questions to consider based on the case study

1. Has Jessica breached confidentiality?
2. How has Jessica acted in a maleficent way?
3. Who benefited from Jessica's actions?
4. How might Jessica approach the situation differently next time?
5. If Jessica was registered as an occupational therapist, what might be the consequences of her actions?

Conclusion

Ethics help health professionals make decisions about what are the right and wrong things to do in both simple and complex situations. Occupational therapists will be faced with making ethical decisions every day of their working lives. All health professionals need to have a strong theoretical understanding of ethics and how they can be used to support their clinical practice. All occupational therapists should be able to articulate an ethical framework based on ethical principles, and then demonstrate practice that meets the expectations of employers and professional and regulatory bodies. In Australia there are two important documents that guide and govern occupational therapy practice—the Code of Ethics for Occupational Therapists and the Occupational Therapy Board of Australia Code of Conduct. It is the responsibility of all occupational therapists to have a working knowledge of how these documents apply to their own specific practice context. Occupational therapists need to be fully aware of their legal responsibilities associated with professional registration and other specific legislation that impacts on their practice. There are significant implications if an occupational therapist engages in unethical behaviours, dubious decision-making or illegal practices.

Summary

- Understanding and upholding ethical principles and relevant laws is critical to the practice of occupational therapy.
- The most common and widely recognised practical implementation of the bioethical principles is the Four Principle Approach.
- The Occupational Therapy Australia Code of Ethics is a transparent disclosure of how practitioners are expected to behave and function in their professional lives.

- Occupational therapists working in Australia have a legal requirement to meet national registration standards to be able to practice occupational therapy. The Occupational Therapy Board of Australia enforces these standards.
- The Occupational Therapy Board of Australia's key role is to protect the public, not to uphold the individual needs of registered occupational therapists.

Review questions

1. What are the ethical principles that can help guide occupational practice?
2. How can a Code of Ethics improve ethical practice in occupational therapy?
3. What is the name of the legislation that is most relevant to occupational therapy practice?
4. Name three other pieces of legislation (either national or state-based) that occupational therapists should be aware of in their practice? Why are these relevant to occupational therapy practice?

References

Australian Health Practitioners Regulatory Agency. (AHPRA). (2014a). *Code of conduct.* https://www.occupationaltherapyboard.gov.au/Codes-Guidelines/Code-of-conduct.aspx

Australian Health Practitioners Regulatory Agency. (AHPRA). (2014b). *Registration.* https://www.ahpra.gov.au/Registration.aspx

Australian Health Practitioners Regulatory Agency. (AHPRA). (2014c). *Guidelines for mandatory notifications.* https://www.occupationaltherapyboard.gov.au/Codes-Guidelines/Guidelines-for-mandatory-notifications.aspx

Beauchamp, T. L., & Childress, J. F. (1994). *Principles of biomedical ethics* (4th edn). Oxford University Press.

Commonwealth of Australia. (1982). *Freedom of Information Act 1982.* Commonwealth of Australia.

Commonwealth of Australia. (1992). *Disability Discrimination Act 1992.* Commonwealth of Australia.

Freegard, H. (2012). Ethics in a nutshell. In H. Freegard, & L. Isted (Eds.), *Ethical practice for health professionals* (pp. 29–45). Cengage Learning.

Health Practitioner Regulation National Law Act 2009 (Qld) (Austl.). https://www.legislation.qld.gov.au/view/html/inforce/current/act-2009-045

Kutchins, H. (1991). The fiduciary relationship: The legal basis for social workers' responsibilities to clients. *Social Work, 36*(2), 106–113. https://doi.org/10.1093/sw/36.2.106

Lohman, H., & Brown, K. (1997). Ethical issues related to managed care: An in-depth discussion of an occupational therapy case study. *Occupational Therapy in Health Care, 10*(4), 1–12. https://doi.org/10.1080/07380579709168827

Occupational Therapy Australia (OTA). (2014). *Code of ethics.* https://otaus.com.au/publicassets/f3bceaea-49ff-e811-a2c2-b75c2fd918c5/OTA%20Code%20of%20Ethics%202014.pdf

8 Occupational therapy in population health and health promotion

Carolynne White, Kate Gledhill and Mong-Lin Yu

Chapter objectives

Upon completion of this chapter, the reader will be able to:

*   Define population health, illness prevention and health promotion.
*   Distinguish between illness prevention and health promotion.
*   Describe how occupational therapists can work in the areas of population health, illness prevention and health promotion.

Key terms

population health; health promotion; prevention; occupational therapy practice; determinants of health; culture; health literacy; equity; health

Introduction

A core aim of occupational therapy practice is to create and facilitate opportunities for people to engage in meaningful occupations, and in doing so, promote health and well-being (World Federation of Occupational Therapists [WFOT], 2012). In contemporary occupational therapy practice, the 'client' is not limited to the individual, but can also include family members and significant others, groups and communities, organisations or populations (Occupational Therapy Board of Australia [OTBA], 2018).

In Australia, people are developing ongoing health conditions earlier in life and the population is getting older (Australian Institue of Health and Welfare [AIHW], 2018). To address these issues and ensure the health system is sustainable, occupational therapists across all areas of practice require a population health perspective that incorporates health promotion and illness prevention. A population health perspective involves changing the focus of occupational therapy from individuals to populations, and implementing strategies at a local, regional and national level to enable people to increase control over (and improve) their health, and its determinants. Occupational therapists bring a unique perspective to population health through their focus on humans as occupational beings who can influence their health, positively or negatively, through what they do in their environment (Wilcock & Hocking, 2015).

This chapter will define health and population health, provide an overview of factors that can influence population health, and describe ways in which the health of populations can be improved. Examples of how occupational therapists can work at a population level will be discussed with a focus on illness prevention and health promotion.

What is health?

'Health' is a familiar term that is often used in everyday communication. However, when people talk about health, they often mean different things. In health care, different models have attempted to describe or define health. In Western health systems, the biomedical model is most often used to understand health. According to the biomedical model, health is an individual's responsibility and refers to an objective biological state characterised by the absence of illness (Germov, 2019). In contrast, the social model defines health as a social construction that is influenced by social factors including a person's living and working conditions, as well as their political and social environments. Therefore, health is seen as a societal responsibility (Germov, 2019). This is especially true for Aboriginal and Torres Strait Islander peoples for whom health means:

> not just the physical well-being of an individual but refers to the social, emotional and cultural well-being of the whole Community in which each individual is able to achieve their full potential as a human being thereby bringing about the total well-being of their Community. It is a whole of life view and includes the cyclical concept of life–death–life.
>
> (National Aboriginal Health Strategy Working Party, 1989)

In 1946, the World Health Organization (WHO) defined health as 'a state of complete physical, mental and social well-being and not merely the absence of disease or infirmity' (WHO, 1946, n.p.). This definition suggests that health is a goal to be achieved. The WHO reviewed this definition in the Ottawa Charter for Health Promotion (WHO, 1986), and instead positioned health as 'a resource for everyday life, not the objective of living. Health is a positive concept emphasizing social and personal resources, as well as physical capacities.' (n.p.) In 1997, WHO committed to develop an international strategy for health, and further affirmed that health is 'a basic human right and is essential for social and economic development' (WHO, 1997, n.p.). The Jakarta Declaration provided an international direction and goal 'to increase health expectancy, and to narrow the gap in health expectancy between countries and groups' (WHO, 1997, n.p.) into the twenty-first century. These historical documents continue to shape our understanding of health and underpin contemporary efforts to improve health at a population level.

What is population health?

Population health refers to 'the health outcomes of a group of individuals, including the distribution of such outcomes within the group' (Kindig & Stoddart, 2003, p. 380). A group can refer to locations of populations such as communities, states or nations, as well as populations that share the same roles, characteristics or experiences, such as students, employees, prisoners, retired adults, people with disability, or any other specified group. In the Occupational Therapy Practice Framework—third edition (OTPF-III), a population also refers to a 'collective of groups of individuals living in a similar locale (e.g., city, state, country) or sharing the same or like characteristics or concerns' (American Occupational Therapy Association [AOTA], 2014, p. S3).

Population health has two key aims. The first aim is to understand patterns of health and disease at the community, state and national level. In Australia, health conditions such as cancer, cardiovascular disease, arthritis and musculoskeletal conditions, mental ill-health and substance use disorders and injuries have a major impact on people's lives and make a substantial contribution to the burden of disease and injury. Burden of disease refers to the loss of health and well-being in a population due to premature mortality, morbidity and disability (Australian Institute of Health and Welfare [AIHW], 2019). The non-fatal burden of disease, measured by the number of years people live with disability, is of particular interest to occupational therapists. In 2015, leading contributors to the non-fatal burden of disease were back pain, anxiety and depressive disorders, osteoarthritis, asthma, chronic obstructive pulmonary disease, rheumatoid arthritis, dementia, hearing loss and coronary heart disease (AIHW, 2019).

The second aim of population health is to identify and address health inequalities to improve the health and well-being of the population. Health inequalities, or disparities, are observable and measurable differences in health status between population groups (AIHW, 2018). The distribution of health and disease in a population follows a social gradient, where people in the lowest socio-economic groups are more likely to live with health conditions and die prematurely than people in the highest socio-economic groups (Wilkinson & Marmot, 2003). For example, the non-fatal burden of disease from musculoskeletal conditions and mental ill-health is higher in lower socio-economic groups compared with higher socio-economic groups (AIHW, 2019). In addition, population groups such as Aboriginal and Torres Strait Islander People, people who reside in rural and remote areas, culturally and linguistically diverse populations, people with disability, members of the lesbian, gay, bisexual, transgender, intersex and queer (LGBTIQ) communities, veterans, and prisoners experience disparities in health status when compared to the general population (AIHW, 2018). To address health inequalities, population health also needs to consider the distribution and accessibility of health services and focus on health equity.

Health equity refers to the rights of people to have access to the health services they need and the resources, capacities and power needed to change or enhance their life circumstances (Keleher & MacDougall, 2016). Health inequities are the unfair and avoidable differences in health status that arise within and between population groups due to the unequal distribution of power, money and resources (Keleher & MacDougall, 2016). Improving the conditions of people's daily lives, such as where people live, play and work, and enabling access to universal health care, are key strategies to achieve health equity (Commission on Social Determinants of Health [CSDH], 2008). The following case study describes how occupational therapists have responded to the physical health inequities experienced by people with mental illness.

Case study: occupational therapy in action—responding to health inequities

People with mental illness experience higher rates of chronic disease and a lower life expectancy in comparison to the general population. Occupational therapists have responded to these inequities at both national and local levels. Nationally,

Occupational Therapy Australia, the professional association representing occupational therapists in Australia, pledged their support for the Equally Well Consensus Statement (National Mental Health Commission, 2016), which aims to raise awareness and support actions to bridge the life expectancy gap between people with mental illness and the general population. As part of their commitment to Equally Well, Occupational Therapy Australia is collecting examples of occupational therapy initiatives that address the physical health of people with mental illness.

In one example, an occupational therapist working in a community health service observed that people with serious mental illness did not use the services available due to systemic factors such as stigma and long waiting lists for primary health care services. The occupational therapist and a health promotion officer designed a quality improvement project to explore and address these systemic barriers and obtained funding from the local Primary Health Network, a government-funded organisation that aims to improve medical services and care coordination for people at risk of poor health outcomes. A needs analysis demonstrated that staff had a limited understanding of the physical health inequities faced by people with mental illness and there were no systems in place to facilitate priority access to primary health care. People with a lived experience of mental illness were employed as consultants to co-design solutions, such as revised care pathways and training and resources for staff to help them understand mental illness, to create a more accessible and supportive health care environment. For lived experience consultants, participation in the project was a meaningful occupation that supported their recovery, while helping to challenge stigma by providing opportunities for formal and informal social interactions between staff and people living with mental illness.

What influences population health?

A combination of factors called determinants influence the health of individuals and populations and can explain differences in health status and outcomes across populations. Determinants that have a positive influence on health are called protective factors, and those that have a negative influence on health are called risk factors (AIHW, 2018). Protective factors, such as eating vegetables and fruit, being physically active and getting enough sleep, help people to maintain good health and well-being and can be effective in preventing and/or managing health conditions. Conversely, risk factors, such as smoking tobacco and using alcohol or other drugs, increase the likelihood of developing chronic disease or can make it difficult to manage health conditions. Risk factors that are within a person's control to change are called modifiable risk factors. For instance, high blood pressure—a leading risk factor for stroke—is considered modifiable as activities such as stopping smoking and engaging in regular physical activity can reduce blood pressure.

What people do each day—understood in population health as their behaviours and lifestyle—can determine health outcomes to a certain extent. However, people's capacity to make choices about what they do in their daily lives is influenced by population determinants that are often beyond their individual control. Since the Ottawa Charter

(WHO, 1986) named education, food, income, peace, shelter, social justice and equity, stable ecosystem and sustainable resources as prerequisites for health, our understanding of the factors that influence health and contribute to illness has developed substantially. Wilkinson and Marmot (2006) identified and collated evidence for ten determinants that are considered to be the root causes of ill health and health inequalities: the social gradient, stress, early life experiences, social exclusion, work, unemployment, social support, addiction, food and transport. Evidence supporting the relationship between the living conditions where people are born, grow, live, work and age (known as the social determinants of health) and their health outcomes is now well established (CSDH, 2008). Over the last 15 years, economic, political, cultural and environmental determinants of health have also been acknowledged (AIHW, 2018). Wilcock and Hocking (2015) argue for human occupation itself to be recognised as a determinant of health, highlighting that many of the prerequisites for health, and indeed the determinants of health, relate to what people do in their daily lives.

The health iceberg model is often used to understand how determinants relate to individual and population-level health outcomes (Talbot & Verrinder, 2017). The iceberg model (see Figure 8.1) indicates that the states of health that you see on the surface,

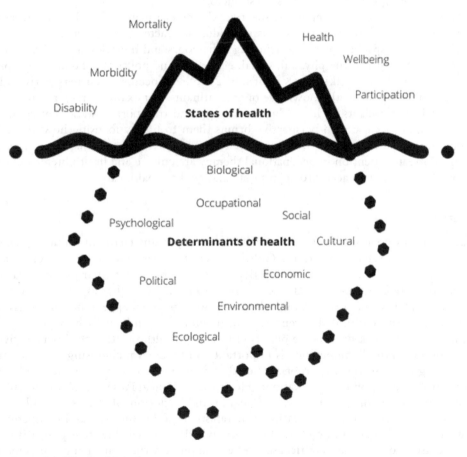

Figure 8.1 The health iceberg.
Source: Adapted from Travis & Ryan (2004). © 1981, 1988, 2004 by Travis, J. W.)

such as morbidity, mortality or quality of life, are merely the tip of the iceberg. Below the surface, multiple determinants contribute to the visible health of an individual. Biological determinants (e.g., genetics and biomedical markers, such as blood pressure or cholesterol) lie just at the waterline. Immediately below the waterline are determinants related to people's occupations, behaviours and lifestyles (e.g., employment, tobacco use, daily routines). Diving deeper, well below the surface, are the psychological, social and cultural determinants (e.g., stress, social inclusion, values, beliefs), which have a significant influence on health. Finally, at the bottom of the iceberg are political, economic, environmental and ecological determinants (e.g., power, money, built and natural environment, climate).

It is important to recognise that these determinants all contribute to health and are interrelated, meaning that they influence each other. For example, at a population level, farmers in rural and remote areas often experience poorer mental health than urban-based professionals. An individual farmer may have a genetic predisposition to depression (biological), which is exacerbated by stress (psychological) related to recent droughts (ecological) and uses alcohol to cope (behavioural). The farmer's ability to seek help for depression may be impacted by a range of determinants including gender norms and stereotypes (cultural), mental health stigma (social), and geographic isolation (environmental), which limits access to services.

From an occupational therapy perspective, the determinants of health can be summarised into: i) person factors, such as individual characteristics, genetics, biomedical markers; ii) occupational factors, including behaviours and lifestyles; and iii) environmental factors, that is, the physical, social, economic and political contexts of people's lives (CSDH, 2008; Wilkinson & Marmot, 2003). An occupational perspective adds depth to population health knowledge of determinants. For example, rather than viewing social determinants such as education, work and transport as static demographic categories, an occupational perspective brings them to life by focusing how and why people do or do not engage in these activities. Two determinants that have recently received greater attention in occupational therapy are culture and health literacy due to their relationship with access to appropriate and quality health care.

Culture

Having an awareness of cultural diversity is an important factor in reducing health inequalities between populations. Culture refers to ideas and meaning, beliefs and knowledge, values and ways of being that are shared by a particular group (Beagan, 2015). Although culture is often used to refer to ethnicity, other aspects of diversity such as gender, sexual orientation, religion, ability, physical appearance and class intersect to create cultural differences. Culture not only influences how individuals view health and seek health care but also influences health practitioners' perspectives. Developing cultural competency is important and involves recognising diversity and delivering the best, most appropriate health care and services to meet the needs of a culturally diverse population (National Health and Medical Research Council, 2006). However, to support the health, well-being and inclusion of diverse populations, Beagan (2015) challenges occupational therapists to go beyond cultural competence, toward cultural safety and cultural humility, which acknowledges that power imbalances exist, and encourages critical self-reflection on how these imbalances are created and maintained.

Health literacy

Health literacy is defined as the abilities of people to gather, understand and utilise information to make appropriate, informed decisions about their health (Australian Commission on Safety and Quality in Health Care [ACSQHC], 2014). Improving health literacy is one important strategy used in population health to enable and empower people to improve their health and prevent illness and disability. Health literacy is influenced by individual factors such as a person's age, education, language, sensory abilities (e.g., eyesight and hearing), geographical location, socio-economic status and cultural background. However, there are also environmental components of health literacy, such as infrastructure, policies, processes, and people and relationships, that impact people's ability to access, understand and use health-related information and services (ACSQHC, 2014). 'Health literacy influences life's occupations as it enables optimal access to and utilization of relevant and meaningful health information and services, and allows informed health decision making and action' (Canadian Association of Occupational Therapists, 2013, p. 1). Occupational therapists have a role in developing an individual's health literacy abilities while also addressing environmental components of health literacy by developing accessible and inclusive policies, programs and resources.

Determinants of health can be addressed together to achieve better health outcomes for populations. The case study gives an example of an intervention that focused on culture and health literacy simultaneously.

Case study: Occupational therapy in action—addressing population determinants

An occupational therapist working in an outpatient oncology unit runs an activity-based 'stress management' group and an 'understanding cancer and recovery' education group, twice a week. He noticed that patients of culturally and linguistically diverse (CALD) backgrounds were under-represented in these groups and observed that among the CALD patients who did attend, few applied the information and skills taught in the group programs in their own lives. The occupational therapist decided to explore the factors that were contributing to the lower attendance rates of CALD patients.

He looked at data from the health service and established that there were differences in oncology consultations between patients who were Australian-born compared to those born overseas. The occupational therapist then started to investigate why this might be the case by exploring the social determinants that were contributing to the lower levels of engagement by CALD patients. Using data from the Australian Bureau of Statistics, he established that there was a higher proportion of people who were born overseas and spoke a language other than English at home in the service's local government area. When he was looking at the literature, he found evidence of cultural differences in the way health professionals interacted with CALD populations. For instance, he learned that doctors spoke more to Anglo-Saxon Australians than to immigrants with interpreters, and spent less time talking about cancer and related issues with immigrants and that immigrants with interpreters spoke to doctors less than Anglo-Saxon Australians (Butow et al., 2011). In addition, the occupational therapist hypothesised that, as many of the patients spoke English as a second language, they may have lower health literacy. To ensure equitable access to the group programs by patients from CALD backgrounds with potentially lower health literacy, the occupational therapist worked with the oncology team to raise their cultural awareness through providing education packages on communication styles with CALD populations. In addition, he co-designed flyers with CALD patients to promote the group programs that had lots of pictures and required minimal reading. The occupational therapist and oncology team also developed content for the sessions that included video clips to illustrate key points. In the sessions, the occupational therapist used the 'teach-back' technique to get group participants to demonstrate their understanding and to reinforce key information. As a result of these measures, the occupational therapist was able to improve the cultural competency of the team as well improve the health literacy of the patients.

Ways of improving population health

Both population health and occupational therapy recognise health and participation as human rights and base interventions on ecological models that focus on what people do in the context of their environment. In both occupational therapy and population health, interventions are guided by shared principles of (a) ethical and evidence-informed practice, (b) social justice and equity, (c) person-centred and collaborative approaches that encourage stakeholder participation in the design and delivery of interventions, (d) tailoring interventions to meet the needs of diverse populations at each lifespan stage, (e) delivering interventions within relevant settings or places, and (f) evaluating the effectiveness of interventions (International Union for Health Promotion and Education, 2016; OTBA, 2018). Ultimately, population health interventions aim to prevent illness and disability and to promote health.

Preventing illness and disability

Preventative approaches often take a biomedical perspective and focus on particular diseases or health conditions. Health protection approaches focus on protecting the population from communicable diseases, such as sexually transmissible infections or coronavirus outbreaks, while prevention approaches focus on chronic health conditions and injuries, such as diabetes or occupational overuse syndrome. From a prevention perspective, the optimal outcome of intervention is the absence of illness or disability, which represents good health. Three levels of prevention are identified: i) primary; ii) secondary; and iii) tertiary (AOTA, 2020).

Primary prevention initiatives are aimed at healthy populations, prior to the development of risk factors and are designed to prevent any progression to a physical or mental health condition. Secondary prevention initiatives target populations who are 'at risk', because they have been exposed to risk factors or are showing early signs or symptoms of a health condition. The aim of secondary prevention is to address risk factors and

---

Case study: Occupational therapy in action—illness and disability prevention

A pair of occupational therapy students was assigned to a project to support the development of children's emotional, behavioural and school readiness skills in a kindergarten setting. The kindergarten was located in an outer suburb, where many of the children were part of low-income, single-parent families. The early childhood educator recognised early life experiences and education as determinants of health and wanted to prevent further disadvantage by creating an environment that supported the children's development and school readiness. After consulting with the early childhood educators, parents, children and teachers and the local primary schools, and reviewing the literature, the students proposed three interventions.

The first intervention was based on primary prevention and involved providing education to educators and parents on young children's emotional and behavioural development and the use of play to enhance young children's early life experiences and prevent behavioural and emotional problems. The second intervention was based on secondary prevention and involved early childhood educators identifying children who have experienced trauma or who are showing signs of developmental delay for further occupational therapy assessment and early intervention. The third intervention was based on tertiary prevention and involved the occupational therapist from the local community health service working directly with children who had been diagnosed with behavioural disorders. The occupational therapist also provided consultations to the educators and parents to extend intervention across home and education environments and share their perspectives on referral processes with students. During the project, the students also created a resource of relevant information booklets and play activities and developed referral pathways in collaboration with the local community health service. An evaluation found that the referral process was simple and clear to the educators and parents, and the education sessions improved parents' understanding of school readiness and increased educators' confidence in identifying children presenting with behavioural and emotional issues.

---

early symptoms to stop or slow the progression of symptoms or disability and, ideally, return individuals to optimal health. Finally, tertiary prevention targets populations who have been diagnosed with an ongoing health condition or disability and refers to interventions to prevent the progression and complications of health conditions and their reoccurrence. The case study provides an example of how primary, secondary and tertiary prevention initiatives can be applied.

Promoting health

The Ottawa Charter (WHO, 1986) defined health promotion as 'a process of enabling people to increase control over, and to improve, their health' (n.p.). The view that health is a resource for life (WHO, 1986) is consistent with occupational therapy's stance that health provides the physical, mental and social capacities that enable people to do what they want, need or are expected to do. Indeed, the OTPF-III (AOTA, 2014) lists health promotion as one of its five intervention approaches.

Health promotion originated in health education, but now goes beyond a focus on individual behaviour and lifestyles to address a wide range of social and environmental determinants. The Ottawa Charter (WHO, 1986) identified five health promotion action areas: i) build healthy public policy; ii) create supportive environments; iii) strengthen community actions; iv) develop personal skills; and v) reorient health services. Developing personal skills and creating supportive environments are central to occupational therapy practice, while the remaining action areas encourage occupational therapists to work with communities to develop policies to create sustained change within health services and other settings. Health promotion initiatives that use combinations of the five actions are more effective than single-track approaches (WHO, 1997). The following case study demonstrates how an occupational therapist used a range of health promotion actions to increase community members' control over their health and well-being.

Case study: Occupational therapy in action—health promotion

A community health service wanted to develop an evidence-based, person-centred approach to working with people who were concerned about their weight. While obesity is an identified risk factor for physical health conditions, clients who accessed the health service also presented with concerns about weight stigma, negative body image and disordered eating. Therefore, to address the clients' concerns in a holistic way, a person-centred approach that recognised people's physical and mental health was needed. An occupational therapist worked with the inter-professional team including a dietitian, health promotion officer, nurse and doctor to review literature, and conduct staff training and consult with community members.

Two approaches to addressing weight were identified in the literature; the weight-normative approach assumes a direct relationship between weight and health, while the weight-inclusive approach views the relationship between weight and health as complex, where one's health is determined more by physical, social and cultural environments and health behaviours, than one's body size (Tylka et al., 2014). After reviewing the evidence for both approaches, and consulting with staff and community members, the community health service decided to adopt a weight-inclusive approach to delivering health care, operationalised by the Health at Every Size® principles (Association for Size Diversity and Health, 2020). To embed this change in practice, the team conducted an audit of the health service and recommended environmental interventions to reduce weight stigma by recognising body diversity in the inclusion policy and creating a supportive environment by upgrading the seating in the waiting area to accommodate people of higher weights and including respectful images of people with various body shapes and sizes in service posters and brochures. Reorienting the focus of health care from weight to well-being led to an increase in referrals, with clients perceiving the service as welcoming and non-judgemental. In addition, the intervention was effective in developing personal skills with clients reporting that they felt more empowered and motivated to participate in activities and occupations to enhance their overall health and well-being.

Occupational therapy's role in fostering health and well-being of individuals, communities and populations

With training in both physical and mental health as well as occupational science, occupational therapy contributes a person-centred perspective and an occupation focus to address health inequalities and improve population health and well-being. Population health approaches are often incorporated into occupational therapists' clinical roles, for instance when conducting quality improvement projects, while others may be employed in a health promotion, illness prevention or population/public health role in a variety of health care, education, workplace and community settings (AOTA, 2020). Adopting a population health approach challenges occupational therapy to adopt a wider lens by focusing on communities and populations, while addressing the broader determinants of participation, health and well-being.

Generic models of practice, such as the Canadian Model of Occupational Performance and Engagement (CMOP-E) (Polatajko et al., 2013), are directly applicable to population health and especially useful for addressing environmental determinants. In addition, specific frameworks have been developed to guide occupational therapy practice with communities and populations:

- Do-Live-Well (Moll et al., 2015) is an occupation-focused, health promotion framework developed to guide interventions and policies at an individual, community and national level. The framework prompts individuals and communities to reflect on how their everyday activities influence health and well-being and explore opportunities to use their time in ways that will promote health and well-being.
- The Community-Centred Practice Framework (Hyett et al., 2019) is a conceptual framework designed to assist occupational therapists to maintain their unique occupation focus in their work with communities. The framework involves exploring community identity and occupations, and identifying assets and barriers, to enable participation within a community.

As these frameworks indicate, population health approaches may incorporate occupation as a means to improve health and well-being, or as an end in itself to support participation and advance occupational justice (AOTA, 2020). Further evaluation of the effectiveness of population health initiatives in occupational therapy has been identified as a research priority (WFOT, 2017). In a population health context, evaluation of process, impact, and outcomes is needed to establish how an intervention is implemented, whether the intervention met its objectives, and its long-term effects on participation, health and well-being (Talbot & Verrinder, 2017).

Conclusion

In this chapter, population health, illness prevention and health promotion were discussed in relation to contemporary occupational therapy practice. Population health, illness prevention and health promotion are related concepts that are integrated in the daily practice of occupational therapy. Occupational therapy and population health share many similarities including:

- a commitment to professional, ethical, and evidence-informed practice;

- an ecological approach that considers people, and what they do, within their environment; and
- working towards equity and social justice.

In addition, occupational therapy contributes a unique occupation focus and a person-centred perspective to population health. The ability to work with communities and populations, as well as individuals and groups, is now specified in the contemporary education of occupational therapists (see also Chapters 6 and 12) and recognised as a required competency for all occupational therapists (OTBA, 2018). Occupational therapy models of practice and emerging practice frameworks provide a solid foundation for addressing determinants of health and supporting the participation, health and well-being of communities and populations.

Summary

- Occupational therapists are increasingly providing services to groups, communities and populations.
- Population health aims to understand patterns of health and disease and identify and address health inequalities.
- There are similarities between occupational therapy and population health approaches in that both focus on the relationships between what people do in their environments and their health and well-being.
- Population health interventions must go beyond individual behaviours and lifestyles to address broader determinants of health, such as culture and health literacy.
- Occupational therapists contribute a person–centred and occupational perspective to population health.

Review questions

1. What is a population and why is it important for occupational therapists to take a population health perspective?
2. What are the key differences between the biomedical model and social model of health?
3. What are the two aims of population health?
4. Which of the social determinants of health identified by Wilkinson and Marmot (2006) relate directly to human occupation?
5. You are working as an occupational health and safety advisor at a large organisation and have been asked to develop a program for employees to prevent occupational overuse injuries. What type of prevention approach would you use and why?
6. Think of a health promotion initiative (e.g. SunSmart, This Girl Can, Movember). Based on the Ottawa Charter (1986), which health promotion actions are used? What occupations do these initiatives involve?

References

American Occupational Therapy Association. (2014). Occupational Therapy Practice Framework: Domain and process, 3rd edition. *American Journal of Occupational Therapy, 68*(Supp. 1), S1–S48. https://doi.org/10.5014/ajot.2014.682006

American Occupational Therapy Association. (2020). Occupational therapy in the promotion of health and well-being. *American Journal of Occupational Therapy, 74,* 7403420010. https://doi.org/10.5014/ajot.2020.743003

Association for Size Diversity and Health. (2020). *HAES(R) principles.* www.sizediversityand health.org

Australian Commission on Safety and Quality in Health Care. (2014). *Health literacy: Taking action to improve safety and quality.* https://www.safetyandquality.gov.au/publications-and-resources/resource-library/health-literacy-taking-action-improve-safety-and-quality

Australian Institute of Health and Welfare. (2018). *Australia's health 2018.* (AUS 221). https://www.aihw.gov.au/reports/australias-health/australias-health-2018/contents/table-of-contents

Australian Institute of Health and Welfare. (2019). *Australian Burden of Disease Study: Impact and causes of illness and death in Australia 2015.* (BOD 22). https://www.aihw.gov.au/reports/burden-of-disease/burden-disease-study-illness-death-2015/contents/table-of-contents

Beagan, B. L. (2015). Approaches to culture and diversity: A critical synthesis of occupational therapy literature. *Canadian Journal of Occupational Therapy, 82*(5), 272–282. https//doi.org/0.1177/0008417414567530

Butow, P., Bell, M., Goldstein, D., Sze, M., Aldridge, L., Abdo, S., Mikhail, M., Dong, S., Iedema, R., Ashgari, R., Hui, R., Eisenbruch, M. (2011). Grappling with cultural differences: Communication between oncologists and immigrant cancer patients with and without interpreters. *Patient Education and Counseling, 84*(3), 398–405. https//doi.org/10.1016/j.pec.2011.01.035

Canadian Association of Occupational Therapists. (2013). *CAOT Position Statement: Enabling health literacy in occupational therapy.* https://caot.in1touch.org/document/3690/E%20-%20Enabling%20Health%20and%20Literacy%20in%20OT.pdf

Commission on Social Determinants of Health. (2008). *Closing the gap in a generation: Health equity through action on the social determinants of health. Final report of the Commission on Social Determinants of Health.* https://apps.who.int/iris/bitstream/handle/10665/43943/9789241563703_eng.pdf;sequence=1

Germov, J. (2019). Imagining health problems as social issues. In J. Germov (Ed.), *Second opinion: An introduction to health sociology* (6th edn, pp. 2–23). Oxford University Press.

Hyett, N., Kenny, A., & Dickson-Swift, V. (2019). Re-imagining occupational therapy clients as communities: Presenting the community-centred practice framework. *Scandinavian Journal of Occupational Therapy, 26*(4), 246–260. https://doi.org/10.1080/11038128.2017.1423374

International Union for Health Promotion and Education. (2016). *Core competencies and professional standards for health promotion.* http://www.iuhpe.org/images/JC-Accreditation/Core_Competencies_Standards_linkE.pdf

Keleher, H., & MacDougall, C. (2016). Concepts of health. In H. Keleher & C. MacDougall (Eds.), *Understanding health* (pp. 3–24). Oxford University Press.

Kindig, D. A., & Stoddart, G. (2003). What is population health? *American Journal of Public Health, 93*(3), 380–383. https://doi.org/10.2105/AJPH.93.3.380

Moll, S. E., Gewurtz, R. E., Krupa, T. M., Law, M. C., Lariviere, N., & Levasseur, M. (2015). 'Do-Live-Well': A Canadian framework for promoting occupation, health, and well-being. *Canadian Journal of Occupational Therapy, 82*(1), 9–23. https://doi.org/10.1177/0008417414545981

National Aboriginal Health Strategy Working Party. (1989). *A national Aboriginal health strategy.* https://www.atns.net.au/agreement.asp?EntityID=757

National Health and Medical Research Council. (2006). *Cultural competency in health: A guide for policy, partnerships and participation.* https://www.nhmrc.gov.au/about-us/publications/cultural-competency-health

National Mental Health Commission. (2016). *Equally Well Consensus Statement: Improving the physical health and well-being of people living with mental illness in Australia.* https://www.mentalhealthcommission.gov.au/Social-Determinants/Equally-well

Occupational Therapy Board of Australia. (2018). *Australian occupational therapy competency standards 2018.* https://www.occupationaltherapyboard.gov.au/Codes-Guidelines/Competencies.aspx

Polatajko, H. J., Davis, J., Stewart, D., Cantin, N., Amoroso, B., Purdie, L., & Zimmerman, D. (2013). Specifying the domain of concern: Occupation as core. In E. Townsend & H. J. Polatajko (Eds.), *Enabling occupation II: Advancing an occupational therapy vision for health, well-being & justice through occupation* (2nd edn, pp. 13–36). Canadian Association of Occupational Therapists.

Talbot, L., & Verrinder, G. (2017). Health promotion in context: Comprehensive primary health care, the new public health and health promotion. In L. Talbot & G. Verrinder (Eds.), *Promoting health: The primary health care approach* (pp. 3–42). Elsevier.

Travis, J. W., & Ryan, R. S. (2004). *Wellness workbook* (3rd edn). Ten Speed Press.

Tylka, T. L., Annunziato, R. A., Burgard, D., Daníelsdóttir, S., Shuman, E., Davis, C., & Calogero, R. M. (2014). The weight-inclusive versus weight-normative approach to health: Evaluating the evidence for prioritizing well-being over weight loss. *Journal of Obesity*, Article ID 983495. https://doi.org/10.1155/2014/983495

Wilcock, A. A., & Hocking, C. (2015). *An occupational perspective of health*. SLACK Inc.

Wilkinson, R., & Marmot, M. (2003). *Social determinants of health: The solid facts*. World Health Organization.

Wilkinson, R., & Marmot, M. (2006). *Social determinants of health* (2nd edn). Oxford University Press.

World Federation of Occupational Therapists. (2012). *Definitions of occupational therapy from member organisations.* http://www.wfot.org/ResourceCentre.aspx

World Federation of Occupational Therapists, Mackenzie, L., Coppola, S., Alvarez, L., Cibule, L., Maltsev, S., Loh, S. Y., Mlambo, T., Ikiugu, M. N., Pihlar, Z., Sriphetcharawut, S., Baptiste, S., & Ledgerd, R. (2017). International occupational therapy research priorities: A delphi study. *OTJR: Occupation, Participation and Health*, *37*(2), 72–81. https://doi.org/10.1177/1539449216687528

World Health Organization. (1946, June 19–22). *Preamble to the constitution of the World Health Organization*. Paper presented at the International Health Conference, New York.

World Health Organization. (1986, November 21). *The Ottawa Charter for Health Promotion*. Paper presented at the First International Conference on Health Promotion, Ottawa. https://www.who.int/healthpromotion/conferences/previous/ottawa/en/

World Health Organization. (1997, July 21–25). *Jakarta declaration on leading health promotion into the 21st Century*. Paper presented at the Fourth International Conference on Health Promotion, Jakarta. http://www.who.int/healthpromotion/conferences/previous/jakarta/declaration/en/

Part II

Professional issues

9 Skills for effective communication in occupational therapy practice

Luke Robinson, Andrea Robinson and Annette Peart

Chapter objectives

Upon completion of this chapter, the reader will be able to:

- Articulate the importance of communication in occupational therapy practice.
- Describe the communication cycle and define the different types of communication (verbal, non-verbal and written) involved.
- Summarise and apply various strategies and frameworks that can assist therapists in developing and refining verbal, non-verbal and written communication skills.
- Outline strategies to build and enhance the therapeutic use of self in occupational therapy service.
- Explain methods to promote effective communication when working with individuals from diverse cultural backgrounds.
- Identify and apply skills, frameworks and strategies to promote effective communication when working in health care and professional teams.

Key terms

communication; therapeutic use of self; therapeutic relationship; rapport building; teamwork, team communication; cross-cultural sensitivity

Introduction

Communication is an integral component of our everyday lives. At its core, communication is the sending and receiving of messages and is a fundamental human right. As occupational therapists, how we communicate using verbal, non-verbal and written messages is essential to the effectiveness of our service provision with clients, their carers or family, colleagues, and other professionals.

Communication is one of the four standards of competent practice expected of Australian occupational therapists (Occupational Therapy Board of Australia, 2018). Therefore, it is fundamental as a practising or student occupational therapist to be aware of the purpose of communication, its key elements, and the skills required for appropriate communication when providing occupational therapy services. Further, it is essential to understand and apply the skills required to work within health care or professional teams and use culturally responsive, safe and relevant communication tools and strategies to ensure the best outcomes for individuals or groups of individuals receiving such services.

This chapter explores the key elements and skills required for effective communication in the context of client interactions, and when working in health care and professional teams. It also defines and explores the concept of the therapeutic use of self when communicating in occupational therapy practice and considerations and strategies to promote effective communication with individuals from diverse cultural backgrounds.

Defining communication

Communication is a complex process involving the purposeful activity of exchanging or transmitting information that is interpreted by one or more individuals or parties (Henderson, 2019). There are five basic elements involved in communication: (1) the sender, (2) the message, (3) the transmission or mode of communication, (4) the receiver, and (5) feedback (Tamparo & Lindh, 2017). As demonstrated in the communication cycle presented in Figure 9.1, communication is a two-way process which can involve various methods of *transmission* (for example, spoken, written or non-verbal) by a *sender*, of a *message* to a *receiver* (for example, client, colleagues). While this view of communication appears straightforward, in reality, a number of factors need to be considered. For example, the ability of multiple messages to be transmitted simultaneously through verbal and non-verbal means, or the ability to involve multiple senders and receivers, must be thought through when describing communication (Wright et al., 2013).

To ensure open, respectful and effective communication when providing occupational therapy services, presenting at team meetings and communicating in other professional contexts, it is important to recognise the two-way nature of communication between the sender and the receiver to ensure mutual understanding (refer Figure 9.1). Generally, misunderstandings or issues in communication between the sender and receiver in health care can result in errors, misdiagnosis, inappropriate treatment, adverse outcomes, and even permanent disability or, in extreme cases, death (Iedema et al., 2015). For example, without a mutual understanding during an occupational performance assessment of a toilet transfer to communicate concerns of *instability*, a client may fall on a therapist leading to potential injury for both parties. In this example, clarifying

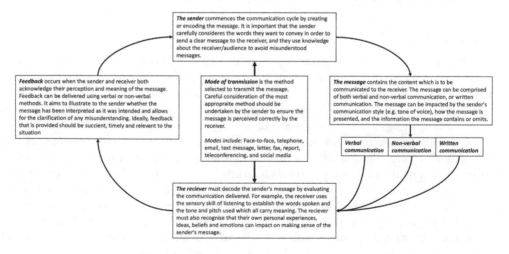

Figure 9.1 The communication cycle.
Source: Adapted from Tamparo and Lindh (2017)

any client concerns about feeling *unsteady, shaky* or *weak in the legs,* or adapting communication to meet the client's needs, can help to reach a mutual understanding and avoid injury for both parties.

Further, it is essential to recognise the inherent power imbalance between a health care professional and the individual(s) receiving health care services and their families and/or carers, and the impact this can have on a communication (Henderson, 2003). Factors which have been shown to lead to feelings of powerlessness in a health care setting include the removal of independence, social status and responsibility, and expression of identity (Purtilo et al., 2014). In response, occupational therapists need to use effective communication skills and strategies to initiate, maintain and end therapeutic relationships with clients and relevant others. This can minimise perceived or actual power imbalance and promote collaborative partnerships (Henderson, 2003).

Types of communication

There are three types of communication appropriate to occupational therapy service provision: verbal, non-verbal and written. Verbal communication is a significant component of occupational therapy service provision and is important in the development of the therapeutic relationship (Allison & Strong, 1994; O'Brien, 2018). Verbal communication is the use of spoken or sign language to transfer a message in the form of information (Henderson, 2019). The construction of phrases and the pitch, tone, volume and speed of speech is used to construct the message transmitted to the receiver.

Non-verbal communication refers to messages transmitted through intentional or unintentional gestures and body language behaviours that occur in addition to, or without, verbal communication (O'Toole, 2016). Non-verbal elements, such as eye contact, facial expression, posture, professional presentation (for example, clothing, personal hygiene), gestures, and the time and place of communication can influence how the receiver interprets and understands the message transmitted by the sender (Henderson, 2019). For example, if a therapist is trying to demonstrate empathy and compassion using verbal communication, but their arms are crossed, and they are looking at the clock on the wall, the receiver may not interpret the therapist as empathic or compassionate. Alternatively, if a therapist is showing excessive direct eye contact, it may appear confrontational, and in some circumstances may be considered culturally inappropriate.

Written communication refers to the use of written sources to communicate information, observations or events (Jefferies et al., 2012). The form of written communication can vary from client service records, team meeting agendas or minutes, instructions, reports, and formal or informal notes. An example of written communication in occupational therapy service provision is documentation that serves as a record or account of verbal communication with clients and accompanying events, or client service records (Henderson, 2019). The purpose of this form of written communication is to communicate information about a client and/or other involved parties, the rationale for occupational therapy service provision, and a chronological record of outcomes or other significant events (Kearney & Laverdure, 2018).

Skill for effective verbal communication

The use of effective language is paramount to ensure that a message is Complete, Clear, Concise, Cohesive and Courteous—an approach referred to as the Five Cs. (Peterson et al., 2010). In addition to the Five Cs, the sender of a message needs to ensure they use language that promotes engagement in the communication cycle (refer Figure 9.1). For example, rather than a therapist saying to a client: 'I need to see you shower yourself' as part of an assessment, an alternative could be: 'as part of my occupational therapy assessment I would like to assess how much you can do for yourself and any risks to your safety while you are having a shower'. Additional skills to promote responsive and appropriate verbal communication are discussed in Table 9.1.

Table 9.1 Skills to promote responsive and appropriate verbal and non-verbal communication

Skill		Description	Purpose
Observation skills		Observation of a person(s) in a given environment noticing their presentation, verbal and non-verbal communication, social skills, tone of voice, behaviour and motor skills (O'Brien, 2018).	Useful when information gathering, determining cognitive or physical capacities, or hypothesis testing.
Active listening skills		Using non-verbal skills, including body language, facial expression, posture, eye contact and gestures to convey interest and understanding (Hazelwood & Shakespeare-Finch, 2011).	Useful to provide encouragement, build therapeutic relationship and trust, ensure accurately recalled information, convey empathy and ensure relevant questions are asked.
Questioning skills	Open-ended questions	Verbal questions that give the person(s) answering control over the information provided and allow the therapist to listen, observe and learn (O'Toole, 2016). Typically involve 'who', 'what', 'where', 'when', 'why' or 'how'.	Useful when the information required is not discreet and may need a thorough discussion of memory, elaboration, opinion, detail and/or description of experiences and feelings. Generally it is less threatening because they allow the person(s) answering to control the information they provide; however, it may be time-consuming or result in unnecessary information.
	Closed-ended questions	Verbal questions used to elicit discrete information, which is short, definite and to the point (O'Toole, 2016). Typically result in 'yes', 'no' or concise answers to check or clarify something.	Useful when information required is discrete or only one answer is desired. These questions demand little of the person(s) and can save time and provide the exact answer without resulting in overthinking or using too many words. They can, however, result in incomplete answers that lack detail or result in wrong conclusions.

Skill		Description	Purpose
Clarifying and facilitating skills	Reflection	Trying to clarify the feelings a person(s) has sent in their message by asking questions in a way that lets the person confirm or reject the interviewer's suggestions based on the discussion so far (Curtin et al., 2017).	Useful to explore and share emotions, convey listening and empathy, explore values and beliefs, build a therapeutic relationship, individualise experiences to allow the person(s) to make sense of information, and encourage in-depth exploration of feelings.
	Paraphrasing	Providing a summary or comment of the person's/persons' own words to show understanding of the message (Curtin et al., 2017)	Useful to confirm understanding and accuracy of information provided, convey empathy, demonstrate active listening, build the therapeutic relationship, and advance the conversation.
	Summarising	Providing a recap or verification of understanding of what the person(s) has said so that both parties are clear at the end of a conversation and to complete an interaction (O'Toole, 2016).	Useful to allow the person(s) to correct interpretation or provide further information, build trust and therapeutic relationship, establish future directions and lay the foundation for collaboration. Also, it is useful during communication when there is a change of theme or large amounts of information have been shared.
	Clarifying	Verifying the person's/persons' message, if it is unclear or needs further elaboration for understanding (Curtin et al., 2017).	Useful to ensure that the interviewer has correctly understood the person's/persons' words, meanings, goals, actions, values or beliefs. It continues to build the therapeutic relationship by deepening trust as feelings are shared and explored.
	Focusing	Helping the person(s) to identify one or more priority issues for exploration and attention (Curtin et al., 2017).	Useful to provide the individual with control of the agenda, ensure client-centred practice by identifying the client's priorities, allow further information to be gathered and given, and allow for articulation of values and beliefs.

Several tools are available to use by occupational therapists when communicating during the therapeutic process. The *Canadian Occupational Performance Measure* (COPM) allows a therapist and client to identify the issues of personal importance to the client and their self-perception of occupational performance over time (Law et al., 1990). The COPM, which focuses on self-care, productivity and leisure occupations, provides therapists with a semi-structured interview schedule to ensure relevant information is collected and the client is an active participant in a two-way communication exchange.

An alternative tool for eliciting a client's perspective of their occupational performance is the use of an *occupational profile*. An occupational profile summarises a client's occupational history and experiences, patterns of daily living, interests, values, habits and needs (AOTA, 2014). By using formal interview techniques and informal conversation, information is gathered to understand what is important and meaningful to the client and identify past experiences and interests to understand the client's current occupational performance issues. Using this approach, therapists and clients can design occupation-based interventions collaboratively. One example of an occupational profile is that based on the Occupational Therapy Practice Framework (AOTA, 2014). In addition to the COPM and the Occupational Profile, the Model of Human Occupation (MOHO) has various dedicated tools to guide communication including, but not limited to, the Occupational Performance History Interview (OPHI-II) which can also assist in communication exchange (Taylor & Kielhofner, 2017).

Another tool which could be considered to assist in effective verbal communication with clients in health care settings is *The Calgary Cambridge Model of History Taking* (CCMHT) (Silverman et al., 2013). This guide, although initially designed for taking a medical history, can be modified for use by occupational therapists when building an occupational profile or the story of a person. Further, it can assist students and therapists in understanding the core elements of conducting successful communicative cycles by exploring five stages (refer to Table 9.2).

Skills for effective non-verbal communication

In occupational therapy service provision, non-verbal communication skills are equally important. Again, a variety of tools are available to occupational therapists to guide effective non-verbal communication. For example, Egan (1975) developed the SOLER model for health care professionals. The model was designed to facilitate active listening (the process of receiving, constructing meaning from, and responding to spoken and/ or non-verbal messages (Egan, 1975; Weger et al., 2014)), by providing prompts and considerations when communicating, and comprises five components:

- **S**quarely: sit squarely (opposite) to the other person.★
- **O**pen posture: adopt a posture where neither arms nor legs are crossed.
- **L**ean towards the other: position the body towards the other person to communicate interest in what they are talking about.★★

★   This position may feel threatening to some people or not feasible due to the environment and, therefore, an angle between chairs may be preferred (Egan, 2007).
★★ This should be done when appropriate and culturally acceptable.

Table 9.2 Use of the *Calgary–Cambridge Model of History Taking* (CCMHT) with an occupational focus

Stage	Actions
1. Initiate the session	Ensure an appropriate environment to engage in the communication cycle, establish initial rapport, and clarify the person's reason for receiving occupational therapy services.
2. Gathering information	Explore the person's occupational profile considering the environments in which they engage in occupations, personal resources, barriers and facilitators to occupational performance in the context of their health and well-being.
3. Providing structure	Make clear to the person the therapeutic process and role of an occupational therapist in the given practice setting. Ensure that the communication cycle flows in a logical and comfortable manner.
4. Building the relationship	Be present with the person and ensure appropriate non-verbal communication is used in response to non-verbal behaviours or cues. Involve the person in the conversation by ensuring open and honest communication. When making plans ensure they are person-centred and incorporate identified occupational performance issues, barriers and facilitators relevant to the person. This is an essential process which requires a shared understanding that will result in shared decision-making.
5. Closing the session	Ensure that the communication cycle ends in a timely and respectful manner. Consider asking the client to paraphrase the key points of discussion. Summarise the key points of what was communicated and clearly articulate any plans relating to further interviews, assessments and/or intervention as appropriate to the person.

Source: Adapted from Baptiste (2017) & Silverman et al. (2013)

- **E**ye contact: use eye contact to project engagement and interest in a conversation, ensuring it is not confrontational or culturally inappropriate.
- **R**elax: avoid fidgeting or demonstrating nervousness.

In response to several limitations of the SOLER model (for example, cultural appropriateness, practice area considerations), several revisions have been proposed including SOLVER, which prompts the sender to **v**ary their voice appropriately, and SURTEY, which allows for cultural variations and prompts the sender to:

- **S**it at an angle to the client;
- **U**ncross legs and arms;
- **R**elax;
- Provide **E**ye contact;
- Give appropriate **T**ouch; and
- Trust **Y**our intuition.

(Stickley, 2011)

It should be noted that many of these models are suited to Western culture and may not accommodate all cultural variations and expectations when communicating (O'Toole, 2016). Additional skills and considerations to promote effective non-verbal communication are discussed in Table 9.1.

When communicating during occupational therapy service provision using verbal or non-verbal methods, it is important to be aware of contextual considerations that may impact on the way the message is transmitted to the receiver. These include client factors, such as a cognitive, motor or psychological impairment; environmental factors, such as noise, lighting or distractions; and ethical considerations, such as the level of privacy available (Acton et al., 1999; Jangland et al., 2009).

Skills for effective written communication

All written health care communication must be accurate, understandable, well-constructed, succinct and professional (Bonk, 2015). Writing high-quality documentation requires commitment, time and practice (Hammoud et al., 2012). O'Toole (2016) proposes five steps to produce accurate, appropriate and quality written communication:

1. Consider the purpose: The purpose should direct the content and inform the focus, details and length.
2. Consider the audience: The content should be written with the specific audience in mind (for example, other health professionals, compensable bodies such as Work-Cover (a compensation system for individuals injured at work), or clients). The writer must also ensure that language used is tailored to the audience (for example, the use of medically focused language or language suitable for people with average literacy levels (Fajardo et al., 2019).
3. Consider ethical requirements: The content should ensure confidentiality and privacy are maintained as required to protect the rights of those discussed in the communication.
4. Consider content and organisation: The content should adhere to the requirements of the organisation and the code of conduct for registered health practitioners (for example, the code outlined by the Occupational Therapy Board of Australia, 2018).
5. Consider professional writing style: The writing style should align to the audience, adhere to relevant legal requirements, and be proofread for grammatical and spelling errors. In addition, the writer should consider the appropriateness of abbreviations (for example, when writing a report for a WorkCover use the full term 'active range of motion' instead of the abbreviation 'AROM' (Sames, 2015).

Various other tools and frameworks are available to guide students and therapists to document written communication in a structured and organised way (Sames, 2015). One example is the SOAP (**S**ubjective – experiences, personal views or feelings of a client; **O**bjective—data from the client encounter such as assessment findings; **A**ssessment—a synthesis of the subjective and objective evidence; and **P**lan—actions to be taken following interaction) note format (Morreale & Borcherding, 2013). While this format is commonly used in acute and sub-acute settings, the basics for composing notes using this format can be adapted and applied in other ways of recording client care (Morreale & Borcherding, 2013). While the SOAP note format provides one option for the documentation of written information, it is essential that the requirements of each practice setting are carefully considered in order to adhere to legal and organisational requirements.

Therapeutic use of self

The therapeutic use of self is another skill that can be used to promote effective communication with clients. The concept of the therapeutic use of self, which dates back to the late 1700s during the moral treatment era, refers to a therapist's interactions with clients and, in particular, how they use their own self (for example, personality, insights, perceptions and judgements) to motivate clients and facilitate the therapeutic process (O'Brien, 2018; Taylor, 2008; 2020). In essence, the therapeutic use of self involves paying attention to the client's needs and responding in a way that promotes the client's goals. This is achieved by building a solid therapeutic relationship during the therapeutic process that is underpinned by mutuality and authenticity to ensure that both parties are present, committed and able to co-participate in a relationship that facilitates the implementation of professional reasoning (Taylor, 2008; Tickle-Degnen, 2014).

To successfully implement therapeutic use of self, a practitioner must first possess a level of self-awareness as to allow a mindful examination of their own role in the intervention/service delivery process (O'Brien, 2018). This involves knowledge of one's own behaviour, emotional responses and their effects that can be projected onto others. Second, they need to learn how to develop trust, provide support, display active listening and empathise by being able to place oneself in the position to understand the client's experience. This can be achieved by showing genuineness, respect, self-disclosure and warmth when communicating with clients, all of which assist in developing and sustaining the therapeutic relationship (McKenna, 2017). Table 9.3 provides examples of how to build and enhance the key skills that are involved in the therapeutic use of self. It is suggested that supervision from a senior therapist be used to deal with issues that arise when developing the skills of the therapeutic use of self, and to provide support, consultation, skill upgrading and opportunities for further development and feedback on personal awareness in the therapeutic process (Burnard, 2005; McKenna, 2017).

Skills for cross-cultural communication

Many societies across the world are characterised by cultural, ethnic and linguistic diversity. Present-day Australia is one of the most multicultural, linguistically and ethnoculturally diverse nations in the world. The 2016 Census of Population and Housing found that more than one-quarter (26 per cent) of Australia's population (6.1 million people) were born overseas, a 1 per cent increase from the previous data collected in 2011 (ABS, 2017). While the most common birthplace of Australians born overseas continues to be England (15 per cent), a jump between the 2011 and 2016 Censuses in the proportion of people born in China (6.0 per cent to 8.3 per cent) and India (5.6 per cent to 7.4 per cent) was observed, highlighting the increasingly multicultural makeup of Australian society.

The 2016 Census reported that there were 300 separately identified languages being spoken in Australian homes, including the languages of the Aboriginal and Torres Strait Islander people (with 10 per cent of the 649,171 Aboriginal and Torres Strait Islander people reporting speaking one of the 150 Australian Indigenous languages at home) and Australian Sign Language (AUSLAN), an important language for the deaf community.

As communication is fundamentally a social process that involves cooperation, negotiation and exchange of meaning, avoiding or neglecting problems between linguistically and culturally different parties in a multicultural society is impossible if only one party is willing or able to modify their linguistic behaviour (Pauwels, 1995; Martin & Nakayama, 2014). In order to achieve culturally competent communication, it is crucial to understand that each person has diverse experiences, worldviews, beliefs, attitudes and values that affect their understanding of power and privilege (O'Toole, 2016).

Table 9.3 Strategies to build and enhance the therapeutic use of self in occupational therapy service delivery

Skill	Strategies to build and enhance
Self-awareness	Keep a reflective journal to document feelings and reactions to life events. The use of Gibbs' (1988) reflective cycle can be helpful in identifying strengths and areas for improvement.
	Ask for feedback to better understand your strengths and areas for improvement.
	Ask for specific feedback about your verbal and non-verbal communication skills.
Developing trust	Follow through with plans and be on time with appointments.
	Be honest and transparent.
	Do not overpromise outcomes that you cannot deliver.
	Maintain confidentiality at all times.
	Use language that is clear, precise and appropriate.
	Ensure client-centred practice.
Developing empathy	Read stories about others who have been through significant life events.
	Participate in activities of other cultures.
	Reflect on the stories of clients, peers and other people.
	Participate in a lived-experience activity (i.e., spend some time in a wheelchair and experience the barriers and challenges faced).
	Try to imagine the injury, condition or circumstances faced from the perspective of the client and/or their family.
Verbal communication	Practise and role-play a variety of interviews to gain experience and feedback.
	Identify the strengths and weaknesses that can form goals for development.
Non-verbal communication	Observe an occasion of service provision and identify the types of non-verbal skills used (use the CCMHT checklist to guide observation).
	Practise expressing your emotions without talking.
	Practise and role-play a variety of interviews to gain experience and feedback.
	Play charades to tune into your style of non-verbal communication.
Active listening	Observe other therapists and recognise the active listening techniques used.
	Practise and role-play a variety of interviews and try to summarise the key points expressed.
	Do not always think about the most apparent or practical solution to a problem in preference to listening to the client's communication.
	Develop techniques to improve listening by setting self-directed goals.
Use of therapeutic modes	Be aware of own preferred therapeutic mode(s), and the importance of adapting modes to best suit the needs of a client(s) in a given moment. The six modes include empathising, collaborating, encouraging, problem-solving, instructing and advocating (Taylor, 2020).

Table 9.4 explores several considerations that can enhance the chances of successful communication between parties when engaged in a therapeutic relationship or when working with individuals or groups of individuals from diverse cultural backgrounds.

Skills for team communication and inter-professional practice

Communication is fundamental to effective teamwork in health care and other professional settings where occupational therapists work. Effective teams in health care, or

Table 9.4 Considerations for cross-cultural communication

Considerations	
Reflect	Apply critical self-awareness by evaluating personal and cultural values, beliefs and traditions. Be aware of your own cultural biases and tendencies to stereotype.
Learn	Investing time to better understand cultural differences and similarities (for example, cultural sensitivity training, films/books).
Respect	Treat all people equally, regardless of difference. Respect should also be given to the environments in which the person lives and works, gender roles and generational relationships relative to different cultural groups.
Privilege	Explore and understand own privilege. Maintain confidentiality as a privileged learner of another person's story.
Do no harm	If for any reason you feel as though you do not have the skills and competency to help another person, refer them on to someone who will be able to provide appropriate care.
Listening	Demonstrate active listening and be aware of non-verbal communication.
Promote social justice	Do not condone discrimination and ethnocentrism by remaining silent.
Social inclusion	Be aware and respect the differences between individualist (places greater value on perceptions of 'self' and 'I', for example, Australia, United Kingdom, United States) and collectivist (places greater value on perceptions of 'we', 'us' or 'the group', for example, China, India and Pakistan) cultures.
High- and low-context cultures	Be aware of the differences between high-context (communication is full of implicit meaning; exemplify the value placed on non-verbal communication) and low-context (does not assume shared background knowledge and understanding; almost everything is explained in words) cultures.
Use of interpreters	Use interpreters (preferably face to face, otherwise consider phone interpreters) when indicated. Ensure that you are prepared, do not ask too many questions at once and direct the communication at the person and not the interpreter to build rapport.

Source: Adapted from Hazelwood & Shakespeare-Finch (2011)

other professional settings, are characterised by trust, respect, collaboration and open communication (Rosenstein & O'Daniel, 2008). The degree of open communication is reflected by a team's ability to communicate clearly, accurately and respectfully, with the freedom to express opinions and to ask questions.

Poor communication within health care organisations is cited as a significant contributing factor in patient safety incidents (Bendaly & Bendaly, 2012). To avoid poor team communication, all health professionals need to develop constructive professional behaviours to communicate with clients and other health professionals involved in the service provision process (Henderson, 2019). In response, several frameworks, such as the *Team Strategies and Tools to Enhance Performance and Patient Safety* (TeamSTEPPs), have been developed to encourage successful team communication and collaboration (Clancy & Tornberg, 2007). This framework focuses on the importance of team structure by recognising the need for individual roles within the team; a structured process where information is clearly and accurately exchanged by team members; a designated leader(s) who can organise the team and review processes; situation monitoring to maintain awareness to support team functioning; and mutual support amongst team members (King et al., 2008).

In addition to the skills explored in the previous sections of this chapter, there are several tools and strategies that therapists can utilise in an attempt to achieve and maintain effective communication within teams and enhance inter-professional practice.

Briefing, monitoring and debriefing

Briefings are a short session before the start of team involvement with a client and provide an opportunity to share the plan, discuss team roles and responsibilities, establish expectations, anticipate outcomes and consider contingencies (Clancy & Tornberg, 2007). A briefing should be viewed as a primer to ensure that the team is united and understands individual roles in the process. After a team has begun its collaboration with the client, they may choose to monitor their plan by having a team huddle, which usually is an ad–hoc meeting to re-establish situational awareness, and review, adjust and reinforce any plans in place. The process of monitoring can occur once or several times during a team's involvement with a client. Following the cessation of the client–team therapeutic relationship, members of a team can debrief about how to improve team performance and effectiveness by discussing lessons learnt and reinforce positive behaviours which lead to team success (Clancy & Tornberg, 2007).

The ISBAR tool

One tool to assist in the transfer of client information and communicating outstanding issues and tasks to a team within a health care setting is the ISBAR handover tool (Thompson et al., 2011). The tool was initially developed to aid communication by offering a pattern of transferred information so errors or omissions in information become clear and avoidable. Use of the ISBAR tool: **I**dentify; **S**ituation; **B**ackground; **A**ssessment and **A**ctions; **R**esponsibility and **R**eferral (refer to Table 9.5) has been shown to substantially improve team communication and result in fewer adverse events (Thompson et al., 2011). This tool is frequently used in multidiscipline medical handover meetings in acute, sub–acute and community settings to ensure a complete picture of health professional involvement and professional reasoning is transparent.

DESC Script and the two–challenge rule

The DESC Script is a template for assertive communication that provides a constructive process for resolving conflicts that can occur within teams (Bower & Bower, 2009).

Table 9.5 Considerations of the ISBAR acronym

	Step	Considerations
I	Identification	Patient, staff members
S	Situation	Symptoms/problem, patient stability/level of concern
B	Background	History of presentation, date of admission and diagnosis, relevant past medical history
A	Assessment and Actions	What are the findings of your assessments/impressions of the situation, what have you done so far?
R	Responsibility and Referral	What you want to be done, interventions underway or that need monitoring, who is responsible for a review and when does it need to occur, and a plan depending on results/outcomes

The script: **D**escribe the specific situation or behaviour using concrete data; **E**xpress the concerns you have and how the situation makes you feel; **S**uggest alternatives and seek agreement; and **C**onsequences should be stated in terms of impact on established team goals, promotes a timely discussion that avoids blaming statements and focuses on *what* is right, rather than *who* is right (Bower & Bower, 2009).

An alternative communication strategy when information conflict exists between team members is the two-challenge rule with the use of the CUS Script (Pian-Smith et al., 2009). The two-challenge rule prompts the user to advocate and assert their statement of concern at least twice using the CUS script [I am **C**oncerned; this makes me **U**ncomfortable; this is a **S**afety issue] in the case where the initial assertion is ignored. If this does not result in a change or is still unacceptable, then the person with the concern should take stronger action by talking to a supervisor or the next person up in the chain of command (Pian-Smith et al., 2009). As issues using this strategy are raised to advocate for a patient/client, this tactic ensures that an expressed concern has been heard, understood and acknowledged.

Case study

Mr Li, a 68-year-old man, who presented with right-sided arm and leg weakness following a stroke, was admitted to the acute stroke unit in a large and busy hospital. The occupational therapist has been referred by the medical team to assess Mr Li's right-sided weakness and investigate his functional independence changes to assist with discharge planning.

The occupational therapist, Sarah, commenced data gathering by reading through the multidisciplinary progress notes documented in the medical record. It is noted in his medical history that Mr Li primarily speaks Mandarin and that he has a long-standing hearing impairment. Sarah organised for a Mandarin interpreter, Jenny, to assist her to complete her occupational therapy assessment. Sarah and Jenny meet with Mr Li and his daughter (Florence), in a four-bedroom within the acute stroke unit. Mr Li was sitting out of bed in a chair on arrival. Following her arrival into the room, Sarah turns the light on and closes the bedside curtains to provide privacy and confidentiality from other patients sharing the room, and to minimise distractions.

Sarah introduces herself, the occupational therapy role and purpose for interaction in the context of Mr Li's presentation following an introduction to Jenny, the interpreter. Directing her communication directly at Mr Li, she asks if it is appropriate for her to sit on the side of his bed to face him during their interaction and also gestures towards the bed as she does this.

She notices that Mr Li is not wearing his hearing aids and asks Florence if he has them with him. Florence proceeds to retrieve the hearing aids from Mr Li's belongings and assists him to fit them in his ears. Sarah invites Florence and Jenny to then sit down next to Mr Li and participate in the assessment with his consent. She also confirms that she is speaking at a suitable volume for him to hear and that he is feeling comfortable in his current environment.

Sarah communicates directly to Mr Li by slowly using short sentences that are translated by Jenny. Sarah uses a combination of both open- and closed-ended questions to develop an occupational profile and establish rapport and a therapeutic relationship with Mr Li.

Mr Li becomes visibly upset when discussing his work role as a shopkeeper. Using her knowledge of non-verbal behaviours and cues, she recognises the need to actively listen to his concerns while also displaying empathy and compassion to his current situation. Sarah provides support and reassurance to Mr Li and explains that the multidisciplinary team are there to help and support him and his family during his recovery.

Following the completion of Mr Li's occupational profile, Sarah conducts a brief functional assessment focused on his ability to complete bed, chair and toilet transfers, walk, and use of his upper limbs in functional tasks. The main occupational performance issues identified by both Sarah and Mr Li were: his need to walk with Sarah's assistance; his difficulty with all transfers and using his right arm to complete basic self-care tasks, including brushing his hair (Mr Li reports great pride in his appearance); his difficulty feeding himself using culturally appropriate utensils (for example, chopsticks); and doing up buttons on his shirt. Sarah discusses possible discharge plans with Mr Li and his daughter. She outlines from their discussions and her assessment; a period of inpatient rehabilitation would be helpful to allow Mr Li to regain strength and functional use of his right hand as well as his independence with walking as he identified returning to work as his primary goal. Towards the end of her assessment, Sarah observes several non-verbal cues from Mr Li that he was becoming fatigued. This included yawning, distractibility, and decreased engagement in the conversation. This prompted Sarah to begin concluding the session.

She asks Mr Li to paraphrase the key points of their discussions to ensure his comprehension of the communication that has taken place during their interaction. Sarah closes the session by summarising the key points to both Mr Li and Florence and outlines her plans for discussing her recommendation with the multidisciplinary team for inpatient rehabilitation. She also obtained Mr Li's consent to return the following day with Jenny to complete a formal cognitive assessment.

Prior to writing her SOAP notes at the nurse's station, Sarah communicates with the speech pathologist (Jim) and provides a verbal ISBAR handover referral after noticing Mr Li may be experiencing some mild communication deficits with evidence of word-finding difficulties. This was also reported by Mr Li, Jenny and Florence. Sarah ensured that in the background section of her ISBAR handover to Jim that Mr Li's primary language was Mandarin, he requires the use of hearing aids and that an interpreter was used successfully.

Conclusion

Communication is an essential skill for effective occupational therapy service delivery in all professional settings. In their professional practice with individuals, their families, groups of people and team members, occupational therapists are required to use verbal, non-verbal and written communication in various ways. Knowledge and application of skills, strategies and frameworks can assist therapists in ensuring that they strive for, and achieve, effective communication with people of all backgrounds, roles in the therapeutic process and, with varying occupational performance capabilities.

Summary

- All occupational therapists are required to possess skills for achieving effective communication.
- Various skills, strategies and frameworks can assist therapists in developing and refining verbal, non-verbal and written communication skills used with individuals receiving occupational therapy services and health professional team members.
- Knowledge of, and strategies to develop, the therapeutic use of self can assist in the therapeutic process by developing a therapeutic relationship.
- Occupational therapists providing services in Australia work with individuals from diverse cultural backgrounds and need to utilise ways to enhance successful communication and understanding between parties.
- Effective communication within teams is a vital component to enhance safety and performance in health care and professional settings.

Review questions

1. What are the five basic elements of the communication cycle?
2. What are two skills or strategies that can assist occupational therapists in achieving effective verbal communication?
3. What are four strategies to build and enhance the therapeutic use of self in occupational therapy service delivery?
4. What are three strategies that occupational therapists should consider to ensure effective communication with individuals from culturally and linguistically diverse backgrounds?
5. When would an occupational therapist consider using the DESC Script, and what does it promote?

References

Acton, G., Mayhew, P., Hopkins, B., & Yauk, S. (1999). Communicating with individuals with dementia the impaired person's perspective. *Journal of Gerontological Nursing, 25*(2), 6–13. https://doi.org/10.3928/0098-9134-19990201-04

Allison, H., & Strong, J. (1994). 'Verbal strategies' used by occupational therapists in direct client encounters. *OTJR: Occupation, Participation and Health, 14*(2), 112–129. https://doi.org/10.1177/153944929401400204

American Occupational Therapy Association. (2014). Occupational Therapy Practice Framework: Domain and process, 3rd edition. *American Journal of Occupational Therapy, 68*(Supp. 1), S1–S48. https://doi.org/10.5014/ajot.2014.682006

Australian Bureau of Statistics. (2017). *Census of population and housing: Reflecting Australia—stories from the Census, 2016.* Cat. no. 2071.0. https://www.abs.gov.au/ausstats/abs@.nsf/mf/2071.0

Baptiste, S. (2017). Communication in occupational therapy practice. In M. Curtin, M. Egan, & J. Adams (Eds.), *Occupational therapy for people experiencing illness, injury or impairment: Promoting occupation and participation* (7th edn, pp. 79–89). Elsevier.

Bendaly, L., & Bendaly, N. (2012). *Improving healthcare team performance: The 7 requirements for excellence in patient care.* Wiley.

Bonk, R. J. (2015). *Writing for today's healthcare audiences.* Broadview Press.

Bower, S. B., & Bower G. H. (2009). *Asserting yourself—updated edition: A practical guide for positive change.* Hachette.

Burnard, P. (2005). *Counselling skills for health professionals* (4th edn). Nelson Thornes.

Clancy, C. M., & Tornberg, D. N. (2007). TeamSTEPPS: Assuring optimal teamwork in clinical settings. *American Journal of Medical Quality, 22*(3), 214–217. https://doi.org/10.1177/1062860607300616

Curtin, M., Egan, M., & Adams, J. (2017). *Occupational therapy for people experiencing illness, injury or impairment: Promoting occupation and participation* (7th edn). Elsevier.

Egan, G. (1975). *The skilled helper: A systematic approach to effective helping.* Brooks/Cole.

Egan, G. (2007). *Skilled helping around the world: Egan's the skilled helper* (8th edn). Thomson Brooks/Cole.

Fajardo, M. A., Weir, K. R., Bonner, C., Gnjidic, D., & Jansen, J. (2019). Availability and readability of patient education materials for deprescribing: An environmental scan. *British Journal of Clinical Pharmacology, 85*(7), 1396–1406. https://doi.org/10.1111/bcp.13912

Gibbs, G. (1988). *Learning by doing: A guide to teaching and learning methods.* Further Education Unit, Oxford Polytechnic.

Hammoud, M. M., Dalrymple, J. L., Christner, J. G., Stewart, R. A., Fisher, J., Margo, K., Ali. I., Briscoe, W., & Pangaro, L. N. (2012). Medical student documentation in electronic health records: A collaborative statement from the Alliance for Clinical Education. *Teaching and Learning in Medicine, 24*(3), 257–266. https://doi.org/10.1080/10401334.2012.692284

Hazelwood, Z., & Shakespeare-Finch, J. (2011). *I'm listening: Communication for health professionals.* Inn Press.

Henderson, A. (2019). *Communication for health care practice.* Oxford University Press.

Henderson, S. (2003). Power imbalance between nurses and patients: A potential inhibitor of partnership in care. *Journal of Clinical Nursing, 12*(4), 501–508. https://doi.org/10.1046/j.1365-2702.2003.00757.x

Iedema, R., Piper, D., & Manidis, M. (2015). *Communicating quality and safety in health care.* Cambridge University Press.

Jangland, E., Gunningberg, L., & Carlsson, M. (2009). Patients' and relatives' complaints about encounters and communication in health care: Evidence for quality improvement. *Patient Education and Counseling, 75*(2), 199–204. https://doi.org/10.1016/j.pec.2008.10.007

Jefferies, D., Johnson, M., & Nicholls, D. (2012). Comparing written and oral approaches to clinical reporting in nursing. *Contemporary Nurse, 42*(1), 129–138. https://doi.org/10.5172/conu.2012.42.1.129

Kearney, K., & Laverdure, P. (2018). Guidelines for documentation of occupational therapy. *American Journal of Occupational Therapy, 72,* 1–7. https//doi.org/10.5014/ajot.2018.72S203

King, H. B., Battles, J., Baker, D. P., Alonso, A., Salas, E., Webster, J., Toomey, L., & Salisbury, M. (2008). TeamSTEPPS™: Team strategies and tools to enhance performance and patient safety. In *Advances in Patient Safety: New directions and alternative approaches (Vol. 3: performance and tools).* Agency for Healthcare Research and Quality (US).

Law, M., Baptiste, S., McColl, M., Opzoomer, A., Polatajko, H., & Pollock, N. (1990). The Canadian Occupational Performance Measure: An outcome measure for occupational therapy. *Canadian Journal of Occupational Therapy, 57*(2), 82–87. https://doi.org/10.1177/000841749005700207

Martin, J. N., & Nakayama, T. K. (2014). *Experiencing intercultural communication: An introduction* (5th edn). McGraw-Hill.

McKenna, J. (2017). Psychosocial support. In M. Curtin, M. Egan, & J. Adams (Eds.), *Occupational therapy for people experiencing illness, injury or impairment* (pp. 416–431). Elsevier.

Morreale, M. J., & Borcherding, S. (2013). *The OTA's guide to documentation: Writing SOAP notes* (3rd edn). SLACK Inc.

O'Brien, J. (2018). *Introduction to occupational therapy* (5th edn). Elsevier.

Occupational Therapy Board of Australia. (2018). *Australian occupational therapy competency standards 2018.* https://www.occupationaltherapyboard.gov.au/codes-guidelines/competencies.aspx

O'Toole, G. (2016). *Communication: Core interpersonal skills for health professionals* (3rd edn). Elsevier.

Pauwels, A. (1995). *Cross-cultural communication in the health sciences: Communicating with migrant patients.* Macmillan Education Australia.

Peterson, A., Kopishke, L., & White, C. (2010). *Legal nurse consulting practices* (3rd edn). CRC Press.

Pian-Smith, M. C. M., Simon, R. D., Minehart, R., Podraza, M., Rudolph, J., Walzer, T., & Raemer, D. (2009). Teaching residents the two-challenge rule: A simulation-based approach to improve education and patient safety. *Simulation in Healthcare: The Journal of the Society for Simulation in Healthcare, 4*(2), 84–91. https//doi.org/10.1097/SIH.0b013e31818cffd3

Purtilo, R., Haddadm A, M., & Doherty, R. F. (2014). *Health professional and patient interaction* (8th edn). Elsevier/Saunders.

Rosenstein, A. H., & O'Daniel, M. (2008). Managing disruptive physician behavior: Impact on staff relationships and patient care. *Neurology, 70*(17), 1564–1570. https//doi.org/10.1212/01. wnl.0000310641.26223.82

Sames, K. (2015). *Documenting occupational therapy practice* (3rd edn). Pearson.

Silverman, J., Kurtz, S. M., & Draper, J. (2013). *Skills for communicating with patients* (3rd edn). Radcliffe Publishing.

Stickley, T. (2011). From SOLER to SURETY for effective non-verbal communication. *Nurse Education in Practice, 11*(6), 395–398. https//doi.org/10.1016/j.nepr.2011.03.021

Tamparo, C. D., & Lindh, W. Q. (2017). *Therapeutic communication for health care professionals* (4th edn). Cengage Learning.

Taylor, R. R. (2008). *The intentional relationship: Occupational therapy and use of self.* F. A. Davis Co.

Taylor, R. R. (2020). *The intentional relationship: Occupational therapy and use of self* (2nd edn). F. A. Davis Co.

Taylor, R. R., & Kielhofner, G. (2017). *Kielhofner's Model of Human Occupation: Theory and application* (5th edn). Lippincott Williams & Wilkins.

Thompson, J. E., Collett, L. W., Langbart, M. J., Purcell, N. J., Boyd, S. M., Yuminaga, Y., Ossolinski, G., Susanto, C., & McCormack, A., (2011). Using the ISBAR handover tool in junior medical officer handover: A study in an Australian tertiary hospital. *Postgraduate Medical Journal, 87*(1027), 340–344. http://dx.doi.org/10.1136/pgmj.2010.105569

Tickle-Dengen, L. (2014). Therapeutic rapport. In M. V. Radomski & C. A. Trombly Latham (Eds.), *Occupational therapy for physical dysfunction* (7th edn, pp. 412–427). Lippincott Williams & Wilkins.

Weger, H., Castle Bell, G., Minei, E. M., & Robinson, M. C. (2014). The relative effectiveness of active listening in initial interactions. *International Journal of Listening, 28*(1), 13–31. https://doi.org/10.1080/10904018.2013.813234

Wright, K. B., Sparks, L., & O'Hair, D. (2013). *Health communication in the 21st century* (2nd edn). Wiley-Blackwell.

10 Working with clients

Client-centred practice

Priscilla Ennals and Ellie Fossey

Chapter objectives

Upon completion of this chapter, the reader will be able to:

- Describe the history and importance of client-centred practice in occupational therapy.
- Define client-centred practice and the key features of this way of working with people.
- Consider the range of factors that occupational therapists need to consider in optimising the client-centred nature of their practice.

Key words

client-centred; collaboration; choice; respect; self-direction; contexts

Overview

Client-centred practice is espoused as central to occupational therapy practice. The 'client' may be an individual, a family, a group, an organisation (e.g., a club, school, workplace), or a whole community. Client perspectives of occupational therapy practices indicate their experiences may be greatly enhanced when a therapist practises in an authentic client-centred manner and negatively impacted when this is not the case. Occupational therapists need to be aware of the influence of power, to listen and communicate effectively, to work in partnership with clients, value their strengths and resilience, and foster choice and hope in these relationships. Contextual factors in the client's situation, the therapist's practice context and broader economic, political and social conditions each impact the use of a client-centred approach.

The history and importance of client-centred practice in occupational therapy

Client-centred occupational therapy practice occurs within a relationship between the client and therapist in which the client is a respected partner, whose unique experiences, values, beliefs and needs are acknowledged and valued, and whose autonomy and choice are respected and fostered (Krupa, 2016; Townsend & Polatajko, 2013). Client-centred practice necessitates developing an understanding of the client within their immediate context, as well as the broader factors influencing their lives and barriers to their participation, for example, economic, political and social inequities (Fleming-Castaldy, 2015). Occupational therapists are not the only health discipline to use this and related terms, with many professionals arguing their approach to care is client/person/family-centred.

The 'client' may be an individual, a family, a group, an organisation (e.g., a club, school, workplace) or a whole community (Townsend & Polatajko, 2013). Family-centred practice extends the idea of the 'client' as being more than the individual, based on the concept that people live, develop and heal in their social contexts, including families of origin and created families, so therapists need to attend to the social networks that surround and support individuals. Family, friends and a wider group of natural supports can be considered, engaged and supported in the therapeutic context. For example, when working with children with disabilities, consideration of parental occupations is important in optimising family quality of life and overall family functioning (Bhopti, 2017). People living with mental illness too identify benefits of family-centred care when they were offered choice and control about who, how, how much and when to include family in their care (Wonders et al., 2019). Communities can also be the focus of intervention, for example, when a community engages an occupational therapist to work in partnership with them to provide an occupational response to a population health issue. Hyett et al. (2019) developed an occupation-focused community-centred practice framework to support community-centred practice, that recommends a four-step process of clarifying who the community client is, what occupations matter to the chosen community, exploring community resources and barriers, and determining strategies for enablement.

The first guidelines for client-centred practice in occupational therapy were published in Canada (Canadian Association of Occupational Therapists, 1991), drawing on the work of humanist psychologist, Carl Rogers (1950). Rodgers's description of working collaboratively with people emphasised that 'clients' are active participants, not passive recipients, of care; a view that fits well with one of occupational therapy's founding principles of *doing with* people, rather than *doing to or for* them (Townsend & Polatajko, 2013). Thus, for over 30 years, led by therapists in Canada, occupational therapists have come to assume that this fit between the theoretical ideas underpinning occupational therapy practice and client-centredness means the practice of occupational therapists is inherently client-centred (World Federation of Occupational Therapists, 2010). Detailed guides to the implementation of a client-centred approach are available (Law, 1998; Sumsion, 2006).

Several well-known practice models describe processes for practising occupational therapy in a client-centred manner, including the Occupational Performance Process Model (OPPM) described in *Enabling Occupation* (Canadian Association of Occupational Therapists, 1997/2002). The more recent Canadian Model of Client-Centred Enablement (Townsend & Polatajko, 2013) identifies enabling skills to support a client-centred approach, such as collaborating, advocating and coaching; and in the Model of Human Occupation (Taylor & Kielhofner, 2017), somewhat similar strategies for enabling change, such as validating, negotiating, coaching and providing support (physical and/ or emotional) are also described. Tools such as the Canadian Occupational Performance Measure (Law et al., 2014) have also been developed to facilitate client-centred practice and outcome measurement. Nevertheless, implementation of client-centred approaches in day-to-day practice continues to be challenging for occupational therapists and colleagues in other health disciplines alike (Sumsion & Law, 2006). Potential barriers have been identified as existing within services, for example, systems, structures, attitudes, prioritisation of safety and risk management, time, and fiscal constraints. Therapists have also described a lack of clear strategies as a barrier.

More recently, the idea that occupational therapy is inherently a client-centred practice has been challenged. This means we need to think critically about our practice, including to pay more critical attention to the power and privilege that therapists hold and to more closely consider our values and assumptions about occupations (Whalley Hammell, 2013a). Furthermore, health consumer movements in recent decades mean health consumers, that is, people who make use of health services and people experiencing disability, have increasingly asserted their rights to participate in health care decision-making, and to engage as partners with health professionals and services (Barnes & Cotterell, 2011). Therefore, rather than assuming our practice is client-centred, occupational therapists need to routinely investigate their clients' perspectives as to whether their practice is experienced as client-centred (Whalley Hammell, 2015). Occupational therapists also need to consider diversity as an essential element of client-centred practice (Kirsh et al., 2006) and to be aware that some cultural groups value collectivism or interdependence ahead of individualism or independence. In an Australian context, Gibson et al. (2015) emphasise the need to draw on a human-rights based approach in partnering with Aboriginal and Torres Strait Islander people. Occupational therapists need to acknowledge both the continuing negative impacts of colonisation, and the strength and resilience of Aboriginal and Torres Strait Islander people; and to practise in ways that emphasise empowerment and self-determination for people and value the interconnectedness within communities. Their paper poses powerful reflective questions relevant to all Australian therapists as they consider what client or community-centred practice means, for example:

> How do you define occupation, participation and meaningful engagement? Is it the same way in which Aboriginal and Torres Strait Islander peoples define it?
>
> How has the Australian history and social contexts shaped your constructs of health and 'everyday practice'?
>
> How does history and everyday practice prevent the acknowledgment, acceptance, or understanding of 'occupations' that are important for Aboriginal and Torres Strait Islander peoples?
>
> (Gibson et al., 2015, p. 216)

Principles of client-centred practice: Illustrative examples

The following examples highlight some of the key principles of client-centred practice and illuminate some the challenges experienced by clients and by therapists in relation to client-centred practice. First, an Australian study investigating client-centred occupational therapy practice from the perspective of people with traumatic brain injury (D'Cruz et al., 2016) illuminates experiences that are client-centred or not:

> Just the whole way she was talking. … She pretty much just put me down in the worst way. … I didn't like her at all and I didn't want to work with her at all because of the way she was to me. (Michael, p. 33)

I'll tell you what I don't like... when someone [therapist] is not sensitive and wants to choose for you. ... It gets you right down to your core ... it feels like ... someone's trespassing with you. (Sam, p. 34)

I think we are trying to achieve the same goal. She's [occupational therapist] got different knowledge to me, so how would you describe it? Collaboration. ... She is not the master of everything. (Kellie, p. 34)

Second, in a Canadian study by Ripat et al. (2014), a student participant reflected on gaining a greater appreciation of the complexity of client-centred practice when the fieldwork supervisor talked through his/her client-centred reasoning process:

I had one educator who was struggling with it [client-centredness] because there was a client with an incomplete spinal cord injury who could sort of walk, and he refused to take a wheelchair when he left the hospital, and so she [said] ... 'I don't know what to do, you know, cause he really needs this, but he won't have it, and so I want to respect what he [wants]' ... really made an impact on me.

(Ripat et al., 2014, p. 7)

These examples show that from a client's perspective, being heard and respected, and having choices is central to client-centred practice, and how therapists can sometimes struggle to enable people to make their own choices.

Definitions and features of client-centred occupational therapy practice

Definitions of client-centred practice in occupational therapy literature have evolved with the development of understanding of what it involves. Two examples are provided in Figure 10.1.

Commonly, definitions of client-centred occupational therapy emphasise respect for clients, supporting clients' involvement in making decisions, recognition of clients' expertise and knowledge, and the need to work in partnership with clients to address their occupational needs (Sumsion & Law, 2006). These ideas highlight that there are a number of features of a client-centred approach, as described in Table 10.1.

Client-centred practice is an approach to providing occupational therapy, which embraces a philosophy of respect for, and partnership with, people receiving services. Client-centred practice recognizes the autonomy of individuals, the need for client choice in making decisions about occupational needs, the strengths clients bring to a therapy encounter, the benefits of client-therapist partnership and the need to ensure that services are accessible and fit the context in which a client lives. (Law et al., 1995, p. 253)

Clients describe client-centred practice as being collaborative practice undertaken by therapists who clearly value and respect their clients, who seek and respect clients' experience and knowledge, who choose closeness over distance and detachment, who create supportive and accepting relationships with clients, and who are kind (Whalley Hammell, 2013b, p. 175)

Figure 10.1 Client-centred practice.

Table 10.1 Features of a client-centred approach

Power	Implementing authentic client-centred practice necessitates an understanding of the influence of power. This includes awareness of one's own power and position as a therapist; the ways in which health professionals and social conditions can disempower people or limit their ability to express their views, make choices and direct their lives. Client-centred practice involves working actively to reduce power inequalities and to support clients to exercise power themselves.
Listening and communicating	Effective listening and communicating is essential to addressing issues of power. For example, using language that the client can understand communicates respect and intent to work in partnership, and provides information that the client needs in an accessible way. Listening is essential to understand clients' lives and situations; clients feel they are valued and respected when they feel listened to. Communicating information effectively to facilitate understanding is essential to enabling clients to make choices and decisions that affect them.
Partnership	Partnership involves working together in a respectful and supportive manner. Characteristics of effective partnership working include: developing an understanding of the other's experience, flexibility, willingness to share knowledge and to negotiate courses of action.
Choice	Choice is a key element of working in partnership. Respect of clients' values, preferences and rights are central to enabling and supporting clients' choice and decision-making. Opportunities for choice can be ensured throughout occupational therapy processes with clients, for example, choices within sessions, choices about interventions, equipment and supports provided, and choices about the focus and goals of occupational therapy services.
Hope	Appreciating the importance of hope, encouragement and fostering a sense of accomplishment is critical in client-centred interactions. People's hopes vary, so that seeking to understand a client's hopes is important; when it is difficult for clients to see progress or that something good will happen, holding hope for clients is also important.
Respect	Respect for clients. Respect for clients' strengths and diversity of experiences and knowledge. Respect for clients' rights to make choices and decisions about their own lives and situations.
Strengths focus	Seeking to understand and deploy the talents, abilities, resources and strengths of a client, family, group or community.

Factors that impact client-centred practice

Contextual factors can play an important role in facilitating or hindering authentic client-centred practice. Thus, both the client's own context and the therapist's practice context can influence how client-centred practice is understood, what it means and how it is implemented. The physical, social, institutional (economic, legal, political) and cultural environment each influence clients' resources and possibilities for participation and so need to be considered in client-centred practice. Similarly, age, gender, language preference, socio-economic status, values, religious and cultural beliefs, and experiences of trauma, disadvantage or discrimination require consideration. Practice contexts in which occupational therapists work, for example, prisons, acute hospitals, community services, schools and private practice also play a role in determining how occupational therapists provide services and the expectations held by clients, families, management and funders within those settings.

The examples below are drawn from published research in Australia. They provide a starting point to think about the kind of issues that arise in different practice settings and contexts.

An Australian grounded theory study explored the experiences of six participants as they recovered and adjusted to life following a stroke (Walder & Molineux, 2019). The findings revealed professional expertise, provision of hope and sharing of information were valued, but participants also identified the need to genuinely partner with therapists in order to feel understood. Avoiding confusion and turmoil required the right information being communicated by therapists at the right time and with an awareness of each person's capacity to process information. The participants emphasised that client-centred practice following stroke requires therapists to understand each client's unique journey and their subjective experience of recovery, and to be willing to adapt therapy in line with fluctuations in fatigue and low motivation.

Emma Gee (2016) contributes to the discussion of client-centredness in her memoir *Reinventing Emma*, a first-person account of a young woman and occupational therapist adapting to life after stroke. With insider knowledge as an occupational therapist, Emma shared her moving journey of personal recovery and identity reclamation as she learned to walk, talk and 'be' again. Emma's recounting of tiny moments in her care and therapy provide insights into the small ways that occupational therapists, and health professionals more generally, can show respect, hope and genuine intentions to partner with people. She also highlights the devastating impact of behaviours—shame, confusion, anger, fear—where the needs of the system or therapist may be prefaced ahead of the needs of the client:

> I suddenly found myself very closed to those who robotically assessed me, assuming that I, the patient, would have nothing to contribute to the process. I needed to feel valued before I could reciprocate and build any rapport with them.
>
> (Gee, 2016, p. 119)

Karen Arblaster and colleagues (Arblaster et al., 2019) have been partnering with people with lived experience of mental ill-health to bring their perspectives on what recovery-oriented mental health practice should look like into the design of occupational therapy pre-registration curriculum. Their work highlights several key concepts relevant to client-centred practice—building on strengths, connecting with hope, using person-centred language rather than language that is professionally framed, and a lifelong effort to understand and partner with people in an authentic and collaborative manner. One of the participants in her study reinforced the need to listen deeply for less visible explanations behind behaviour, and to consider how past and current power differences might be influencing behaviour:

> Once [clinicians] have a deeper understanding of trauma and ... these horrendous life experiences that people may have been through, and ... understand ... that behaviour is a communication and coping strategy, then often the way they approach people and their willingness to enable dignity changes.
>
> (Arblaster et al., 2019, p. 679)

Summary

- Client–centred practice is espoused as central to occupational therapy practice.
- Evidence-based practice supports using a client-centred approach in occupational therapy.
- The 'client' may be an individual, a family, a group, an organisation (e.g., a club, school, workplace) or a whole community.
- Client perspectives of occupational therapy practices indicate their experiences may be greatly enhanced when a therapist practises in an authentic client-centred manner and negatively impacted when this is not the case.
- Awareness of the influence of power, effective listening and communicating, working through building partnerships with clients, and fostering choice and hope are key elements of an authentic client-centred practice.
- Contextual factors in the client's situation, the therapist's practice context and broader economic, political and social conditions each impact the use of a client-centred approach.
- Being curious about the diverse cultural context of each client is an essential underpinning of client-centred practice.

Review questions

1. What are the origins of client-centred practice in occupational therapy?
2. Why is client-centred practice important in occupational therapy?
3. What is client-centred practice and what are some of its key features?
4. What factors may influence the implementation of a client-centred approach in practice?
5. What values, knowledge and skills help to optimise the client-centred nature of an occupational therapist's practice?

References

Arblaster, K., Mackenzie, L., Gill, K., Willis, K., & Matthews, L. (2019). Capabilities for recovery-oriented practice in mental health occupational therapy: A thematic analysis of lived experience perspectives. *British Journal of Occupational Therapy, 82*(11), 675–684. https://journals.sagepub.com/doi/10.1177/0308022619866129

Barnes, M., & Cotterell, P. (2011). *Critical perspectives on user involvement*: Policy Press.

Bhopti, A. (2017). Promoting the occupations of parents of children with disability in early childhood intervention services: Building stronger families and communities. *Australian Occupational Therapy Journal, 64*(5), 419–422. https://doi.org/10.1111/1440-1630.12297

Canadian Association of Occupational Therapists. (1991). *Occupational therapy guidelines for client-centred practice*. CAOT Publications ACE.

Canadian Association of Occupational Therapists. (1997/2002). *Enabling occupation: An occupational therapy perspective*. CAOT Publications ACE.

D'Cruz, K., Howie, L., & Lentin, P. (2016). Client-centred practice: Perspectives of persons with a traumatic brain injury. *Scandinavian Journal of Occupational Therapy, 23*(1), 30–38. https://doi.org/10.3109/11038128.2015.1057521

Fleming-Castaldy, R. P. (2015). A macro perspective for client-centred practice in curricula: Critique and teaching methods. *Scandinavian Journal of Occupational Therapy, 22*(4), 267–276. https://doi.org/10.3109/11038128.2015.1013984

Gee, E. (2016). *Reinventing Emma. The inspirational story of a young stroke survivor*. Openbook Creative.

Gibson, C., Butler, C., Henaway, C., Dudgeon, P., & Curtin, M. (2015). Indigenous peoples and human rights: Some considerations for the occupational therapy profession in Australia. *Australian Occupational Therapy Journal, 62*(3), 214–218. https://onlinelibrary.wiley.com/doi/abs/10.1111/1440-1630.12185

Hyett, N., Kenny, A., & Dickson-Swift, V. (2019). Re-imagining occupational therapy clients as communities: Presenting the community-centred practice framework. *Scandinavian Journal of Occupational Therapy, 26*(4), 246–260. https://doi.org/10.1080/11038128.2017.1423374

Kirsh, B., Trentham, B., & Cole, S. (2006). Diversity in occupational therapy: Experiences of consumers who identify as minority group members. *Australian Occupational Therapy Journal, 53*(4), 302–313. https://doi.org/10.1111/j.1440-1630.2006.00576.x

Krupa, T. (2016). Canadian triple model framework for enabling occupation. In T. Krupa, B. Kirsh, D. Pitts, & E. Fossey (Eds.), *Bruce and Borgs' psychosocial frames of reference: Theories, models and approaches for occupation-based practice* (4th edn, pp. 123–133). SLACK Inc.

Law, M. (1998). *Client-centred occupational therapy.* SLACK Inc.

Law, M., Baptiste, S., Carswell, A., McColl, M. A., Polatajko, H., & Pollock, N. (2014). *The Canadian Occupational Performance Measure (COPM)* (5th edn). CAOT Publications ACE.

Law, M., Baptiste, S., & Mills, J. (1995). Client-centred practice: What does it mean and does it make a difference? *Canadian Journal of Occupational Therapy, 62*(5), 250–257. https://doi.org/10.1177/000841749506200504

Ripat, J., Wener, P., Dobinson, K., & Yamamoto, C. (2014). Internalizing client-centredness in occupational therapy students. *Journal of Research in Interprofessional Practice and Education, 4*(2). http://dx.doi.org/10.22230/jripe.2014v4n2a173

Rogers, C. R. (1950). A current formulation of client-centred therapy. *Social Services Research, 24*(4), 442–450. https://doi.org/10.1086/638020

Sumsion, T. (2006). *Client-centred practice in occupational therapy: A guide to implementation.* Churchill Livingstone Elsevier.

Sumsion, T., & Law, M. (2006). A review of evidence on conceptual elements informing client-centred practice. *Canadian Journal of Occupational Therapy, 73*(3), 153–162. https://doi.org/10.1177/000841740607300303

Taylor, R. R., & Kielhofner, G. (2017). *Kielhofner's model of human occupation: Theory and application* (5th edn). Lippincott Williams & Wilkins.

Townsend, E., & Polatajko, H. (2013). *Enabling occupation II: Advancing occupational therapy vision for health, well-being and justice through occupation* (2nd edn). CAOT Publications ACE.

Walder, K., & Molineux, M. (2019). Listening to the client voice—a constructivist grounded theory study of the experiences of client-centred practice after stroke. *Australian Occupational Therapy Journal, 67*(2), 100–109. https://doi.org/10.1111/1440-1630.12627

Whalley Hammell, K. R. (2013a). Client-centred occupational therapy in Canada: Refocusing on core values. *Canadian Journal of Occupational Therapy, 80*(3), 141–149. https://doi.org/10.1177/0008417413497906

Whalley Hammell, K. R. (2013b). Client-centred practice in occupational therapy: Critical reflections. *Scandinavian Journal of Occupational Therapy, 20*(3), 174–181. https://doi.org/10.3109/11038128.2012.752032

Whalley Hammell, K. R. (2015). Client-centred occupational therapy: The importance of critical perspectives. *Scandinavian Journal of Occupational Therapy, 22*(4), 237–243. https://doi.org/10.3109/11038128.2015.1004103

Wonders, L., Honey, A., & Hancock, N. (2019). Family inclusion in mental health service planning and delivery: Consumers' perspectives. *Community Mental Health Journal, 55*(2), 318–330. https://doi.org/10.1007/s10597-018-0292-2

World Federation of Occupational Therapists. (2010). *Position statement on client-centredness in occupational therapy.* https://www.wfot.org/resources/client-centredness-in-occupational-therapy

11 Decolonising occupational therapy through a strengths-based approach

Jade Ryall, Tirritpa Ritchie, Corrine Butler, Ashleigh Ryan and Chontel Gibson

Chapter objectives

Upon completion of this chapter, the reader will be able to:

- Apply the six key dimensions of Gibson et al.'s (2020a) strengths-based approach.
- Discuss ways to listen respectfully to a person, such as 'hearing' how the person experiences health, well-being and occupations.
- Describe appropriate communication skills that allow the person to engage in the therapeutic journey.
- Propose how an occupational therapist might build authentic partnerships, such as responding to power imbalances.
- Reflect critically on Australian contexts, such as political, professional, social and historical contexts.
- Apply a human rights-based approach.
- Evaluate occupational therapy processes and outcomes using a strengths-based approach.

Key terms

Aboriginal and Torres Strait Islander people; self-determination; human rights; communication; decolonisation; strengths-based approach

Introduction

This chapter introduces a strengths-based approach that was originally developed by Aboriginal people, and then adapted by five members of the National Aboriginal and Torres Strait Islander Occupational Therapy Network (NATSIOTN) for use within occupational therapy courses. Strengths-based approaches are foundational to occupational therapy, and they are often viewed as being synonymous with client-centred approaches. Strengths-based approaches are of particular importance when working with Aboriginal and Torres Strait Islander people, because among many things, they counterbalance negative stereotypes that are portrayed about Aboriginal and Torres Strait Islander people (Fogarty et al., 2018).

Strengths-based approaches can bring Indigenous knowledges into the fore, providing some counterbalance to historical exclusion of the leadership, science and experiences of Indigenous people within the profession. Both the stereotypes and exclusion of Indigenous peoples are often linked to the colonisation process, and as such, we promote a decolonising lens. A decolonising lens encourages occupational therapists to critically reflect on broader contexts, including colonisation. These critical reflections can facilitate occupational therapists to better understand themselves, their profession, the society that they live in, and then most importantly guide any action that is required to break down power imbalances with people who access services (Gibson, 2020). Fogarty et al. (2018) outline the multiple types of strengths-based approaches that have been used in the context of Aboriginal and Torres Strait Islander health.

In this chapter, we (the Aboriginal occupational therapy authors) provide one strengths-based approach, which was initially developed with Elders and older Aboriginal people living in NSW and encapsulates many of the other strengths-based approaches outlined in Fogarty et al. (2018) and Gibson et al. (2020a). In this chapter, we build on Gibson et al.'s (2020a) work and we do so by focusing on occupational therapy practice and bringing more First Nation's knowledges into sight. Although the strengths-based approach in this chapter focuses on occupational therapists working with Aboriginal and Torres Strait Islander people, it may be used with all communities, including non-Indigenous communities.

Strengths-based approach

Many health professions, including occupational therapy, use strengths-based approaches; however, very few professionals can articulate how their strengths-based philosophies underpin practice (Gibson et al., 2020b). Furthermore, strengths-based approaches are problematic when they focus solely on the person's strengths, resources and responsibilities, without understanding how contexts, like politics, professional frameworks and more influence the person and their access to health care (Fogarty et al., 2018).

It is important to understand how health professionals' values, beliefs and world views influence accessible health care. Gibson et al.'s (2020a) strengths-based approach illustrated six key dimensions to support social, health and well-being services for Aboriginal and Torres Strait Islander people. We will now use Gibson et al.'s (2020a) six key dimensions and demonstrate how each dimension could be applied in occupational therapy.

Dimension 1: Listening respectfully to the person

Listening respectfully to what a person says demonstrates the occupational therapist's commitment to understanding and connecting with the person. This commitment includes understanding the person's experiences, the relationship between past and present, and their hopes for the future. It is important to listen with interest and compassion and consider where the person's story begins. A person's story begins at a different time to the referral. The referral information is crucial because it can often set the tone for the therapeutic relationship, influencing what is heard, and perhaps, more importantly, what is not heard. Barker and Buchanan-Barker (2005a), explain that 'some people often find it difficult to assert their own story, finding themselves instead, framed by the stories written by others in their professional records'. When listening to or reading the referral information, ask yourself questions like: When or how has this information been gathered? Whose words are privileged? Whose perspective is being shared and valued in the referral information?

When an occupational therapist commences a therapeutic relationship, it is vital to develop a connection with the person. A key aspect of connecting is listening to what the person is willing to share about themselves, their lived expertise, and their knowledge. Time will allow the therapist to listen deeply. Many Aboriginal scholars highlight the importance of deep listening. Miriam-Rose Ungunmerr-Baumann (2002) explained deep listening as a spiritual journey, whereby listening to our inner self is essential. Uncle Lewis Yerloburka O'Brien explained deep listening as being able to use multiple ways of viewing life to look at a complex situation (LIME Network, 2017).

Dennis McDermott explained that listening requires some action from the therapist or person (LIME Network, 2017). In occupational therapy, deep listening should include reflecting on how the occupational therapy lens may not necessarily privilege the person and their lived experiences, but instead, it may privilege Western ideologies (Gibson et al., 2020a). For example, there are distinct differences between Indigenous and Western conceptualisations of health, disability and occupations, yet the lens of occupational therapy can be biased, often favouring Western ways of knowing, being and doing (Gibson et al., 2020a; Gibson et al., 2020b). Deep listening skills, along with the other skills highlighted in the dimension, provide some of the foundational skills for working with all communities.

Dimension 2: Using appropriate communication skills

Communicate in a way that conveys value in and respect for the person. Appropriate communication skills include occupational therapists using 'generic interview skills', like actively listening, asking open-ended questions, and promoting strengths-based language. Examples of active listening skills include paying attention to the person, using facial expressions and gestures such as smiling or nodding, reserving judgement, summarising what you hear, and seeking clarification about what you are hearing. Open-ended questions encourage the person to explore and express themselves in an open and non-leading manner. Some open-ended questions include: What are the things that are important to you? How do you usually do X? and How do you like to spend your time?

Applying these skills can create the space required for people to lead the conversation and share the parts of their story that are most defining to them and their social and emotional well-being. This can help the occupational therapist to begin to learn the unique cultural, social, historical and political contexts the person may be speaking and acting from and within. Strengths-based assessments are conversational and purposeful (Francis, 2014). They are also specific, detailed, and individualised to the person (Francis, 2014). Some Aboriginal and Torres Strait Islander communities have communication protocols, like not looking people directly in the eye or not asking direct questions. It is impossible to always know all of the communication protocols that you will need as an occupational therapist. However, you can learn local community protocols by taking the time to build rapport and then, learn from the community, including community who work within your service or other services.

Offer your knowledge and expertise in a way that supports the person to make informed decisions about their health and health care. Support informed decision-making by exploring with the person their current strengths, abilities, options, opportunities and the possible benefits and limitations of any options. Learn about what solutions or directions that the person wishes to take, respecting their right to decide what they need, and recognising that any decision needs to belong to and make sense to the person (Barker et al., 2005b). This person-led approach to practise is meaningful when working with Aboriginal and Torres Strait Islander people. Cultural knowledge, practices and protocols play a central role in decision-making around social and emotional well-being needs for Aboriginal and Torres Strait Islander peoples. A person may make choices that the occupational therapist does not understand. In these instances, seek to learn what is motivating the person's decision, remain supportive, and continue to keep the person informed of all options and opportunities available.

Dimension 3: Building authentic partnerships

Authentic partnerships refer to developing relationships between two or more people which are trusting, meaningful and equal (Corrigan & Burton, 2014). Key partners may include occupational therapists, other service providers and, most importantly, relevant Aboriginal and Torres Strait Islander people. Family members, Elders, community members and community organisations, such as Local Land Councils and Aboriginal Health Services, are often crucial partners. Authentic partnerships provide opportunities for building and extending relationships, valuing and privileging diverse world views, developing reflexive and responsive services, facilitating cultural competency and, importantly, supporting a human rights approach (Taylor & Thompson, 2011). Partnerships may expand the occupational therapists' understandings of Aboriginal and Torres Strait Islander people's expressions and experiences of health, well-being and occupations (Gibson et al., 2015). Corrigan and Burton's (2014) three-pronged partnership approach is one example of how occupational therapists might want to consider when building and strengthening partnerships with Aboriginal and Torres Strait Islander people. The three-pronged approach includes preparation, action and maintenance.

Preparation

Preparation is key for all successful and authentic partnerships. Preparation requires occupational therapists to critically reflect and develop an understanding of the Australian context. Perhaps, more importantly, and further explored below, is that occupational therapists reflect on their positionality, status and contextual factors. This involves reflecting on current ways of knowing, being and doing, and continually evaluating if these approaches are appropriate when working with Aboriginal and Torres Strait Islander people. Occupational therapists must be committed to respecting, understanding and incorporating diverse voices that will stem from these partnerships. This commitment may include learning about the community, community perspectives and beliefs, and local histories, like prior relationships between Aboriginal and Torres Strait Islander people and service providers.

There is a long history of services not doing the right thing by communities, and it is important to understand and work towards healing any wrongs of the past, even if you were not directly involved in past experiences. For example, government officials, including their service providers, acted in ways that compromised the safety of Aboriginal and Torres Strait Islander people. This long history still lingers today. Building authentic partnerships allows service providers and Aboriginal and Torres Strait Islander people space where they can get to know each other and build common ground. Preparation is critical before action, and it is critical to continue to prepare during the action phase of partnership development.

Action

Taking affirmative action to commence and continue the partnership is essential. Take the time to get to know the community or even multiple communities that are within the confines of your service boundary. Discuss the multiple ways that business can be done and be ready to create new ways of working. Develop shared partnership goals, shared communication processes and shared accountability for all partnership outcomes. It is just as important to share partnership successes as it is any partnership challenges (Gibson et al., 2015). Work through any conflict and differences. Sometimes, occupational therapists may work in a service that will not change the way it conducts business to accommodate a human rights-based approach. If this is the case, then the occupational therapist will need to decide on the action they will take (or not take). Actions may include advocating for change, leaving the workplace to find another workplace that is aligned with your values, or accepting a less than desirable status quo in partnership arrangements. Many Aboriginal and Torres Strait Islander people are skilled at seeing and/or working out how organisations influence relationships between the community members and service providers. Consequently, Aboriginal and Torres Strait Islander people may be sceptical about forming a relationship with an individual therapist and/or their organisation.

Maintenance

The maintenance phase is essential, and the duration of the partnership, and therefore maintenance phase, may vary. Being consistent and reliable is important. Continue to be present and follow up on any promises made. Demonstrate integrity by doing what you say, even when no one else is present. If things change and you cannot do what you promised, then go back to your partner to discuss and find another way forward. Recognise and address any signs that may indicate a breakdown in the partnership (Corrigan & Burton, 2014). Signs may include but are not limited to decreased attendance at meetings or therapy sessions, and reduced sharing of resources and personal information. Common pitfalls for health service providers who form partnerships with Aboriginal and Torres Strait Islander people include the health service provider assuming the role of the leader or decision-maker; being unable to navigate or reflect on one's personal beliefs; discrediting and devaluing community members; not including community perspectives; not fulfilling promises; and, finally, projecting a 'mission day' approach. (Note that the mission days refer to a period where churches and/or religious affiliates provided housing and education to Aboriginal and Torres Strait Islander people.) Although some Aboriginal people may have used the missions as an avenue to escape the harsh realities of a colonising country, many Aboriginal people were often forcibly removed from their families and placed in missions. In these missions, Aboriginal people were forced to practise Christian ideals and had limited opportunities to practise their own culture.

Dimension 4: Critically reflecting on Australia's political, social and historical contexts

Critical reflection refers to the ability to design, analyse, evaluate and re-adjust practice, with the aim of improving professional outcomes (Lyons, 2010). Lyons (2010) argues that while critical reflections help individuals to make meaning of experiences, they are just that, experiences. As individuals, we experience the world in unique ways, and therefore, we need to consider theory and culturally diverse experiences that extend beyond individual experiences. In Australia, health professionals face many barriers when exploring diverse theories and experiences. Barriers stem from the political, social and historical contexts, like being raised and socialised in a colonised country. This firmly entrenched colonial context can prevent health professionals from easily engaging and using Aboriginal and Torres Strait Islander health philosophies.

It is challenging to break down the barriers that allow critical reflections. Accepting critical reflection as a life-long journey that requires hard work is helpful. Hard work involves many things, but of importance is moving through discomfort, and then taking necessary action. Like a rigorous exercise program, critical reflection needs to occur regularly, with a team of people who have diverse experiences and in a forever evolving process to avoid stagnation. For this dimension, we will present three examples where we illustrate how we use theory or diverse experiences to critically reflect.

Example 1: Critically reflecting while listening in a therapeutic conversation

During a therapeutic conversation, try to become aware of when your values and beliefs are influencing what you hear. You might notice the urge to give advice or give the person a summary of what you would do in their situation. You might notice that you start saying things such as, 'I don't think you should feel like that …', 'If it were me, I would …', or 'I think the most important thing right now is …'. You might be thinking, 'I do not know why the person is so worried about X' or 'I do not understand why they want to do it that way'. Notice these thoughts or questions, recognise how your values and beliefs are influencing what you are hearing, and return to listening to the person's story.

Example 2: Advance Australia Fair—fair for all or just a select few?

To reflect critically on Australia's political, social and historical contexts, we require an understanding of colonisation on a global scale. Australia's colonisation commenced during a period often misrepresented by its name, called the 'Age of Discovery or Exploration'. During that period, Western European people sent ships to 'explore' new routes for financial wealth and provide respite from a burgeoning capitalist system. In practice, this resulted in Western European people conquering, subjugating or ransacking the land and any other items of subjective worth (Kendi, 2016). As a nation, we have never unpacked what this means for all Australians. For example, who has ownership over lands? Whose farming practices are used? How were the traditional owners of country treated when the forced takeover of land occurred? How many First Nations people had access to education and/or their pay cheques? How does the colonising process continue to inform the relationships between non-Indigenous people with Aboriginal and Torres Strait Islander people? These questions and others may lead you to a place of investigation that uncovers the historical inaccuracies and propaganda taught in the Australian education system.

Example 3: Colonisation and occupations in Australia

Maori Occupational Therapist Isla Emery-Whittington, with Ben Te Maro (2018) highlighted the pervading historical legacy of colonialism in occupational therapy. For example, Emery-Whittington illustrated that the British philosopher John Locke, credited as being the father of both capitalism and occupational sciences, practised in ways that were considered racist (Emery-Whittington & Te Maro, 2018). One racist ideology held by Locke was his belief that Indigenous people could not possess intellectual capacity because they did not show any desire to fully utilise the land (Emery-Whittington & Te Maro, 2018). Scholars like Bruce Pascoe (2014) prove this and similar claims made by European people to be false by illustrating the sophisticated and eco-friendly land management practices that allowed Aboriginal people to thrive. Although these land practices were recorded in the European explorers' journals, the same authors of these journals concluded that Aboriginal people were unable to look after their own lands. Falsehoods about Aboriginal people such as this continue to influence contemporary life, politics and services, including occupational therapy. In the future, we anticipate that the profession will delve more deeply into some of the oppressive ideologies from bygone eras, which are still pervasive, and then critically examine how these bygone eras continue to influence contemporary occupational therapy practice.

Occupational therapists have frameworks that may facilitate the examination of the relationship between colonisation and occupations, as well as privilege Indigenous peoples' voices. However, perspectives dominating discourses about occupations continue to be based on Western and Judaeo-Christian ideologies and this restricts the applicability across cultures (Hocking, 2009). In more recent years, occupational therapy scholars are contributing to the literature by exploring and expanding beyond Western and Judaeo-Christian ideologies. Iwama (2006) illustrated how occupations are culturally grounded. Ramugondo and Kronenberg (2015) moved away from the individualistic approach of occupations by focusing on collective occupations, which include families, communities and societies. In collective occupations, the relationships between individuals are on a continuum, ranging between liberating and oppressive, and these relationships determine participation in occupations (Ramugondo & Kronenberg, 2015). Emery-Whittington's decolonising occupations offers a framework to critique colonisation and the impact on occupations, not just in New Zealand, but globally too. Gibson's (2020) conceptualisation of cultural occupations shines a light on occupations that strengthen cultural well-being and cultural integrity, especially in Aboriginal and Torres Strait Islander communities. In essence, the concept of occupations continues to evolve and be informed by pluralistic cultural paradigms. However, despite some efforts within occupational therapy and occupational science, there is much more work to be undertaken to support the critique of colonisation, cultural diversity and privileging of Indigenous peoples' perspectives.

Dimension 5: Applying a human rights–based approach

The Declaration on the Rights of Indigenous Peoples (from here on called 'The Declaration') affirms the minimum standards for the survival, dignity, security and well-being of Indigenous peoples worldwide. The Declaration covers all areas of human rights as they relate to Indigenous peoples. The Australian Human Rights Commission developed a Community Guide to the UN Declaration on the Rights of Indigenous People that helps Aboriginal and Torres Strait Islander people navigate partnership arrangements and advocate for their needs (Australian Human Rights Commission, 2010). The fundamental and foundational human rights of Indigenous peoples are categorised into four principles: self-determination, participation in decision-making, respect for and protection of culture and finally, equality and non-discrimination (Australian Human Rights Commission, 2010). We will use these four principles in this strengths-based approach to illustrate how the dimension of human rights can be applied in occupational therapy.

Self-determination

Self-determination refers to Aboriginal and Torres Strait Islander people having the freedom to live well, to determine what it means to live well, and to live according to one's values and beliefs (Australian Human Rights Commission, 2010, p. 24). This means that Aboriginal and Torres Strait Islander people should participate in any decisions that affect them. In occupational therapy practice, you may want to consider how you and your service ensure that Aboriginal and Torres Strait Islander people are part of all relevant decision-making processes (Gibson et al., 2015). For example, in practice, ensure people are free to make decisions without being coerced, are provided with all relevant information promptly, and the information is provided in a respectful way that makes sense. At a service level, ensure that you engage with all relevant communities and ensure that a collective voice does not override individual choices in practice. Furthermore, consider how broader processes, like automatic referrals to other services, may deny the person of an informed and prior consent or that a strict time limit for initial assessments may not allow appropriate time to connect with the person. There are multiple ways to ensure self-determination occurs, and it is best to work with local communities and individuals to discuss how this should occur locally.

Participation in decision-making

Aboriginal and Torres Strait Islander people have a right to participate and lead any decisions that affect them (Australian Human Rights Commission, 2010, p. 40). As stated above, occupational therapists hold a duty to consult and partner with Aboriginal and Torres Strait Islander people whenever a decision will affect an individual or community. For example, when developing group programs, consult with local Elders and relevant community groups to ensure a need exists, and that co-design of the program can occur. Each community will have its ideas about decision-making structures and practices, and you can assist in uncovering or co-developing these via long-standing partnerships. Importantly, diverse governance structures and practices exist within what you might view as on community, and as such, develop flexible and multiple partnership arrangements, so all needs are met.

Respect for and protection of culture

The Declaration asserts Aboriginal and Torres Strait Islander people's rights to language, culture and spiritual identity (Australian Human Rights Commission, 2010, p. 30). This should include rights to country, resources and knowledge. To respect culture, occupational therapists should work with the person and community to understand which cultural connections are important. Cultural connections refer to any connection that strengthens culture, and this may mean a cultural connection to the land, to family, to community and culture (Gee et al., 2014). For example, someone in long-term rehabilitation may need a one-day or two-day pass to go back to country or rehabilitation may include being on country and participating in relevant occupations that strengthen cultural connections. Cultural connections will vary, and sometimes, due to colonisation and other factors, some cultural connections may not be practised.

Equality and non-discrimination

Equality refers to people having the right to be free and being considered equal to all other groups of people (Australian Human Rights Commission, 2010, p. 20). Non-discrimination refers to no one being denied their rights because of factors such as race, colour, sex, language, religion, political or other opinions, national or social origin, property or birth (UN Human Rights Committee, 1989). However, in Australia, inequality and discrimination exist. For example, social determinants are not distributed equally between population groups and this influences who can or perhaps more importantly, who cannot participate in some occupations. Racism and discrimination are critical social determinants that negatively affect Aboriginal and Torres Strait Islander people. To promote equality and non-discrimination, occupational therapists need to understand that racism and discrimination are systemic, which means they exist within our profession and the organisations that employ occupational therapists. It is important for occupational therapists to take an anti-racist stance by being accountable for recognising and responding to all forms of racism. For example, occupational therapists could advocate for more equitable and just environments, deliver accessible and equitable services, and understand how racism, like racial microaggressions, might prevent people from participating in occupations that are supportive of their health and well-being (Emery-Whittington & Te Maro, 2018; Gibson et al., 2020a; Grullon et al., 2018).

Dimension 6: Evaluating occupational therapy processes and outcomes

Effective evaluation with Aboriginal and Torres Strait Islander people is based on three fundamental premises: a continuum of evaluation, facilitating consumer empowerment and decolonising evaluation procedures.

Continuum of evaluation

The evaluation process involves not just evaluating the intervention provided, but also how it sits within the broader program, the context of the profession and the context of colonisation. Evaluation works best when there are shared objectives, performance indicators or benchmarks (Hunt, 2013a). Working with the person and community to guide the evaluation purpose and outcomes is essential. Furthermore, it is crucial to understand any baseline data that is available or that can be collected; the method of evaluation; the relationships between all key stakeholders in the evaluation; and, finally, the time required to conduct a rigorous evaluation. Failing to involve Aboriginal and Torres Strait Islander people in an appropriate evaluation may lead to the evaluation process not being viable or accepted by the Aboriginal and Torres Strait Islander community (Muir & Dean, 2017).

Facilitating consumer empowerment

A human rights approach to evaluation is necessary, and it means involving Aboriginal and Torres Strait Islander people in all aspects of occupational therapy processes. Occupational therapists should work with Aboriginal and Torres Strait Islander people and community to identify an evaluation process that is based on free, prior and informed consent. Occupational therapists can achieve this by having agreed outcomes with Aboriginal and Torres Strait Islander people about what they want to achieve, partner roles and responsibilities, and visible indicators of an evaluation process that meets identified outcomes (Hunt, 2013b). Occupational therapists can share the 'power' and decision-making processes, as well as foster mutual trust (Hunt, 2013b). Community consultation and participation is an essential component in the design, data collection and reporting phase of evaluation (Muir & Dean, 2017). Facilitating consumer empowerment will support interventions and programs that are more likely to be focused on the outcomes and goals of Aboriginal and Torres Strait Islander people.

Decolonising evaluation processes

To determine the effectiveness of the occupational therapy process, it is important to ask, 'What difference does our program make for the people we deliver services with?' Evaluation with Aboriginal and Torres Strait Islander people is about self-determination, empowering Aboriginal and Torres Strait Islander families to identify for themselves and exercise opportunities to live well, according to Aboriginal and Torres Strait Islander values and beliefs. To do this, occupational therapists need to reshape accountabilities and organisational structures that support better evaluation. Innovative strategies need to be used to enable people to participate meaningfully (Nimegeer et al., 2011, in Hunt, 2013a). Evaluation processes fail all key parties when they: i) do not address power inequalities; ii) expect Indigenous people to function in Western bureaucratic processes; and iii) favour Western knowledge over Indigenous knowledges (Hunt, 2013a). Review and evaluation should assess partnership processes and partnership outcomes, which supports the partnership to adapt and operate effectively (Bailey & Hunt, 2012). Aboriginal and Torres Strait Islander people's involvement in evaluation acknowledges that Aboriginal and Torres Strait Islander people are the best people to decide how to address issues faced by Aboriginal and Torres Strait Islander communities (Australian Human Rights Commission, 2010, p. 41), and Williams' (2018) Ngaa-bi-nya Aboriginal and Torres Strait Islander program evaluation framework provides an exemplar that individuals and organisations can use.

Conclusion

In this chapter, we provided a deep and complex strengths-based approach, which can be applied in occupational therapy. Although the focus of the strengths-based approach in this chapter was used in the context of Aboriginal and Torres Strait Islander people, it can be used more broadly.

Summary

In summary, this strengths-based approach revealed that:

- Connecting with Aboriginal and Torres Strait Islander people can be achieved by listening respectfully, using appropriate communication skills and building authentic partnerships.
- During critical reflections, it essential to understand how values, beliefs and worldviews influence occupational therapy. Seeking to understand colonisation and other information that is not readily available within the discipline will potentially diversify the occupational therapy lens.
- Taking affirmative action means undertaking a multitude of activities that reduce the power imbalances resulting from colonisation and ongoing oppressive policies.
- Applying a human rights-based approach and culturally responsive evaluation process forms the basis of affirmative actions.

Review questions

1. How might you use each of the strengths-based dimensions in practice?
2. How can you broaden your understanding of the Australian political, historical and social contexts so that you can deepen your critical reflections?
3. How might you use Aboriginal and Torres Strait Islander people's science, practice and leadership to become aware of your gaps in knowledge?
4. What strategies and actions will you take if you are employed in a workplace that will not allow you to operationalise a strengths-based approach?
5. Why is a decolonising lens essential to use in a strengths-based approach?

References

Australian Government. (n.d.). *Rights of equality and non-discrimination*. Attorney-General's Department. https://www.ag.gov.au/RightsAndProtections/HumanRights/Human-rights-scrutiny/PublicSectorGuidanceSheets/Pages/Rightsofequalityandnondiscrimination.aspx

Australian Human Rights Commission. (2010). *The community guide to the UN Declaration on the Rights of Indigenous Peoples*. AHRC. https://humanrights.gov.au/declaration_indigenous/downloads/declaration_guide2010.%20pdf

Bailey, S., & Hunt, J. (2012). Successful partnerships are the key to improving Aboriginal health. *NSW Public Health Bulletin, 23*(4), 48–51. http://dx.doi.org/10.1071/NB11057

Barker, P., & Buchanan-Barker, P. (2005a). *The Tidal Model: A guide for mental health professionals* (p. 11). Brunner-Routledge. http://www.tidal-model.com/

Barker, P., & Buchanan-Barker, P. (2005b). *The Tidal Model: A guide for mental health professionals* (p. 208). Brunner-Routledge. http://www.tidal-model.com/

Corrigan, N., & Burton, J. (2014). *Partnership training manual: Creating change through partnerships*. Secretariat of National Aboriginal and Islander Child Care (SNAICC). https://www.snaicc.org.au/wp-content/uploads/2015/12/03346.pdf

Emery-Whittington, I., & Te Maro, B. (2018). Decolonising occupation: Causing social change to help our ancestors rest and our descendants thrive. *New Zealand Journal of Occupational Therapy, 65*(1), 12–19. https://search.informit.com.au/documentSummary;dn=779745338782955;res=IELHEA

Fogarty, W., Lovell, M., Langenberg, J., & Heron, M-J. (2018). *Deficit discourse and strengths-based approaches: Changing the narrative of Aboriginal and Torres Strait Islander health and wellbeing*.

The Lowitja Institute. https://www.lowitja.org.au/page/services/resources/Cultural-and-social-determinants/racism/deficit-discourse-strengths-based

Francis, A. (2014). Strengths-based assessments and recovery in mental health: Reflections from practice. *International Journal of Social Work and Human Services Practice, 2*, 264–271. https://doi.org/10.13189/ijrh.2014.020610

Gee, G., Dudgeon, P., Schultz, C., Hart, A., & Kelly, K. (2014). Aboriginal and Torres Strait Islander social and emotional wellbeing. In N. Purdie, P. Dudgeon, & R. Walker (Eds.), *Working together: Aboriginal and Torres Strait Islander mental health and wellbeing—principles and practice* (2nd edn, pp. 55–68). ACER.

Gibson, C. (2020). When the river runs dry: Leadership, decolonisation and healing in occupational therapy. *New Zealand Journal of Occupational Therapy Te Hautaka Whakaora Ngangahau o Aotearoa, 67*(1), 11–20.

Gibson, C., Butler, C., Henaway, C., Dudgeon, P., & Curtin, M. (2015). Indigenous peoples and human rights: Some considerations for the occupational therapy profession in Australia. *Australian Occupational Therapy Journal, 62*(3) 214–218. https://doi.org/10.1111/1440-1630.12185

Gibson, C., Crockett, J., Dudgeon, P., Bernoth, M., & Lincoln, M. (2020a). Sharing and valuing older Aboriginal people's voices about social and emotional wellbeing services: A strength-based approach for service providers. *Aging & Mental Health, 24*(3), 481–488. https://doi.org/10.1080/13607863.2018.1544220

Gibson, C., Chatfeild, K., O'Neill-Baker, B., Newman, T., & Steele, A. (2020b). Gulburra (to understand): Aboriginal Ability Linker's person-centred care approach. *Disability and Rehabilitation*, 1–7. https://doi.org/10.1080/09638288.2020.1713236

Grullon, E., Hunnicutt, C., Morrison, M., Langford, O., & Whaley, M. M. (2018). A need for occupational justice: The impact of racial microaggression on occupations, wellness, and health promotion. *OCCUPATION: A Medium of Inquiry for Students, Faculty & Other Practitioners Advocating for Health through Occupational Studies, 3*(1), Article 4. https://nsuworks.nova.edu/occupation/vol3/iss1/4

Hocking, C. (2009). The challenge of occupation: Describing the things people do. *Journal of Occupational Science, 16*(3), 140–150. https://doi.org/10.1080/14427591.2009.9686655

Hunt, J. (2013a). *Engaging with Indigenous Australia: Exploring the conditions for effective relationships with Aboriginal and Torres Strait Islander communities.* Issues paper no. 5 produced for the Closing the Gap Clearinghouse. Australian Institute for Health and Welfare. https://www.aihw.gov.au/getmedia/7d54eac8-4c95-4de1-91bb-0d6b1cf348e2/ctgc-ip05.pdf.aspx?inline=true

Hunt, J. (2013b). *Engagement with Indigenous communities in key sectors.* Resource sheet no. 23 produced for the Closing the Gap Clearinghouse. Australian Institute for Health and Welfare. https://www.aihw.gov.au/getmedia/c3d74d39-0ded-4196-b221-cc4240d8ec90/ctgc-rs23.pdf.aspx?inline=true

Iwama, M. (2006). *The Kawa model: Culturally relevant occupational therapy.* Churchill Livingstone.

Kendi, I. X. (2016). *Stamped from the beginning: The definitive history of racist ideas in America.* Random House.

LIME Network. (2017). *Ngara … Deep Listening … Seeing 'Two Ways' What can Indigenous knowledge, mindfulness and observational skills training bring to medical practice?* Poche Centre for Indigenous Health and Well-Being. http://www.limenetwork.net.au/wp-content/uploads/2017/10/seminar03-programme.pdf

Lyons, N. (Ed.). (2010). *Handbook of reflection and reflective inquiry: Mapping a way of knowing for professional reflective inquiry.* Springer Science & Business Media.

Muir, S., & Dean., A. (2017). Evaluating the outcomes of programs for Indigenous families and communities. AIFS. https://aifs.gov.au/cfca/publications/evaluating-outcomes-programs-indigenous-families-and-communities

Pascoe, B. (2014). *Dark emu: Black seeds: Agriculture or accident?* Magabala Books.

Ramugondo, E. L. (2015). Occupational consciousness. *Journal of Occupational Science, 22*(4), 488–501. https://doi.org/10.1080/14427591.2015.1042516

Ramugondo, E. L., & Kronenberg, F. (2015). Explaining collective occupations from a human relations perspective: Bridging the individual-collective dichotomy. *Journal of Occupational Science, 22*(1), 3–16. https://doi.org/10.1080/14427591.2013.781920

Taylor, K. P., & Thompson, S. C. (2011). Closing the (service) gap: Exploring partnerships between Aboriginal and mainstream health services. *Australian Health Review, 35*(3), 297–308. https://doi.org/10.1071/AH10936

Ungunmerr-Baumann, M-R. (2002). *Dadirri—a Reflection.* Emmaus Productions. https://libguides.msben.nsw.edu.au/ld.php?content_id=47905834

UN Human Rights Committee (HRC). (1989). *CCPR General Comment No. 18: Non-discrimination.* https://www.refworld.org/docid/453883fa8.html

Wilcock, A., & Townsend, E. (2014). Occupational justice. In B. A. Boyt Schell, G. Gillen, & M. E. Scaffa (Eds.), *Willard & Spackman's occupational therapy* (12th edn). Lippincott Williams & Wilkins.

Williams, M. (2018). Ngaa-bi-nya Aboriginal and Torres Strait Islander program evaluation framework. *Evaluation Journal of Australasia, 18*(1), 6–20. https://doi.org/10.1177/1035719X18760141

12 Occupational science in Australia

Mandy Stanley, Matthew Molineux and Gail Whiteford

Chapter objectives

Upon completion of this chapter, the reader will be able to:

- Define occupational science.
- Identify key concepts within occupational science.
- Describe the history of occupational science in Australia.
- Identify the contribution of Australian occupational scientists.
- Describe the relationship between occupational science and occupational therapy.

Key terms

occupational science; occupational balance; occupational deprivation; occupational adaptation

Introduction

The initial development of occupational science as a discipline is formally acknowledged as occurring at the University of Southern California (USC) under the stewardship of its Elizabeth Yerxa, and subsequently Florence Clark who became the inaugural Chair of Occupational Science (Pierce, 2014). The first doctoral program commenced at USC in 1989 with seven students. Students recall the experience as an exciting time of exploration with a strong sense of creating a science of occupation (Pierce, 2014).

It was a period of intensive scholarly development. One of the collaborations driving that development was between Elizabeth Yerxa and Ann Wilcock, who were both interested in understanding the rich, situated and complex nature of occupation. Indeed, when Elizabeth and Ann met for the first time at the World Federation of Occupational Therapists congress in Melbourne in 1990, they immediately recognised the synchronicity of their work. Subsequently, Ann developed and taught the first course in occupational science in Australia at the University of South Australia in 1992 and later published her groundbreaking text titled *An Occupational Perspective of Health* in 1998.

Many of the current leaders in occupational science in Australasia were students in those early classes. They were exposed to a vast array of readings including, for example, works by Bronowski and Marx, and they were encouraged to develop their ideas on how to understand the complex phenomenon called *occupation*. All the students had occupational therapy backgrounds and found that the richness of the area for scholarship fuelled their interest and passion for occupation as a phenomenon of interest.

In 1993, Wilcock launched the *Journal of Occupational Science* with the aim of publishing research related to the occupational nature of human beings. Her vision for the journal was to bring together the work of people from a range of backgrounds including, but not exclusively, occupational therapy, such as human geography, anthropology, sociology, public health and organisational psychology, who had a common interest in what people do and intersections with health and well-being.

From those early days, the journal has gone on to make a significant contribution to the development of the corpus of research on occupation internationally. The journal had its editorial office based at the University of South Australia for over 20 years before signing with the publishing house Taylor and Francis, reflecting the growth in the journal in that time. It remains the only journal in occupational science and is held in high regard, enjoying a reputation for publishing articles of high quality. Currently, the *Journal of Occupational Science* has an international editorial and advisory board and receives submissions from all over the world. Australians and New Zealanders have had significant input to the development of the journal. The contribution of New Zealand academic Professor Clare Hocking as editor of the journal through those developments over time cannot be overstated.

Australian occupational scientists have also made significant contributions to the development of occupational science across the world through their involvement in establishing the Australasian Society of Occupational Scientists (ASOS) and the International Society for Occupational Science (ISOS), particularly Dr Alison Wicks, who has held leadership positions in both organisations. For a full description of the development and impact of ASOS and ISOS, we recommend readers review Wicks' chapter in Whiteford and Hocking's book, *Occupational science: Society, inclusion, participation* (2012).

Occupational science: A brief review

In this section we present a brief overview of three key concepts within occupational science: the occupational nature of humans; occupational balance; and occupational deprivation. We also present the concept of occupational adaptation through a discussion of loneliness from research undertaken by Stanley et al. (2010).

The occupational nature of humans

One of the most significant Australian contributions to occupational science has been Ann Wilcock's original work on the occupational nature of humans and the occupational brain. Wilcock (1993; 1995; Wilcock & Hocking, 2015) drew on literature from evolutionary science and anthropology to put forward the idea that engagement in occupation was the mechanism for people to fulfil their basic needs and thus survive. Further, occupational engagement enabled people to achieve health and well-being and the ability to reach their potential and thrive. Wilcock argued that because of the advanced evolution of the human brain and its ability to integrate and adapt, humans have an innate need to engage in occupations that are shaped by the socio-cultural context in which they are performed.

Occupational balance

One of the more developed concepts within occupational science is that of occupational balance. The notion of occupational balance was part of the very beginnings of the occupational therapy profession posited by Adolf Meyer (1922/1977), based on his extensive observations of patients in long-term institutional environments. Early ideas of occupational balance were that individuals needed to achieve a balance of work, rest and play to have a balanced lifestyle and thus health and well-being. This fairly simplistic conceptualisation can be questioned by thinking about people who are healthy who do not have a balance of work, sleep and leisure, such as those retired from paid employment. There has been considerable theoretical development of the concept with Matuska and Christiansen (2008) arguing that the balance is between desired and actual patterns of occupation to meet basic needs as well as having satisfactory social relationships and occupations that give meaning, and challenge and contribute to a sense of self. Further development of the concept remains with regard to moving beyond individuals in Western societies (Wagman et al., 2015).

Occupational deprivation

As a concept, occupational deprivation has gained traction internationally as consideration is given to the many forces that can prevent people—individuals, families and communities—from engaging in occupations. Drawing on Wilcock's (1993) earlier work, Whiteford defined occupational deprivation as 'a state of prolonged preclusion from engagement in occupations of necessity and/or meaning due to factors which stand outside the control of the individual' (Whiteford, 2004, p. 305). Whiteford went on to examine how occupational deprivation was experienced by people who have gone through refugee processes (Whiteford, 2005) and, most recently, worked with Aakifah Suleman in extrapolating occupational deprivation to understandings of the impacts of forced migration (Suleman & Whiteford, 2013). In a future which clearly has many challenges including climate change, pandemics, workplace reforms, labour shifting and increasing numbers of people in forced migration around the globe, there is a lot of scope (and, perhaps, a moral argument) to continue investigating occupational deprivation and its impacts on health and well-being.

Occupational adaptation

Occupational adaptation according to Nayar and Stanley (2015) is the overcoming of occupational challenges presented by occupational disruption or transition across the lifespan which involve reconstruction of one's occupational identity and mastery of the environment, and is negotiated through engagement in occupation. To understand occupational adaptation as a concept, let us consider Mary and her story of loneliness:

Mary is 88 years old and recently was hospitalised for several weeks for major surgery and experienced a number of complications following the surgery. This episode of ill health followed quite closely the death of her long-term partner. Her children live interstate and telephone regularly; however, they were concerned for Mary and convinced her to move in to a smaller unit after coming out of hospital rather than return to her large family home. Mary says she is feeling very lonely as she is not as mobile as she used to be, has moved away from her friends and neighbours and has not made new connections in her community. She has experienced a number of major changes in the last six months. She is reluctant to reveal to her family that she feels lonely as she doesn't want to be a burden.

For Mary to experience health and well-being it is necessary to go through a process of occupational adaptation. In Mary's current situation there is a mismatch between the demands of the environment and Mary's capacity to engage in social occupations to enable her to address loneliness. Mary decides to ask her neighbours to her unit for a coffee and discovers that she shares an interest in the same football team as one of her neighbours. She also rings an old friend and asks if she would mind coming to pick her up and take her to the church service they used to attend together each week. Slowly she uses engagement in occupations to re-connect, build relationships with others and in time adapt to her situation.

From the story about Mary we can see that occupational adaptation is necessary after a change such as bereavement, loss or ill health. Other occupational transitions that might precipitate the need for occupational adaptation include becoming a parent for the first time or acquiring a disability such as stroke (Walder & Molineux, 2017; Williams & Murray, 2013). A conceptual analysis of occupational adaptation concluded that conceptually it is not fully mature, which limits the clinical utility (Walder et al., 2019). Occupational scientists need to rise to the challenge of better defining the concept and developing it theoretically. People experiencing major occupational transitions may need assistance from someone like an occupational therapist if they don't have the resources to make the adaptations themselves as Mary was able to.

Relationship between occupational science and occupational therapy practice

While occupational science originated from within occupational therapy, the relationship between them is neither i) generally well understood; nor ii) well communicated. This scenario is fuelled by the lack of agreement internationally about what the relationship *should* be (Molineux, 2010). Some authors have been critical of occupational science, arguing that the research efforts within occupational science would reduce available research funding to establish the effectiveness of occupational therapy interventions (Morley et al., 2011). The emergence of occupational science alienated some occupational therapy clinicians as they were unfamiliar with the language and the new concepts and theories (Whiteford et al., 2000).

Currently, differing views are held with regard to the relationship between occupational science and occupational therapy. Many occupational therapists believe that occupational science is the unique domain of occupational therapists and that the two are so closely related they cannot be separated. Still others (including Wilcock, 1993) have argued that all occupational therapists should be occupational scientists but that occupational science is open to and enriched by multidisciplinary contributors.

In some countries—such as the United States—there are PhD and master's programs in occupational science. In Australia and New Zealand, however, there are no programs of study leading to a formal qualification in occupational science. Some academic occupational therapy departments include occupational science in the title but generally occupational science knowledge is incorporated within the entry-level occupational therapy curriculum. Few programs offer specific courses in occupational science, and in this respect occupational science and occupational therapy have continued to inform each other. As to whether or not this is problematic may be a matter of some conjecture, but as Pierce (2014) cogently suggests: 'It is no longer necessary to argue why one vision of occupational science may be better than another. Clearly, occupational science has multiple intents.' (p. 7)

Our view, which has admittedly been influenced by Wilcock over time, is that knowledge generated within occupational science provides the knowledge base that informs occupational therapy practice. Clearly, this is important if occupational therapists are to claim their domain *as* occupation and their expertise *in* occupation.

Case study: Forensic mental health—occupational science translated into occupational therapy

I first came across the concept of occupational deprivation when I was at university. Our readings were focused on occupational justice and occupational deprivation. At that time, my understanding of occupational deprivation was that it occurs when people are unable to take part in meaningful occupations, due to factors that are outside their control, and that this could lead to isolation, a lack of self-identity and a sense of hopelessness.

However, it wasn't until I first started working in the forensic hospital I realised that occupational deprivation could be a real risk. I knew that occupational deprivation arises from external circumstances, which prevent the individual from using his or her capacities to their fullest, and that this could lead to failure of maintaining health. I was able to see—right in front of me—the patients I was working with experiencing occupational deprivation. The patients had very low levels of motivation, the way they looked at themselves as contributing members in society was impacted and, as a result, the confidence that they had in themselves in being able to reintegrate back into the community was diminishing. As well as losing confidence, the patients' feelings of competence and their sense of self-efficacy (derived from the 'doing' of occupations) were being severely eroded. This was due to both the restrictive nature of the forensic hospital and the fact that many of the existing programs had a psycho-educational basis rather than a focus on occupation. Seeing this, and reflecting on what I knew about occupational justice and occupational deprivation, ignited my motivation to do something. So, using this motivation, I developed the Op Shop program.

The Op Shop program was initially developed by me and three other therapists. Through quality improvement initiatives we identified limited opportunities for the patients to engage in productive and skill-building occupations within the forensic hospital. As occupational therapists working in mental health services, we understood fully that barriers to employment exist for forensic mental health service users and that it is imperative that employment needs are addressed at the earliest possible stages in recovery. Barriers to employment may include the stigma associated with a mental health condition, a fragmented employment history, out-of-date skills, a lack of confidence and low self-esteem. What we also realised was that this environment was depriving the patients of opportunities to engage in meaningful roles—for example, as a team leader or as an inventory controller—through which these areas could be addressed. Because of this lack of opportunities, it was clear that we were leaving the patients at a great risk of occupational deprivation.

Occupational science sees people as occupational beings, and explores the relationship between occupation and identities, particularly during disruptions that change 'ways of doing'. This is very true for the patients in forensic settings; the process of a highly restrictive hospitalisation process and environment in which opportunities to participate in occupations are often curtailed impacts negatively on identity. Think about it—in society people always ask, 'what do you do?' So what do you respond when you don't 'do' anything? We really wanted to provide a space and an opportunity in which the patients could participate in something real, learn some skills and maybe even make a contribution to others. Again, based on the understandings of occupation gained from occupational science research, we knew this would be the most powerful approach to assisting the patients' return to successful community living.

So, given that we wanted this to be a real opportunity, the roles we created in the Op Shop were set up to be just like open employment. An advertisement was designed which stated the applicants must write an application letter addressing the selection criteria and provide this letter to their unit occupational therapist. Assistance was given to any patients who required it to complete the application or wished for further guidance, to ensure that all patients could apply—whatever their current state of health. Overall, we tried to design it so that roles could be tailored to applicants according to their existing skill level. This ensured we were creating a program as similar to open employment as possible, that is, a space in which people work together in a variety of roles with differing demands.

After the Op Shop project team evaluated the applications, the applicants were offered an interview, with the project team as the interview panel. However, the 'job interview' was also combined into an orientation to the Op Shop program, and a chance for the patient to ask the team further questions about what they would be doing, how it was run, etc. This was important because the roles they were going into were designed to be those that would build on their strengths and through which they could learn new skills and feel part of something important. At the time of development, it was the single most significant occupational opportunity in the forensic hospital and we were affirmed in our view of its potential value when a large number of patients applied.

Operationally, the Op Shop had one outlet: a large, open plan-room, with female and male bathrooms which served as change rooms. The Op Shop layout included male and female clothes separated on different display tables, and all items were organised into gender, sizes and categories, such as T-shirts, pants, jumpers, accessories, etc. This ensured there were a range of activities and roles designed for the patients—now actively in the occupation of volunteer—including sorting, preparation and set-up, tidying up, cleaning and customer service. Overall, the Op Shop program is like any community shop in that it provides a variety of roles and responsibilities for the workers/volunteers, while providing a valuable service.

In essence, it has been powerful in demonstrating the link between meaning and motivation and over time we saw that for the patients such an opportunity to engage in the occupations associated with worker/volunteer roles, minimised occupational disruption during their hospitalisation in the short term, and occupational deprivation in the long term. Individuals were able to develop and maintain skills in areas that were either lacking or absent, potentially increasing their chances of employment following discharge. Furthermore, and most importantly, the increase in their sense of hope, pride, self-efficacy, self-identity and social skills was extremely evident. The patient volunteers shared things like:

- it makes you feel good… it's enjoyable—that you can do something for somebody
- the restrictions can be so depriving and debilitating here in the hospital, that you can never do anything for someone else
- I want to try and get a career when I get out, and this helps with putting me in a position where I have to work with people, so I know I can do that when I leave

Or, as one young male volunteer put it perfectly for me: '[the Op Shop] makes me feel involved and trusted'.

Indeed, such comments, made me take a step back and in doing so I was able to see the extreme difference between when an individual is deprived of occupations, and how they are as people when they are engaged in occupation. I reflected:

> As an occupational therapist working in the forensic hospital, I am prov-ing how it has everything to do with us. How the concepts of occupational science, occupational justice and occupational deprivation can be brought through to practise in a really powerful way. We recognise the right of people with different needs to engage in occupations, and we know how this impacts on their health and well-being. By running this program every month, people have the opportunity to participate in occupations they haven't engaged in in a long time or even develop new occupations. At the end of the day, we are here for the patients, and if we don't provide them with the opportunities to participate—to be included and engage in something meaningful to them—then how are we helping their recovery?

Included with permission from Emma Todd, previously Occupational Therapist, Justice and Forensic Mental Health, NSW Health and currently Occupational Ther-apist, Mental Health Intensive Care Unit, Prince of Wales Hospital, NSW Health.

The future of occupational science

As occupational science matures it has grown in depth and scope of scholarship. Pierce (2014) points to studies that have found that occupational science publications quadru-pled between 1990 and 2000, and that between 1996 and 2006 not only did the number of articles increase dramatically, but the research approaches used and the foci of the research also diversified significantly. Interestingly, given the ongoing debates about interdisciplinarity in occupational science, so too has the number of articles by authors outside occupational therapy.

Despite this numerical increase in publications, what is evident from a deeper analysis is that the origins of the authors are largely Western countries and tend to reflect the cultural, philosophical and linguistic traditions of those countries. To really be of great-est value and relevance, there needs to be a greater diversity of perspectives reflected in the literature (Hocking, 2012; Kinsella, 2012). An excellent example of this in recent times is represented by the work of Galvaan (2012). Set in a township in South Africa in which residents experience disadvantage every day, Galvaan employed observation, interviews and the use of disposable cameras in capturing images of engagement in everyday occupations of a group of young people. She critically examined what occupational choice means in diminished environments, alongside what resilience and adaptation might similarly mean in such environments.

Such research has a great deal of salience. For occupational science to fulfil its potential then, there also needs to be a move from the focus on individual engagement in occupation—an orientation arguably influenced by occupational therapy's relationship to biomedicine—to consideration of occupational engagement by collectives, communities and populations. This does seem to be increasingly addressed by researchers such as Pereira (see Pereira & Whiteford, 2013), Laliberte Rudman (2012), Dennhardt (see Dennhardt & Laliberte Rudman, 2012), Ramugondo and Kronenberg (2015) and very possibly heralds yet another stage in the genesis of a discipline whose potential is yet to be fully realised.

Conclusion

Australia has made a significant contribution to the development of occupational science over time and has been a leader in the advancement of the discipline. The contribution made by a number of scholars who have variously provided important inputs on conceptual, philosophical and pragmatic issues has furthered understandings of the important relationship between occupational science and occupational therapy. A number of key occupational science concepts have been developed through a range of research approaches in a variety of contexts. Occupational science continues to evolve in Australia and internationally.

Summary

- Occupational science is the study of occupation as a complex, situated phenomenon.
- Occupational science and occupational therapy have an important relationship as understanding occupation is a requisite to enabling it.
- Australian scholars, led by Ann Wilcock, have made a unique and important contribution to the development over time.
- Occupational science will be strengthened by greater diversity of researchers globally and a more pluralistic epistemic foundation.

Review questions

1. When did occupational science begin in Australia and who was the originator?
2. Using the definition provided, make a list of examples of occupational deprivation other than that discussed in the chapter.
3. How do you define occupational adaptation?
4. How would you describe your understanding of the relationship between occupational science and occupational therapy?

References

Dennhardt, S., & Laliberte Rudman, D. (2012). When occupation goes wrong: A critical reflection on risk discourse and their relevance in shaping occupation. In G. Whiteford & C. Hocking (Eds.), *Occupational science: Society, inclusion, participation* (pp. 117–136). Wiley-Blackwell.

Galvaan, R. (2012). Occupational choice: The significance of socioeconomic and political factors. In G. Whiteford & C. Hocking (Eds.), *Occupational science: Society, inclusion, participation* (pp. 152–162). Wiley-Blackwell.

Hocking, C. (2012). Occupations through the looking glass: Reflecting on occupational scientists' ontological assumptions. In G. Whiteford & C. Hocking (Eds.), *Occupational science: Society, inclusion, participation* (pp. 54–66). Wiley-Blackwell.

Kinsella, E. A. (2012). Knowledge paradigms in occupational science: Pluralistic perspectives. In G. Whiteford & C. Hocking (Eds.), *Occupational science: Society, inclusion, participation.* (pp. 67–85) Wiley-Blackwell.

Laliberte Rudman, D. (2012). Governing through occupation: Shaping expectations and possibilities. In G. Whiteford & C. Hocking (Eds.), *Occupational science: Society, inclusion, participation* (pp. 100–116). Wiley-Blackwell.

Matuska, K., & Christiansen, C. (2008). A proposed model of lifestyle balance. *Journal of Occupational Science, 15*(1), 9–19. https://doi.org/10.1080/14427591.2008.9686602

Meyer, A. (1977). The philosophy of occupation therapy. Reprinted from the Archives of Occupational Therapy, Volume 1, pp. 1–10, 1922. *American Journal of Occupational Therapy, 31*(10), 639–642.

Molineux, M. (2010). Occupational science and occupational therapy: Occupation at center stage. In C. Christiansen & E. Townsend (Eds.), *Introduction to Occupation: The art and science of living* (2nd edn, pp. 359–383). Prentice Hall.

Morley, M., Atwal, A., & Spiliotopoulou, G. (2011). Has occupational science taken away the occupational therapy evidence base? A debate. *British Journal of Occupational Therapy, 74*(10), 494–497. https://doi.org/10.4276/030802211X13182481842065

Nayar, S., & Stanley, M. (2015). Occupational adaptation as a social process in everyday life. *Journal of Occupational Science, 22*(1), 26–28. https://doi.org/10.1080/14427591.2014.882251

Pereira, R., & Whiteford, G. (2013). Understanding social inclusion as an international discourse: Implications for enabling participation. *British Journal of Occupational Therapy, 76*(2), 112–115. https://doi.org/10.4276/030802213X13603244419392

Pierce, D. (2014). *Occupational science for occupational therapy.* SLACK Inc.

Ramugondo, E., & Kronenberg, F. (2015). Explaining collection occupation from a human relations perspective. Bridging the individual collective dichotomy. *Journal of Occupational Science, 22*(1), 3–16. https://doi.org/10.1080/14427591.2013.781920#

Stanley, M., Moyle, W., Ballantyne, A., Jaworski, K., Corlis, M., Oxlade, D., Stoll, A., & Young, B. (2010). 'Nowadays you don't even see your neighbours': Understanding loneliness in the everyday lives of older Australians. *Health and Social Care in the Community, 18*(4), 407–414. https://doi.org/10.1111/j.1365-2524.2010.00923.x

Suleman, A., & Whiteford, G. (2013). Understanding occupational transitions in forced migration: The importance of life skills in early refugee resettlement. *Journal of Occupational Science, 20*(2), 201–210. https://doi.org/10.1080/14427591.2012.755908

Wagman, P., Hakansson, C., & Jonsson, H. (2015). Occupational balance: A scoping review of current research and identified knowledge gaps. *Journal of Occupational Science, 22*(2), 160–169. https://doi.org/10.1080/14427591.2014.986512

Walder, K., & Molineux, M. (2017). Occupational adaptation and identity reconstruction: A grounded theory synthesis of qualitative studies exploring adults' experiences of adjustment to chronic disease, major illness and injury. *Journal of Occupational Science, 24*(2), 225–243. https://doi.org/10.1080/14427591.2016.1269240

Walder, K., Molineux, M., Bissett, M., & Whiteford, G. (2019). Occupational adaptation—analysing the maturity and understanding of the concept through concept analysis. *Scandinavian Journal of Occupational Therapy*, *28*(1), 26–40. https//doi.org/10.1080/11038128.2019.1695931

Whiteford, G. (2004). When people cannot participate. In C. Christiansen & E. Townsend (Eds.), *Occupation: The art and science of living* (pp. 221–242). Prentice Hall.

Whiteford, G. (2005). Understanding the occupational deprivation of refugees: Case study from Kosovo. *Canadian Journal of Occupational Therapy*, *72*(2), 78–87. https://doi.org/10.1177/000841740507200202

Whiteford, G., Townsend, E., & Hocking C. (2000). Reflections on a renaissance of occupation. *Canadian Journal of Occupational Therapy*, *67*(1), 61–69. https://doi.org/10.1177/000841740006700109

Wicks, A. (2012). The International Society for Occupational Science: A critique of its role in facilitating the development of occupational science through international networks and intercultural dialogue. In G. Whiteford & C. Hocking (Eds.), *Occupational science: Society, inclusion, participation* (pp. 163–183). Wiley-Blackwell.

Wilcock, A. A. (1993). A theory of the human need for occupation. *Journal of Occupational Science: Australia*, *1*(1), 17–24. https://doi.org/10.1080/14427591.1993.9686375

Wilcock, A. A. (1995). The occupational brain: A theory of human nature. *Journal of Occupational Science*, *2*(2), 68–72. https://doi.org/10.1080/14427591.1995.9686397

Wilcock, A. A., & Hocking, C. (2015). *An occupational perspective of health* (3rd edn). SLACK Inc.

Williams, S., & Murray, C. (2013). The experience of engaging in occupation following stroke: A qualitative meta-synthesis. *British Journal of Occupational Therapy*, *76*(8), 370–378. https://doi.org/10.4276/030802213X13757040168351

13 The education of occupational therapists in Australia

Academic and practice education

Louise Farnworth, Mary Kennedy-Jones and Mong-Lin Yu

Chapter objectives

Upon completion of this chapter, the reader will be able to:

- Relate the history and scope of occupational therapy education in Australia.
- Describe the mechanism of accreditation of educational programs including the Accreditation Standards for Entry-level Occupational Therapy Education programs (2018), WFOT Minimum Standards for the education of occupational therapists (2016) and the Australian Occupational Therapy competency standards (2018). This includes the specific requirements for educational programs to address Aboriginal and Torres Strait Islander practice, inter-professional education and consumer involvement.
- Highlight practice education in contemporary occupational therapy programs including the use of innovative models of student supervision to accommodate growing numbers of students studying to become occupational therapists and how placement availability can be improved by providing funding to agencies.
- Discuss contemporary issues in occupational therapy education in Australia.

Key terms

education; training; accreditation; registration; practice education; minimum standards; competency

History of occupational therapy education in Australia

In 1942, the first occupational therapy program in Australia was established in New South Wales. In 1947, a second training program opened in Victoria (Anderson & Bell, 1988). Subsequently, courses in occupational therapy were established in Queensland in 1950, Western Australia in 1961 and a decade later in South Australia. A diploma level qualification was awarded at the end of two and a half years of study. All occupational therapy curricula at the time included studies in psychiatry, psychology, anatomy, physiology, medical and surgical conditions, occupational therapy theory and clinical practice. Also included were skills in arts and crafts, for example, weaving, pottery and woodwork. The length of the courses soon increased to three years; then, by the early 1970s all occupational therapy entry level educational programs in Australia changed to three and a half or four-year baccalaureate level degrees.

The new century led to changes internationally in the entry level of occupational therapy education. Coulthard (2002) argued that this was necessary as the environments in which occupational therapists were required to work were more demanding, practice decisions had to be supported by evidence and occupational therapists were required to work independently. It also was consistent with changes to entry-level education in other health disciplines such as physiotherapy. The occupational therapy professional associations in the United States and Canada approved raising the occupational therapy entry to practice level to a master's degree. This provided the impetus for the development of a graduate-entry master's (GEM) in occupational therapy in 2000 at the University of Sydney in addition to the baccalaureate degree. Several Australian universities soon followed by introducing a graduate-entry master's degree (GEM), as well as many also maintaining a bachelor's degree level intake.

Occupational therapy education in Australia today

Occupational therapy as a career option has become increasingly popular. Since the 1990s, there has been rapid growth in the number of occupational therapy programs, as well as an increase in the number of students accepted each year into these programs. Universities have developed new programs to attract quality students to their university. To illustrate, in 1991 there were five occupational therapy educational programs, all bachelor's level. Currently, there are over 20 universities that offer courses in occupational therapy across six states and territories of Australia—South Australia, Victoria, New South Wales, Western Australia and Queensland, and the Australian Capital Territory. One university has campuses in three states and two have programs on different campuses, including both metropolitan and rural campuses. This growth in the number of programs continues.

While in the United States, there are now doctoral entry-level programs, the relevant levels in Australia are bachelor, bachelor with honours and Graduate entry master's (GEM). Until 2012, both the baccalaureate (including honours), and master's level of entry to the profession were regarded as equally meeting the professional educational accreditation standards in Australia albeit with different academic outcomes in line with the Higher Education Standards Framework (2015), including meeting the requirements of the Australian Qualifications Framework (AQF, 2013) levels. According to the AQF, the purpose of the bachelor's (level 7) degree qualifies individuals to apply a broad and coherent body of knowledge in a range of contexts to undertake professional work, and provides a pathway for further learning, usually within three years. The bachelor's (honours) (level 8) degree additionally requires graduates to plan and execute a project, or piece of research, requiring a year of study following the three-year bachelor's degree, or for occupational therapy, usually a project is embedded within a four-year program. The GEM (level 9) qualification requires individuals to demonstrate a higher level of mastery of theoretical knowledge and critical reflection, and to be able to deal with complex information, problems and concepts so as to be able to contribute to professional practice or scholarship.

Students in GEM programs must first meet both university and professional prerequisite bachelor level studies. Generally, the GEM degree is from two to two and a half years in duration but often with accelerated learning (more academic weeks per year). All entry-level programs must demonstrate that graduates have met the expected 1,000 hours of fieldwork across the program. In Australia, most occupational therapy programs are still at bachelor or bachelor honours levels. An increasing number of universities offer the GEM. Some universities have both bachelor and GEM programs.

Occupational therapy education programs standards

Now you know that there are over 20 occupational therapy programs in Australia and that some are at different academic levels, how do you know that your occupational therapy educational program will qualify you to be able to register for practice as an occupational therapist and for you to be able to compete equitably for employment with graduates from other programs? The following outlines the different levels of governance to ensure that every Australian occupational therapy program meets minimum professional standards.

World Federation of Occupational Therapists

Chapter 4 outlines that the World Federation of Occupational Therapists (WFOT) is the international body representing occupational therapists. The WFOT provides an international benchmark for occupational therapy education to ensure the quality of education programs globally, and graduation from a WFOT-approved program supports international mobility of graduates. WFOT therefore has needed to develop standards that are reflective of the dynamic qualities of occupational therapy education worldwide. These are known as the WFOT *Minimum Standards for the Education of Occupational Therapists* (Revised) (2016). Australian occupational therapy education programs meet, and generally exceed, these Standards by undertaking a continual approval and re-approval process. Depending on the length of the program, the WFOT re-approval process takes place every 5–7 years.

The educational program accreditation process: Occupational Therapy Council of Australia Ltd

Programs of study leading to an entry-level qualification in occupational therapy must be accredited by the Occupational Therapy Council of Australia Ltd (OTC). The OTC is the body appointed by the Occupational Therapy Board of Australia (OTBA) to assess and accredit Australian occupational therapy education programs as part of the accreditation functions under the *Health Practitioner Regulation National Law Act 2009* (National Law). The OTC undertakes an initial accreditation assessment of new programs prior to the first intake of students. The standards are used to assess whether a program of study, and the education provider (university) that delivers the program of study, provide those people who complete the program with the knowledge, skills and professional attributes necessary to practise the profession in Australia in a competent and ethical manner.

The *Accreditation standards for entry-level occupational therapy education programs* (OTC, 2018) reflect contemporary views on measuring quality in education, in particular with a focus on assessing outcomes, and incorporate the *WFOT Minimum Standards for the Education of Occupational Therapists* (2016). The updated Accreditation Standards (2018) came into effect in January 2020 and comprise five domains (see Table 13.1). Each domain includes a standard statement that is supported by a number of criteria. The criteria are indicators, which set out expectations that an accredited program must meet.

Table 13.1 Accreditation standards domains

Domain	Standard statement
Public safety	Assuring public safety is paramount in program design and implementation.
Academic governance and quality assurance	Academic governance and quality improvement systems are effective in developing and delivering sustainable, high-quality occupational therapy education.
Program of study	Program design, delivery and resourcing enable students to achieve the required occupational therapy learning outcomes, attributes and competencies.
The student experience	Students are provided with equitable and timely access to information and support relevant to their occupational therapy program.
Assessment	Graduates have demonstrated achievement of all program learning outcomes, including the requirements for safe, ethical and competent occupational therapy practice.

The university completes a detailed self-assessment document demonstrating how the program meets the Accreditation Standards, and an independent review of the self-assessment documentation is undertaken by a two- or three-person team of national assessors appointed by the OTC National Accreditation Assessor Panel prior to a 2–3-day site visit conducted at the university. The site visit enables the assessment team to assess how the program functions, gain information from key stakeholders, and validate or refute the information presented in the submission.

As a student, new graduate or practitioner, you may have the opportunity to be part of the accreditation process as a key stakeholder for the educational program. You also will be contributing to the program accreditation when you provide critical and reflective feedback on your student learning experiences, and when you act in leadership roles, such as being a student representative. These activities are aspects of the accreditation process that demonstrate the overall standard of governance of the program.

If the OTC is reasonably satisfied the program meets the accreditation standards, or will meet the accreditation standards within a reasonable time with the imposition of conditions, the program will be accredited by the OTC. The OTC then monitors the program and the education provider to ensure the occupational therapy program, and the university, continue to meet the accreditation standards with reaccreditation within a five-year cycle.

Occupational Therapy Australia, the professional association, has the responsibility for accrediting programs to determine if they meet the World Federation of Occupational Therapists (WFOT) Standards. The OTC and Occupational Therapy Australia have an agreement whereby the OTC provides accreditation reports to Occupational Therapy Australia who then determines whether or not a program meets the WFOT minimum standards and can be listed as WFOT-approved (see also Chapter 4).

A fully accredited program means worldwide recognition of the standard of occupational therapy education. Further, students who graduate from an accredited program are eligible to apply with Australian Health Practitioners Regulation Agency (AHPRA) for registration to practise in Australia. Subject to additional national requirements, graduates become eligible to apply to practise in other countries.

The standards are dynamic so over time they have been modified in response to changing community expectations and population health needs. On reading Chapter 6 you will be aware that occupational therapy professional values have an historical basis that are largely influenced by the values and philosophy developed over time. The values and philosophy of the profession provides the foundation for occupational therapy theory that is used to translate knowledge that guides practice. These values and philosophy also underpin the standards of practice that are assessed through the program accreditation. You should be able to see congruence between the philosophy and values of occupational therapy in the models of practice and assessments of occupational performance that you have been studying. Additionally, occupational therapy curricula need to accommodate contextual variations and changes as ideas that come from professional and educational research findings, practice and experience.

More recently, there has been a significant increase in the practice contexts in which occupational therapists engage. Therefore, the Australian entry-level educational standards (OTC, 2018) aim to recognise the changing nature of educational program design, content, as well as regional, national and international differences that now exist in occupational therapy practice. For this reason, the Australian occupational therapy educational standards reflect the influence of both the WFOT's *Minimum Standards for the Education of Occupational Therapists* (2016) as well the Australian context.

The current Australian accreditation standards (OTBA, 2018) address the growing range of practice contexts that employ occupational therapists and the three main policy developments in the health care sector. The first of these policy developments is the standards specifically acknowledging the need for occupational therapists to enhance their cultural responsiveness and capabilities for practice, in particular with Aboriginal and Torres Strait Islander populations and, more broadly, across other cultural groups. Evidence indicates that Aboriginal and Torres Strait Islander peoples are more likely to access health services where, among other things, providers communicate respectfully, and have awareness of underlying social issues and culture. All programs of study are required to include student learning outcomes that are guided by *The Aboriginal and Torres Strait Islander Health Curriculum Framework* (Department of Health, 2014). Additionally, universities are strongly encouraged to enrol students from underrepresented groups such as Aboriginal and Torres Strait Islander peoples to address the gap in representation of Aboriginal and Torres Strait Islanders practising as occupational therapists.

The second policy development is the need for the application of inter-professional learning for collaborative client-centred practice education in health professional preparation programs. Community health organisations are large and complex, and comprise a range of allied health professionals. Often continuity of care is not provided, with clients seeing new and different staff at each visit. For example, Stewart (2017) highlighted that ineffective inter-professional communication led to the majority of the complaints from clients as a consequence of receiving contradictory and mixed messages from health practitioners. As a result, the need for good teamwork, including communication and collaboration between health professionals, is paramount.

Inter-professional education (IPE) is defined as an intervention where the members of more than one health or social care profession, or both, learn interactively together, for the explicit purpose of improving inter-professional collaboration or the health/well-being of patients/clients, or both (Reeves et al., 2013). This learning should occur during and after qualification as a health professional and comprise attitudes, knowledge and skills needed to work together effectively. Importantly, communication and collaboration amongst team members are regarded as critical skills needed to ensure client safety. To do this, many universities incorporate practice scenarios with teams of health professional students simultaneously, sometimes with simulated clients. Some universities have health professional student clinics. The student team includes a range of health professionals who will be given a complex clinical scenario, and the learning for students is organised around solving a common set of problems (Hall & Weaver, 2001). Each discipline takes account of the other's contribution and works towards a holistic approach to manage a client's complex health needs while maintaining their specialised role, and maintaining continuous communication with every other team member.

The third policy development concerns the collaboration and consultation with key stakeholders including the perspectives of consumers/service users/clients to inform the design, delivery and evaluation of the program. Cooper and Spencer-Dawe (2006) argued that service users (consumers) should be considered as important contributors to IPE for health students. While it is usual in a program to have the involvement of consumers to talk with students about their lived experience, what is different in the revised standards is the involvement of consumers in the broader aspect of program development and assessment to help ensure authenticity and relevancy. Once exposed more fully to a consumer perspective, students are more likely to apply the principles of teamwork and place the consumer at the centre of the caring process. This helps students to link the theory with real life.

The Australian Occupational Therapy Competency Standards

While educational programs are accredited, graduates of programs also need to be able to meet the *Australian Occupational Therapy Competency Standards* (Occupational Therapy Board of Australia, 2018) commissioned by the Occupational Therapy Board of Australia (OTBA) through the Australian Health Practitioner Regulation Agency (AHPRA, 2013). These became effective from 2019. They describe the standards understood and applied to practice for competent practice by occupational therapists for registration and for regulation by the OTBA. This includes all new graduates from entry-level programs. The current competency standards represent a broadening of the previous *Australian Minimum Competency Standards for New Graduate Occupational Therapists* (Occupational Therapy Australia, 2010).

The competency standards outline professional behaviours all occupational therapists should demonstrate to practise safely and ethically. They affect occupational therapists working across all practice settings, including research, education, management and other roles not involving direct contact with clients. Educational programs must be able to ensure that new graduates are able to meet these competency standards. If not yet fully met, new graduates also need to identify any further continuing professional development activities that will be required to practise as a new therapist. The practice behaviours are not presented in order of importance. Rather, every standard and behaviour is considered to be equally important and together describe competent practice.

The four standards are:

- Professionalism: practice that is ethical, safe, lawful and accountable; supports client health and well-being through occupation; and consideration of the person and their environment;

- Knowledge and learning: knowledge, skills and behaviours in practice are informed by relevant and contemporary theory, practice knowledge and evidence, and are maintained and developed by ongoing professional development and learning;
- Occupational therapy process and practice: practice acknowledges the relationship between health, well-being and human occupation, and their practice is client-centred for individuals, groups, communities and populations; and, finally,
- Communication: occupational therapists practise with open, responsive and appropriate communication to maximise the occupational performance and engagement of clients and relevant others.

Australian Health Practitioners Regulation Agency (AHPRA)

The main role of AHPRA (the registration and regulation authority) is to protect the public (see also Chapter 4). One of the ways AHPRA does this is by making sure that only practitioners who have the skills and qualifications to provide safe care to the Australian community are registered to practise their profession. Under the National Law, the university is responsible for ensuring that all occupational therapy students enrolled in an approved program of study, or who are undertaking a period of clinical training, are registered with AHPRA to protect the public's safety in much the same way that health practitioners must be registered. For example, universities are mandated to report to AHPRA any matters related to a student's health and well-being that may have an impact on public safety. Universities will encourage students with health challenges to self-report to the professional practice coordinator if they have doubts about their ability to perform effectively on placement. This enables AHPRA to act on student impairment matters or when there is a conviction of a serious nature that may impact on public safety.

Practice education

Practice education is a major component of occupational therapy education. It enables students to integrate knowledge, professional reasoning and professional behaviours within practice, and to develop knowledge, skills and attitudes to the level of competence required of qualifying occupational therapists (WFOT, 2016). It is also a component of the program that can lead to the development of new practice areas through innovative models of supervision (Rodger et al., 2007).

To be accredited, students in entry-level educational programs are expected to complete a minimum of 1,000 hours of practice placements (Holmes et al., 2010), which can be distributed in every year of the curriculum, to ensure integration of theory to practice. During these hours, students should experience a variety of placement opportunities with a range of people who have different occupational needs, and in different contexts, including approaches with individuals, communities/groups and populations and people of different ages, gender and ethnicity, health conditions and delivery settings.

Both the Australian accreditation standards (OTC, 2018) and the WFOT Minimum Standards (WFOT, 2016) specify that occupational therapy practice is more than at the level of individuals or groups, and should include working at societal levels in the areas of health promotion and community development. In addition, changes within the health and human service sectors have impacted on health care services and delivery, and therefore occupational therapy practice. Some of these practices are described in this book. To be able to further develop this occupational therapy scope of practice, educational programs must address usual as well as emerging areas of practice through academic studies and practice education.

Innovative models of student supervision

Student supervision models in practice education are not limited to 1:1 student–therapist and nor do they require an on-site occupational therapist supervisor. Innovative practice education models have arisen to enable the demands of current and future practice to be met, as well as accommodating the rapidly growing number of students. Innovative placements incorporate peer-assisted learning, utilise shared supervision, and provide experiences across multiple clinical area/sites.

Project placements (see Chapter 28) can also be offered as part of the practice education program. Project placements can include quality assurance, service development, capacity building, community development and project management activities (Fortune & McKinstry, 2012). Students are able to use their problem-solving skills, creativity and initiative, as well as build skills in clinical reasoning, client-centred practice and professional and personal development during these placements (Overton et al., 2009). Additional benefits of project placements are to address health and well-being service gaps, but also the potential to develop a wider, more current, employment base, and new practice niches for graduates of occupational therapy programs.

University-supported placements (also referred as long-arm supervision placements) are increasingly used to enable practice education to occur in areas that may become future occupational therapy practice. Supervision is provided by university-employed supervisor/s via multiple supervision methods (e.g., site visits, phone calls, emails, teleconferences), in combination with university-developed tutorials, workbooks, and online resources and activities (see, for example, Dancza et al., 2016). Many universities expect that students will have a range of supervision experiences to best use professional training resources, plus giving students exposure to a fuller range of contemporary practice education.

Simulation is also used to increase practice education capacity and quality. The Australian accreditation standards allow for up to 20 per cent of the 1,000 hours of practice education to include simulation activities embedded within an academic program. Simulation activities include written case studies, role play and use of standardised patients (Rodger et al., 2010). To contribute to practice education hours, simulation activities need to be authentic with a high level of complexity, and evaluated using practice education protocols such as the Student Practice Evaluation Form—Revised Edition (Imms et al., 2018; Rodger et al., 2010). Imms et al. (2018) found that a simulated placement experience was considered to provide an equivalent learning experience to a usual placement.

The significance of classroom activities in preparing students for professional practice cannot be underestimated. The study of human occupation and its relationship to health and well-being forms the foundational theoretical lens based on values and philosophy (Taylor & Kielhofner, 2017; Townsend & Polatajko, 2013) through which all occupational therapists view the practice world. This perspective is what differentiates occupational therapists from other health professionals, and professionals from technicians. Yet this is probably the most conceptually difficult aspect for students to embrace in an occupational therapy curriculum. Students need to learn about and understand concepts such as occupational analysis; the impact of the environment, including the physical, built world and the social environment; how people use their time; and the importance of meaning and purpose of occupations for health and well-being. Additionally, students need to be able to effectively incorporate occupationally focused language and practices to enact their unique professional role.

Funding of practice education

An increasing issue for universities is the funding of practice education. In Australia, universities receive funding from the Commonwealth through the Commonwealth Grant Scheme, based on the number of the Commonwealth-supported places taken up to a set limit (Department of Education, 2014) and student contributions. Practice education is supported by this funding as part of an occupational therapy program. Funding in Australia varies across states, universities and health organisations; however, the costs are commonly shared by universities and health care providers. There has been a history of health care providers offering placements for free at their own costs to support practice education in recognition of the value of training a future occupational therapy workforce. However, with no funding coming to health care organisations to offer placements, some states have moved to a billable placement system to increase health training capacity. For example, Placeright in Victoria provides a state-wide online platform to plan and coordinate health placements, and sets maximum chargeable fees to guide public health services and education providers in establishing placement fees (Health Victoria, 2019). South Australia also commenced using Placeright in 2019 and started charging for placements. The rollout of NDIS also facilitates the increase of health organisations charging placement fees to fund placements.

Student Practice Evaluation Form (SPEF-R)

Practice education in all occupational therapy programs in Australia is evaluated using the Student Practice Evaluation Form—Revised Edition (SPEF-R) (University of Queensland, 2008). This is a criterion referenced assessment that emphasises formative and summative feedback for students undertaking part- or full-time professional practice placements, including project-related placements (see www.uq.edu.au/spef).

Professional development groups that support occupational therapy educators

The Australian and New Zealand Occupational Therapy Fieldwork Academic group (ANZOTFA)

ANZOTFA was formed to encourage the universities and the professional association in the first instance, to work together to facilitate the provision of sufficient placements. Its members are the fieldwork academics at the universities who provide occupational therapy education in Australia and New Zealand. The group also provides a leadership role in continuing professional development related to the scholarship of fieldwork (practice-based) learning.

The Australian and New Zealand Council of Occupational Therapy educators (ANZCOTE)

ANZCOTE comprises the head of the program from each university that offers courses in occupational therapy. This group meets annually to consider national and international curriculum developments, including alignment with the AQF (2013) and occupational therapy workforce developments. Workforce discussions are held in conjunction with the national occupational therapy professional association OTA.

Challenges and opportunities for occupational therapy education

As discussed, occupational therapy has been undergoing major developments in the level of entry to the field and the focus of practice leading to extended scope of practice such as project-related work. For occupational therapy educators, ongoing questions are: What is core and what added curriculum should be included to take advantage of new health service delivery developments? What level of education is best able to achieve this?

One specific opportunity for occupational therapists has come about with full implementation in 2019–2020 of the National Disability Insurance Scheme (NDIS). First proposed by the Productivity Commission (2011), the NDIS is part of a ten-year National Disability Strategy designed to build inclusion of all Australians (Commonwealth of Australia, 2011; Callaway & Tregloan, 2018). Theoretically, occupational therapists are well positioned to provide NDIS-funded services, but to do so requires therapists to have diverse skills that prepare them to fulfil a range of positions. These positions are in holistic, participation-focused assessment, health promotion, community development and research (Productivity Commission, 2011; Russi, 2014). While the aims of the scheme are to provide lifelong goal-directed planning and funded supports for people with significant and permanent disabilities, in the early stages of implementation many issues with the Scheme were identified (Parliament of Australia & Tune, 2019, see the Tune Report Australian Government 2019).

In addition to these early implementation issues, the NDIS has required therapists to develop a new language and a new way of arguing for the needs of NDIS recipients to fit the types of funding available. Assessments used for NDIS planning may be philosophically challenging to occupational therapists who require new skills that go beyond their entry-level-accredited program. There is a challenge for therapists to keep up to date with the regular changes to the scheme rules and operational guidelines, and to consider the interface between the NDIS and other systems including the defined funding responsibilities of each.

The NDIS holds much potential for occupational therapists and the scheme participants with whom these professionals work, but also may be challenging to be able to assist people with disabilities and their families to harness the available opportunities. It necessitates occupational therapy curriculum redesign to provide learning that enables graduates to be competitive when working in the NDIS, while also reflecting the profession's core values, expertise and philosophies (Barclay et al., 2019).

Related to this is another dilemma in occupational therapy education concerning what is considered core curriculum to be work ready on graduation. Fortune et al. (2013) questioned whether occupational therapy graduates are adequately prepared for super complex environments. For occupational therapy curricula, which are already overcrowded, will there be space for the addition of new skills to enable occupational therapists to work in new and developing roles? Examples of new and emerging areas for occupational therapy practice are outlined in later chapters in this book. As you progress through your education, think about how your program is equipping you to be work ready. Questions still arise related to whether advanced educational outcomes attained from GEM programs better suit occupational therapists undertaking work such as that required in NDIS practice, or is a four-year bachelor's or honours degree entry program sufficiently able to prepare graduates for complex positions?

The question regarding the minimum standard for entry into the profession of occupational therapy in Australia remains. Should the status quo remain and there be multiple educational entry points including bachelor's and graduate entry master's degrees (Farnworth et al., 2010)? While intuitively it may appear that a master's level qualification may lead to enhanced academic, research, education and practice outcomes, there is little evidence yet to demonstrate that the level of education makes a significant difference to graduate readiness to practice.

Conclusion

The education of occupational therapy students in Australia is an important and ongoing issue. Students complete a combination of academic, classroom-based education plus 1,000 hours of practice education. This has led to the development of new practices. In Australia, occupational therapy education is offered at an undergraduate level and a graduate-entry master's level. The number of occupational therapy education programs in Australia continues to grow and ongoing challenges to source sufficient, quality practice education opportunities exist. The level and scope of occupational therapy entry-to-practice education is of a high standard and is well regarded internationally.

Summary

- Entry-to-practice education for the occupational therapy profession is currently offered via two streams in Australia: the baccalaureate degree or the graduate–entry master's level.
- Programs of study leading to a qualification in occupational therapy must be accredited by the Occupational Therapy Council of Australia Ltd (OTC).
- The World Federation of Occupational Therapists expects 1,000 hours of practice education as a requirement for all entry-level occupational therapy educational programs.
- Students who graduate from an accredited occupational therapy program are eligible to apply with Australian Health Practitioners Regulation Agency (AHPRA) for registration to practise in Australia.
- Practice education is evaluated using the Student Practice Evaluation Form— Revised Edition (SPEF-R) across Australia.
- In a practice world that is changing with technology, development of interprofessional practice opportunities and greater complexity with the health system, occupational therapy education needs to be both responsive and adaptive.

Review questions

1. What are the different levels of occupational therapy education in Australia and what is the difference?
2. In Australia, what types of practice education can fulfil the 1,000 hours?
3. What is professional accreditation and who accredits occupational therapy entry-level programs in Australia?
4. What has led to the development of new innovative practice education models and how effective are they?

References

Anderson, B., & Bell, J. (1988). *Occupational therapy: Its place in Australia's history.* Association of Occupational Therapists.

Australian Health Practitioner Regulation Agency. (2013). *Quality framework for the accreditation function.* http://www.ahpra.gov.au/Legislation-and-Publications/AHPRA-Publications.aspx#accreditation

Australian Qualifications Framework. (2013). *Australian Qualifications Framework.* https://www.aqf.edu.au/

Barclay, L., Callaway, L., & Pope, K. (2019). Perspectives of individuals receiving occupational therapy services through the National Disability Insurance Scheme: Implications for occupational therapy educators. *Australian Occupational Therapy Journal, 67*(1), 39–48. https://doi.org/10.1111/1440-1630.12620

Callaway, L., & Tregloan, K. (2018). Government perspectives on housing, technology and support design within Australia's National Disability Strategy. *Australian Journal of Social Issues, 53*(3), 206–222. https://doi.org/10.1002/ajs4.40

Commonwealth of Australia. (2011). *2010–2020 National Disability Strategy; An initiative of the Council of Australian Governments.* Commonwealth of Australia. https://www.dss.gov.au/sites/default/files/documents/05_2012/national_disability_strategy_2010_2020.pdf

Cooper, H., & Spencer-Dawe, E. (2006) Involving service users in interprofessional education: Narrowing the gap between theory and practice. *Journal of Interprofessional Care, 20*(6), 603–617. https://doi.org/10.1080/13561820601029767

Coulthard, M. (2002). Preparing occupational therapists for practice today and into the future. *Canadian Journal of Occupational Therapy, 69*(5), 253–260. https://doi.org/10.1177/000841740206900501

Dancza, K., Copley, S., Rodger, S., & Moran, M. (2016). The development of a theory-informed workbook as an additional support for students on role-emerging placements. *British Journal of Occupational Therapy, 79*(4), 235–243. https://doi.org/10.1177/0308022615612806

Department of Education. (2014). *Commonwealth grant scheme guidelines 2012.* https://www.legislation.gov.au/Details/F2014C00829

Department of Health. (2014). *Aboriginal and Torres Strait Islander Health Curriculum Framework.* https://www1.health.gov.au/internet/main/publishing.nsf/Content/aboriginal-torres-strait-islander-health-curriculum-framework

Farnworth, L. J., Rodger, S., Curtin, M., Brown, G. T., & Gilbert Hunt, S. (2010). Occupational therapy entry-level education in Australia: Which path(s) to take? *Australian Occupational Therapy Journal, 57*(4), 233–238. https//doi.org/10.1111/j.1440-1630.2010.00862.x

Fortune, T., & McKinstry, C. (2012). Project-based fieldwork: Perspectives of graduate entry students and project sponsors. *Australian Occupational Therapy Journal, 59*(4), 265–275. https://doi.org/10.1111/j.1440-1630.2012.01026.x

Fortune, T., Ryan, S., & Adamson, L. (2013). Transition to practice in supercomplex environments: Are occupational therapy graduates adequately prepared? *Australian Occupational Therapy Journal, 60*(3), 217–220. https://doi.org/10.1111/1440-1630.12010

Hall, P., & Weaver, L. (2001). Interdisciplinary education and teamwork: A long and winding road. *Health Education, 35*(9), 867–875. https://doi.org/10.1046/j.1365-2923.2001.00919.x

Health Practitioner Regulation National Law Act 2009. https://www.legislation.qld.gov.au/view/pdf/inforce/current/act-2009-045

Health Victoria. (2019). *Placeright.* https://www2.health.vic.gov.au/health-workforce/education-and-training/student-placement-partnerships/placeright

Higher Education Standards Framework (Threshold Standards). (2015). https://www.legislation.gov.au/Details/F2015L01639/Explanatory%20Statement/Text

Holmes, J. D., Bossers, A. M., Polatajko, H. J., Drynan, D. P., Gallagher, M., O'Sullivan, C. M., Slade, A. L., Stier, J. J, Storr, C. A., & Denney, J. L. (2010). 1000 fieldwork hours: Analysis of multisite evidence. *Canadian Journal of Occupational Therapy, 77*(3), 135–143. https://doi.org/10.2182/cjot.2010.77.3.2

Imms, C., Froude, E., Chu, E. M. Y., Sheppard, L., Darzins, S., Guinea, S., Gospodarevskaya, E., Carter, R., Symmons, M. A., Penman, M., Nicola-Richmond, K., Gilbert Hunt, S., Gribble, N., Ashby, S., & Mathieu, E. (2018). Simulated versus traditional occupational therapy placements: A randomised controlled trial. *Australian Occupational Therapy Journal, 65*(6), 556–564. https://doi.org/10.1111/1440-1630.12513

Occupational Therapy Australia. (2010). *Australian Minimum Competency Standards for New Graduate Occupational Therapists.* http://www.otaus.com.au/sitebuilder/aboutus/knowledge/asset/files/16/australian_minimum_ competency_standards_for_new_grad_occupational_therapists.pdf

Occupational Therapy Board of Australia. (2018). *Australian Occupational Therapy Competency Standards.* https://www.occupationaltherapyboard.gov.au/codes-guidelines/competencies.aspx

Occupational Therapy Council of Australia. (2018). *Accreditation Standards for Australian Entry-level Occupational Therapy Education Programs.* https://www.otcouncil.com.au/wp-content/uploads/OTC-Accred-Stds-Dec2018-effective-Jan2020.pdf

Overton, A., Clark, M., & Thomas, Y. (2009) A review of non-traditional occupational therapy practice placement education: A focus on role-emerging and project placements. *British Journal of Occupational Therapy, 72*(7), 294–301. https://doi.org/10.1177/030802260907200704

Parliament of Australia & Tune, D. (2019). *Review of the National Disability Insurance Scheme Act 2013; Removing red tape and implementing the NDIS participant service guarantee.* Government of Australia. https://www.dss.gov.au/sites/default/files/documents/01_2020/ndis-act-review-final-accessibility-and-prepared-publishing1.pdf

Productivity Commission. (2011). *Disability care and support.* https://www.pc.gov.au/inquiries/completed/disability

Reeves, S., Perrier, L., Goldman, J., Freeth, D., & Zwarenstein, M. (2013) Interprofessional education: Effects on professional practice and healthcare outcomes. *Cochrane Database of Systematic Reviews, 3.* CD002213. https//doi.org/10.1002/14651858.CD002213.pub3

Rodger, S., Bennett, S., Fitzgerald, C. & Neads, P. (2010). *Use of simulated learning activities in occupational therapy curriculum.* Health Workforce Australia.

Rodger, S., Thomas, Y., Dickson, D., McBryde, C., Broadbridge, J., Hawkins, R., & Edwards, A. (2007). Putting students to work: Valuing fieldwork placements as a mechanism for recruitment and shaping the future occupational therapy workforce. *Australian Occupational Therapy Journal, 54*(s1), S94–S97. https://doi.org/10.1111/j.1440-1630.2007.00691.x

Russi, M. V. (2014). NDIS and occupational therapy: Compatible in intention and purpose from a consumer perspective. *Australian Occupational Therapy Journal, 61*, 364–370. https://doi.org/10.1111/1440-1630.12138

Stewart, M. (2017). Stuck in the middle: The impact of collaborative interprofessional communication on patient expectations. *Shoulder and Elbow, 10*(1), 66–72. https://doi.org/10.1177/1758573217735325

Taylor, R. R., & Kielhofner, G. (2017). *Kielhofner's Model of Human Occupation: Theory and application* (5th edn). Lippincott Williams & Wilkins.

Townsend, E., & Polatajko, H. (2013). *Enabling occupation II: Advancing occupational therapy vision for health, well-being and justice through occupation* (2nd edn). CAOT Publications ACE.

University of Queensland. (2008). *Student Practice Evaluation Form—Revised Edition (SPEF-R)*. https://spef-r.shrs.uq.edu.au/

World Federation of Occupational Therapists. (2016). *Minimum Standards for the Education of Occupational Therapists (Revised 2016)*. https://www.wfot.org/assets/resources/COPYRIGHTED-World-Federation-of-Occupational-Therapists-Minimum-Standards-for-the-Education-of-Occupational-Therapists-2016a.pdf#:~:text=The%20World%20Federation%20of%20Occupational%20Therapists%20%28WFOT%29%20Minimum,quality%20assurance%20for%20development%20beyond%20the%20levels%20specified

14 Research in occupational therapy

Helen Bourke-Taylor, Ted Brown and Lisa O'Brien

Chapter objectives

Upon completion of this chapter, the reader will be able to:

- Describe the contribution that research makes to underpin and justify occupational therapy education and practice in Australia.
- Explain the purpose of different methodologies commonly used by occupational therapy researchers.
- Highlight the importance of becoming an informed and skilled research consumer as an occupational therapy student and professional.

Key terms

research; evidence–based practice; qualitative research; quantitative research

Introduction

Research has a non-negotiable place within the field of occupational therapy. There are three key reasons why occupational therapists and students need to recognise and understand the importance of research within the field: professional, legal and ethical obligations/requirements.

From a competency perspective, new graduates must possess attributes that include the ability to incorporate high-level research evidence and reasoning into professional practice, maintain competency as a practitioner through lifelong learning and professional development activities, and contribute to the development and evaluation of services; all of which rely on the application of research skills (Occupational Therapy Australia, 2010). From a legal perspective, registration within Australia requires practitioners to maintain current knowledge and be capable of deciding what actions are most appropriate within their clinical practice. Registration of occupational therapists with the Australian Health Practitioner Regulation Agency (AHPRA) and the Occupational Therapy Board of Australia (OTBA) is about protecting members of the public and consumers of health care services from harmful, incompetent or unethical practice.

AHPRA mandates that occupational therapists must keep up to date with research evidence in their field of practice and provide services that are evidence-based. To be competent, registered occupational therapists in Australia requires the mastery of research skills appropriate to practice so that the services provided do more than just prevent harm. As described by Moyers (2010, p. 476), occupational therapists:

> need to focus on preventing harm by ensuring that our clients are not seriously injured during implementation of services due to practitioner neglect or malpractice due to poor risk management ... in addition, harm results when our clients receive ineffective intervention or intervention not as effective as an alternative method in improving occupational performance and participation in daily life. Harm also results from occupational therapy population or organization-based services that are poorly designed, implemented and evaluated. The harm that occurs relates to the cost-benefit of services in terms of expenditures made for poor outcomes.

Occupational therapists can assume different roles as they incorporate research into practice. Cusick and Kielhofner (2006) defined these as:

- research *producer*, involving active engagement in research that produces new knowledge for the field and beyond;
- research *collaborator*, involving being part of research as a participant, adviser, co-investigator, provider of intervention or evaluation, data collector or co-author;
- research *consumer*, providing evidence-based, informed practice with clients, programs, populations or organisations; and
- research *advocate*, involving active identification of knowledge gaps, generation of research questions, lobbying to lead investigation or evaluation of an issue that is known to be underserved and under-researched.

Both new and experienced occupational therapists need to be actively engaged in all of these roles. Occupational therapy as a profession has moved into a phase where many clinicians conduct, produce, and consume research, with some becoming expert *clinician researchers*.

History of occupational therapy research

Occupational therapy education programs in Australia were offered initially at the certificate and diploma level in the 1940s, 1950s and early 1960s by independent education providers or colleges. In the late 1960s and early 1970s, entry-level occupational therapy education moved into the university sector which enabled the initial development of a more formal and systematic body of knowledge.

Dedicated occupational therapy journals were established in Canada (*Canadian Journal of Occupational Therapy*) in 1933, in the United Kingdom (*British Journal of Occupational Therapy*) in 1938, in the United States (*American Journal of Occupational Therapy*) in 1946, and in Australia (*Australian Occupational Therapy Journal*) in 1952. The *Occupational Therapy Journal of Research*, the first journal dedicated to publishing occupational therapy-specific research, was established in 1980. Research foundations that exclusively promote and fund occupational therapy research were established in the United States (1965), Canada (1983), United Kingdom (2001) and more recently in Australia (2012).

Up until the mid-1960s, occupational therapists were mainly a profession of *knowledge borrowers* of research from other fields (e.g., medicine, biomechanics, anatomy, psychology, education). However, advancement in research production has resulted in the profession becoming *knowledge generators*. Another important shift in the profession was the development of occupation-specific theories, models and practice frameworks, providing a foundation for occupation-focused research within the discipline.

Occupational therapists in Australia made an important contribution to evidence-based practice (EBP) by creating and further expanding the OTseeker database, which is accessed by occupational therapists from around the world. This contains abstracts of systematic reviews, randomised controlled trials and other resources relevant to occupational therapy interventions. Another significant development within the Australian occupational therapy discipline was the establishment of the Occupational Therapy Australia Research Foundation (OTARF) which was officially registered as a charity in 2012. The mandate of the OTARF is to grow the research capacity—individually and collectively—of the members of OT Australia through a range of activities including grant provision, education and mentoring. The Occupational Therapy Australia Research Foundation aims to promote occupational therapy research specifically related to Australian practice, policy and education, and offers small grants, awards and scholarships, and access to various projects that contribute to this aim.

In 2017, the Occupational Therapy Australia Research Academy was started with the mandate of recognising scholars in the occupational therapy profession and enhancing research capacity building in the discipline as well as profiling the contribution of occupational therapy researchers and scholars nationally and internationally. Inductees are made a Fellow of the Occupational Therapy Australia Research Academy (FOTARA). Fourteen inaugural Fellows of the Research Academy were announced at the OTAUS 2017 national conference in Perth, Western Australisa and a further six were named at the 2019 national conference in Sydney, New South Wales.

Occupational therapy research in Australia continues to make great strides. Current and future students have enormous opportunities to assist the profession to further consolidate our position as key *knowledge producers*. Within an occupational therapy entry-to-practice degree, students learn research method and evidence-based practice skills and apply these in practice education contexts and to specific projects. Honours programs, postgraduate research thesis-based master's and doctoral degrees enable students to learn and actively participate in the generation and publication of new and original knowledge. Clinicians may complete higher degrees and subsequently remain *research collaborators and producers* in their professional roles as *clinician researchers*. Occupational therapists who work in university education programs are expected to be both educators and research *knowledge producers* by the nature of where they are employed.

Diversity and breadth of research in occupational therapy

With any research, the first step involves identifying the question to be answered; the second is to decide which research design is the best fit to answer the question posed. For example, if you want to know how effective a specific treatment (e.g., orthoses for treating wrist contractures after a stroke) is compared to no intervention, you might conduct a randomised controlled trial (see Lannin et al., 2007). If you want to gain insights about older Australians' experiences of acute hospitalisation, you might conduct a qualitative study involving in-depth interviews with older people who have been hospitalised (see Cheah & Presnell, 2011).

Evaluating complex occupational therapy interventions (i.e., those that have multiple components) can be challenging and researchers must be careful to select the appropriate design, comparison group/s and outcome measures. To guide researchers, the Medical Research Council (UK) has developed a framework for the development and evaluation of complex interventions (Craig et al., 2008; 2019). Another essential aspect of occupational therapy research is including the consumer or client's perspective. The most effective research includes consumers as co-researchers, with meaningful engagement across all stages including research design (Bagley et al., 2016). This may make translation and application of findings more effective (Pizzo et al., 2015).

There are many different research design methodologies offering a range of ways to contribute to our professional knowledge. It is vital for occupational therapists to understand the different methodologies so that, when examining research, they can critique the design and rigour in the study so that translation to practice may be achieved. This section will outline the most commonly used methodologies in occupational therapy research and provide brief examples from within the profession (see Table 14.1). It is important to note that, after a study has been designed and before any participant recruitment and data collection is allowed to occur, it is necessary for the project to undergo a thorough assessment and gain approval from a human ethics review board. Ethics approval is never granted unless the rights, vulnerabilities, risks, dignity and interests of the participants involved in the study are considered.

Table 14.1 Examples of occupational therapy research and different research designs

Research method	Brief definition	Example of occupational therapy research	Summary of study
Quantitative			
Systematic review	A systematic review is a critical assessment and combined evaluation of the available evidence (usually RCTs or clinically controlled studies) on a particular assessment or intervention. It is usually focused on a clinical question, and aims to identify, appraise, select and synthesise all high-quality research evidence relevant to that question.	Cole, T. et al. (2019). Effectiveness of interventions to improve therapy adherence in people with upper limb conditions: A systematic review. *Journal of Hand Therapy, 32*(2), 175–183.	This review aimed to determine the effectiveness of interventions to improve treatment adherence in people with upper limb conditions and to report on outcome measures used when reporting adherence. It carefully selected and appraised the quality of all eligible trials according to specific criteria. Results were extracted from each study and pooled for meta-analysis where possible. The authors concluded that behavioural approaches may help to achieve adherence in chronic conditions; however, there is insufficient evidence for any adherence interventions in acute conditions. They also recommended reliable valid measures of adherence for future research.

Research method	Brief definition	Example of occupational therapy research	Summary of study
Randomised Control Trial (RCT)	A planned experiment comparing the efficacy of an intervention against that of a 'control'. Participants are randomly allocated and groups are comparable at baseline; therefore, differences in outcomes after treatment can be attributed to the true effects of the treatment that the experimental group received with confidence.	James, S. et al. (2015). Randomized controlled trial of web-based multimodal therapy for unilateral cerebral palsy to improve occupational performance. *Developmental Medicine & Child Neurology, 57(6),* 530–538.	This matched-pairs waitlist-control randomised controlled trial aimed to evaluate the effectiveness of a web-based therapy program in children with unilateral cerebral palsy on occupational performance, upper limb function, and visual perception. The intervention group demonstrated significantly greater post-intervention scores than the comparison group on most measures, but they were not clinically meaningful. There were no differences between groups on measures of impaired upper limb function.
Cohort study	A cohort is any group of people who are similar in some way (e.g., have the same condition and were treated with a particular therapy) and followed over time. Researchers measure what happens to a group that were exposed to a specific variable and then compare them to a similar group that has not been exposed to that variable. They can be prospective (the researcher collects data at a future date after exposure) or retrospective (the researcher collects data from past records to see if an outcome happened).	Rosenwax, L. et al. (2015). Community-based palliative care is associated with reduced emergency department use by people with dementia in their last year of life: A retrospective cohort study. *Palliative Medicine, 29(8),* 727–736.	The aim of this study was to describe patterns in the use of hospital emergency departments in the last year of life by people who died with dementia and whether this was modified by use of community-based palliative care. The researchers compared records of all people living in Western Australia who died with dementia in a two-year period (dementia cohort; $N = 5261$) with a comparative cohort of decedents without dementia who died from other conditions amenable to palliative care ($N = 2685$). Researchers found that > 70% of both the dementia and comparative cohorts attended hospital emergency departments in the last year of life, but only 6 per cent of the dementia cohort used community-based palliative care compared to 26 per cent of the comparative cohort. They concluded that

(Continued)

Research method	Brief definition	Example of occupational therapy research	Summary of study
			community-based palliative care of people who die with or of dementia is relatively infrequent but associated with significant reductions in hospital emergency department use in the last year of life, particularly in the final weeks.
Single Subject Experimental Design (SCED)	One participant (or unit, e.g., a hospital ward) is studied in an experiment in which the person (or unit) acts as their own control. Measurement of the outcome variables is repeated at different times, usually at baseline and after the intervention, to determine whether the outcome has been affected by the delivered intervention.	Hayner, K. A. et al. (2012). Effectiveness of the California Tri-Pull Taping method for shoulder subluxation poststroke: A single-subject ABA design. *American Journal of Occupational Therapy, 66,* 727–736.	This study evaluated the effectiveness of the California Tri-Pull Taping method for clients with post-stroke inferior subluxation of the glenohumeral joint. It involved ten participants who were followed for nine weeks using an interrupted time series quasi-experimental single-subject ABA design to examine shoulder pain, activities of daily living (ADL) function, active range of motion, tape comfort and subluxation.

Qualitative

Grounded theory	This theory is constructed through the analysis of data. Data are the stories told through in-depth interviewing and other collected data. This inductive methodology requires a systematic and objective analysis of peoples' experiences to derive a theoretical framework or model.	Crawford, E. et al. (2016). The structural-personal interaction: Occupational deprivation and asylum seekers in Australia. *Journal of Occupational Science, 23*(3), 321–338.	This study examined asylum seekers' experiences in Australia using constructivist grounded theory. Researchers combined field notes from ten months of weekly participant observation, 11 formal interviews, 34 survey responses and four policy documents to identify a substantive theory: the Structural-Personal Interaction (SPI). The SPI explains how occupational deprivation arises from an interaction between social structures (citizenship status and policy) and the asylum seekers' personal characteristics.

Research method	Brief definition	Example of occupational therapy research	Summary of study
Phenomenology	Phenomenological researchers are interested in the way people experience their world, and how best to understand their experiences.	Lim, J. et al. (2016). Experiences of international students from Asian backgrounds studying occupational therapy in Australia. *Australian Occupational Therapy Journal*, *63*(5), 303–211.	This study aimed to explore and describe the experiences of international students from Asian backgrounds studying occupational therapy in Australia. A phenomenological approach involving in-depth interviews with eight participants was used, and data were analysed using hermeneutic (i.e. interpretive rather than purely descriptive) methods. The researchers found that OT theory was seen as compatible with participants' home cultures; however, application was seen as problematic due to the structural and cultural differences between health care systems. The students had made adaptations to fit in as occupational therapy students in Australia, but continued to see themselves as different. These adaptations also changed how they saw themselves in relation to their home culture, raising concerns about the effort required to fit back in and belong again.
Ethnography	A thorough method for constructing knowledge and understanding about the shared culture and experience of a group of people called 'key informants'.	Haines, C. et al. (2010). Participation in the risk-taking occupation of skateboarding. *Journal of Occupational Science*, *17*(4), 239–245.	This study used in-depth interviews with seven active skateboarders to describe the values, behaviours, beliefs and attitudes to injury in order to understand the meaning and identity derived from the occupation. The authors presented a chronology of participation in this risk-taking occupation and highlight that the core values of freedom and striving to achieve one's best outweigh the risk of injury inherent to participation in the occupation.

(Continued)

Research method	Brief definition	Example of occupational therapy research	Summary of study
Narrative	A narrative study takes the form of an account, over time, of an event, action or experience that is experienced by a person or group. A narrative study draws on multiple data sources and may be a collection of stories that compare lived experience or may shed light on some aspect of the person or identity of the person participating. This method may study life course experience in a time-captured period or across time. Narratives originate in the social science and humanities.	Hewitt, A. et al. (2010). Retirement: What will you do? A narrative inquiry of occupation based planning for retirement: Implications for practice. *Australian Occupational Therapy Journal*, 57, 8–15.	This retrospective narrative study involved the experience of four older people's decision to plan for the activities they would undertake once retired, the planning process and subsequent experience of retirement. Paradigmatic-type narrative analysis led to the development of categories and subsequent themes to reveal the participants' experiences of these issues: environmental influences (families, finances), the planning process and retirement experiences. Application to the role of occupational therapists in successfully planning for retirement were presented.
Participatory Action Research (PAR)	PAR usually involves a process in which a group of researchers actively reflect on a problem that they encounter in everyday practice. After identifying and critically examining the key issues, the researchers form a strategy or plan to improve the situation. The next stage of the research process is to implement the plan and, after a period of time,	Kramer-Roy, D. et al. (2012). Supporting ethnic minority families with disabled children: Learning from Pakistani families. *British Journal of Occupational Therapy*, 75(10), 442–448.	This study aimed to describe the support needs of six Pakistani families with disabled children in the United Kingdom. After an exploratory phase of individual interviews and activities, three action research groups (women, men, and non-disabled siblings) were formed; each group then engaged in their own research activities. They found that a lack of belonging in their community affected families' well-being, and that faith was an important, mostly positive, aspect of their sense of being.

Research method	Brief definition	Example of occupational therapy research	Summary of study
	evaluate its impact (i.e., what changes were made?). This reflection–action–evaluation cycle may be repeated several times, leading to deeper knowledge and evolution of practice.		
Psychometric	Overview of multiple psychometric evaluations— reliability and validity (see Chapter 25)	Hodges, A. et al. (2018). Evaluating the psychometric quality of school connectedness measures: A systematic review. *PLoS ONE, 13*(9), e0203373.	This was a systematic review of 19 journal articles detailing the psychometric properties of self-report measures of affective, cognitive and behavioural aspects of 15 school connectedness for students aged six to 14 years. Conducted by occupational therapists interested in a sense of school connectedness experienced by young children with autism, this article systematically and thoroughly critiqued recently published studies that evaluated the psychometric properties defined by COSMIN.).

Qualitative research

Qualitative research 'fundamentally depends on watching people in their own territory and interacting with them in their own language on their own terms' (Miller & Kirk, 1986, p. 9). Its methodologies aim to develop an 'understanding of the meaning and experience dimensions of human lives and their social worlds' (Fossey et al., 2002, p. 717).

Qualitative research is attractive to occupational therapists as it is, by its very nature, client-centred, providing evidence of the ways people live and experience an aspect of life where there would otherwise perhaps only be numerical findings. Data collection can involve any of the following approaches alone or in combination: interviews (individual or group); structured or unstructured observation; researcher self-reflection; and document analysis, including text, photographs or journals. There are many different design frameworks in qualitative research, including (but not limited to) phenomenology, ethnography, grounded theory, narrative, case study and participatory action research (see Table 14.1 for more explanation and examples).

Quantitative research

Chapter 15 has additional information regarding evidence-based practice. The basic strategy in quantitative research is to compare groups of people according to an outcome of interest. Study designs can be broadly classified as either *experimental* or *non-experimental* (also known as *observational*). The purpose of conducting the research can also be used to classify it as either *descriptive* or *analytical*. Figure 14.1 illustrates these classifications and the relative strength of the evidence derived from each study design.

Beginning with experimental studies, the most scientifically rigorous design is the randomised controlled trial (RCT). The main advantage of this design is that random assignment tends to make the groups comparable both in terms of measured characteristics and characteristics that were not or could not be measured (Cox & Reid, 2000). The disadvantages include the ethical issues associated with conducting an experiment where participants do not get to choose their own treatment. Similarly, RCTs are costly, labour-intensive, time-consuming, and complex to conduct. The RCT design is not always feasible for some occupational therapy intervention approaches or client groups due to the ethical and practical considerations related to care and/or service delivery. Chapter 15 provides more information about evaluating interventions and accumulating evidence.

Other types of experimental studies include the single case experimental design (SCED) and multiple baseline design, both involving measuring change within a person or group by comparing them to themselves after intervention and over time (Evans et al., 2014). In SCEDs, measurement is repeated at predetermined times to detect whether the intervention affects the outcome variables of interest.

When it is not ethical or feasible to conduct an experiment (for example, when the intervention could involve risk, the condition is rare, or outcomes take a long time to become evident), the effects of treatments can be examined using an observational study. It is possible to identify cause-and-effect relationships in cohort and case–control studies by comparing outcomes in treated and control groups (Rosenbaum, 2002). Another

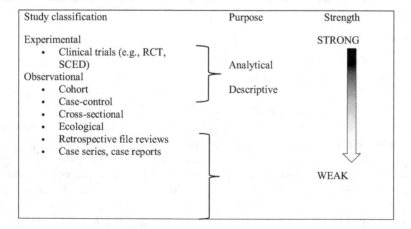

Figure 14.1 Classification, purpose and strength of evidence for different research designs.
Note: (RCT = Randomised controlled trial; SCED = Single case experimental design)

observational design frequently used in occupational therapy is the cross-sectional study where data is collected at one point in time from a sample of people. This is a quick and inexpensive way to measure the prevalence of a particular phenomenon, and is often used for an initial exploration of a hypothesis. Disadvantages include difficulties recruiting a representative sample, and inability to draw causal inferences from the data, as there is no temporal relationship between exposure and outcome.

Mixed methods

Mixed methods provide researchers with multiple ways of seeing and understanding participants' perspectives and effective elements of interventions or situations. This is described as 'triangulation of data' which means that the mixed methods design provides a triangular view of the issue under investigation through multiple types of overlapping data that confirm and explain the phenomenon under study (i.e., data available in numbers and words). It is a research approach where 'a researcher or team of researchers combines elements of qualitative and quantitative approaches (e.g., use of qualitative viewpoints, data collection, analysis, inference techniques) for the purposes of breadth and depth of understanding and corroboration' (Creswell & Plano Clark, 2011, p. 5). There may be multiple phases of a study. Researchers employing such methods are driven to answer questions about 'how many', 'how effective', 'how common', as well as how people experience health and life situations.

Mixed methods can be used to design an instrument or measurement tool, with the qualitative component determining which aspects are important to people (Creswell, 2014). Creswell and Plano Clark (2011) discuss several commonly used mixed methods designs including the convergent design, where researchers collect both types of data at the same time within the same project and merge findings, and sequential styles, where one type of data is collected first followed by the other. For example, the explanatory sequential design involves collecting quantitative data in phase 1 of the study, followed by qualitative data in phase 2 of the study. The qualitative study further explores findings from phase 1 and gathers participants' contextual and real-life experiences to explain relationships that were revealed in the initial study (Creswell & Plano Clark, 2011). In contrast, an exploratory mixed methods study will investigate the topic using a qualitative study in phase 1; phase 2 then builds on phase 1 to quantitatively explore or evaluate the issue under study (Creswell & Plano Clark, 2011). The exploratory design may be used when researchers are developing instruments in phase 2. Phase 1 of such a model informs the content of the instrument that is then tested in phase 2. This method of instrument design is called an instrument development variant (Creswell & Plano Clark, 2011).

Assessment, evaluation, reliability and validity

Measurement of the variables involved in a research project requires the use of psychometrically sound measurement tools (Brown, 2012). Chapter 25 has more information about assessment in occupational therapy. The research underpinning sound measurement tools is another body of research within the occupational therapy profession. In clinical practice, occupational therapists need to be conversant with the research evidence supporting the use of the assessment tools and outcome measures that they select to use with clients. For example, occupational therapists routinely assess clients and evaluate progress using established clinical measurement tools.

The terms assessment and evaluation are used inconsistently and interchangeably in the literature, leading to some confusion about what they actually mean. The definitions used here are consistent with the Occupational Therapy Practice Framework—third edition (OTPF-III; AOTA, 2017). *Assessment* involves information gathering, relative to some known objective or goal. *Evaluation* is 'the process of obtaining and interpreting data necessary for intervention. This includes planning for and documenting the evaluation process and results' (AOTA, 2005, p. 663). Evaluation is a process that involves administering assessments, interpreting the findings, and formulating hypotheses about what might work in intervention based on the results of the assessments (Mulligan, 2003).

When selecting an outcome measure or assessment tool, researchers and clinicians need to consult a standardised framework to ensure that the tool is reliable, valid, responsive and clinically useful. A previous lack of consensus on terminology and definitions of measurement properties created confusion over relevant properties and what they actually represent. An international consensus for the definition of these terms has been reached through the COSMIN (COnsensus-based Standards for the selection of health Measurement INstruments) initiative (Mokkink et al., 2018a; 2018b). The standardisation of measurement terminology included in the COSMIN provides a complete picture of how properties relate to one another. Researchers in occupational therapy have demonstrated that they find the COSMIN useful when evaluating the properties of measures as evidenced by a special issue on measurement in the *Australian Occupational Therapy Journal* in October 2018.

Reliability refers to the ability of a test to collect data consistently or the 'degree to which the measurement is free from measurement error' (Mokkink et al., 2010). Specific subtypes of reliability include internal consistency, correlations between subscales and total scale score, test–retest reliability, intra-rater reliability, inter-rater reliability and split-half reliability. Usually a test needs to have established validity before its reliability can be investigated.

Validity refers to how well the items of a test represent the construct, attribute or dimension it purports to measure. Subtypes of validity include content validity, criterion validity, and construct validity (Mokkink et al., 2010).

Responsiveness denotes the ability of an 'instrument to detect change over time in the construct to be measured' while *interpretability* is how meaningful change is clinically (Mokkink et al., 2010). It is important to understand these concepts when selecting assessment tools for use in occupational therapy practice as well as research. See Chapter 25 for more information.

Evidence-based practice and research

Evidence-based practice (EBP) refers to the use of research findings to underpin health care practitioners' decision-making and clinical reasoning. Chapter 15 provides specific information about EBP; hence this chapter provides an overview. EBP considers the best available evidence, the clinician's prior experience, and the preferences and expectations of the client/patient and family (Sackett et al., 1996). Occupational therapists must therefore be skilled at sourcing, critiquing, translating and applying research evidence to back up their day-to-day professional practice. Therapists also need to be skilled at explaining the best evidence using terminology that clients and families will understand.

Therapists draw on their own clinical experience when collaborating with the client and family to apply evidence. Therapists attend continuing education events such as short courses, seminars, symposiums and conferences to hear about the latest evidence and advancements in their field. They can also access professional publications such as books, journals, websites and publications. The Cochrane Collaboration publishes high-quality systematic reviews and meta-analyses so that the public and professionals can readily access information that has already been synthesised and summarised. One source of occupational therapy specific journals is OTDBase and one database that critiques and rates the quality of studies is OTseeker. Other credible databases that occupational therapists often refer to for evidence are listed in Table 14.2.

Relationship between occupational therapy research and EBP

The relationship between occupational therapy research and EBP is cyclical and interlinked. When occupational therapists complete a study and publish the findings, this contributes to the overall body of profession-specific knowledge. Occupational therapists who are searching the literature can then access, critique and apply this new knowledge. If a clinician comes up with a question and searches the relevant databases but cannot find any evidence (or the existing evidence sourced is insufficient), then this can lead to the generation of further research questions that need to be answered. In sum, research provides the evidence that therapists can refer to but EBP can also generate further research questions that require investigation in the future.

Table 14.2 Key databases and specific occupational therapy and allied health examples

Databases	*EBP-specific databases*
• CINAHL Plus: Cumulative Index to Nursing and Allied Health Literature • PsycInfo • OVID Emcare • MEDLINE • Proquest • AMED: Allied and complementary medicine • SCOPUS • ERIC: Education Resources Information Center • Embase • DARE: Database of Abstracts of Reviews of Effectiveness	• OTseeker: http://www.otseeker.com/default.aspx • OT-CATS: http://www.otcats.com • Evidence Exchange for OT Critically Appraised Topics: http://www.aota.org/Practice/Researchers/Evidence-Exchange.aspx • Centre for Evidence-Based Rehabilitation: http://www.srs-mcmaster.ca/Default.aspx?tabid=630 • Joanna Briggs Institute (Australia): http://www.joannabriggs.edu.au • Centre for Evidence-Based Medicine (Canada): http://www.cebm.utoronto.ca • Centre for Evidence-Based Medicine (UK): http://www.cebm.net • Centre for Evidence- Based Mental Health: http://www.cebmh.com • Cochrane Collaboration: http://www.cochrane.org • PEDro—Physiotherapy Evidence Database: http://www.pedro.org.au • PsycBITE: http://www.PsycBITE.com • Rehab+: http://plus.mcmaster.ca/rehab • speechBITE: http://www.speechbite.com

In practice, however, it's important to be aware that some practitioners are resistant to EBP (Cusick & Kielhofner, 2006; Hoffman et al., 2010). Research has shown that even when occupational therapists learn to peruse evidence and have improved knowledge of the research pertaining to a clinical area, many retain non-research informed strategies with regard to decision-making in clinical practice (Campbell et al., 2013).

Funding occupational therapy research in Australia

There are several sources of research funding in Australia, including government, institutional, private/corporate and philanthropic. The most common types of grants include scholarships for postgraduate study; travel grants to visit another research centre or attend conferences; project grants and fellowships. Fellowships are often targeted at those who have completed doctoral studies.

For novice researchers, it is helpful to search databases such as the one provided on the Health Practitioner Research page of Queensland Health's website (https://www.health.qld.gov.au/hpresearch) to find grants that are appropriate to the applicant's skills and qualifications. Some large institutions (such as universities, hospitals, not-for-profit agencies, private companies, non-governmental organisations, employers or charitable foundations) have grants aimed at helping early career researchers to get started. Those pursuing a research career can also register with grant search databases such as Research Professional (www.researchprofessional.com) to get regular emails regarding grants that fit their profile and interests.

For occupational therapists working in organisations that offer direct services to clients such as schools, not-for-profit organisations or community centres, there are a large number of philanthropic grants available to fund research. The primary intent of such funding is to benefit a group of under-served Australians in need. Philanthropic trusts and funding bodies prefer and select programs and research projects that have a high translation impact, meaning that real people will benefit in the short and long term.

For experienced researchers, the main sources of funding include the Australian Research Council (ARC) and the National Health and Medical Research Council (NHMRC). Both have individual researcher-support schemes (such as post-graduate scholarships or Investigator grants) and project grant funding. Both the ARC and NHMRC are very competitive funding schemes and the success rates for applications to both are low. Another source of funding for tertiary level education research is the federal government Office for Learning and Teaching (OLT) grant program.

Conclusion

This chapter introduced an exciting part of your future professional life. Acquiring the skill to develop a research question, design a study or search for evidence to answer a clinical question is essential. Occupational therapy is a unique discipline and our central concern is occupation, based on our philosophical and theoretical foundations. This means that our primary intentions are to improve the client's capacity to participate in the daily occupation that they want, need and are required to participate in (Gustafsson et al., 2014). This is the essential focus of application of evidence—will this intervention/program/service improve the client's occupational performance?

The new generation of occupational therapists must develop advanced understanding and skills in critical evaluation of research, and choose to actively apply their knowledge for the benefit of consumers. The future of our profession as a scientifically sound discipline is relying on you to make your unique contribution as a research producer, collaborator, consumer or advocate.

Summary

- It is imperative that all occupational therapy students and practitioners are informed consumers and users of research evidence.
- Occupational therapy as a profession has moved from a field of knowledge borrowers to a dynamic profession of knowledge generators.
- Occupational therapists often undertake quantitative, qualitative and mixed methods research studies.
- The validity and reliability of assessment tools are important to ensure that meaning and relevant data can be generated.

Review questions

1. Explain three ways that exploratory research differs from efficacy research and justify the need for both types of research in the occupational therapy profession.
2. What type of research provides occupational therapists with knowledge about lived experience and informs client-centred practice?
3. Do new graduate occupational therapists need to be able to evaluate the strengths and limitations of published research that relates to their clients? Explain and justify your answer.

References

American Occupational Therapy Association (AOTA). (2005). Standards of practice for occupational therapy. *American Journal of Occupational Therapy, 59*, 663–665. https://doi.org/10.5014/ajot.59.6.663

American Occupational Therapy Association (AOTA). (2017). Occupational Therapy Practice Framework: Domain and Process, 3rd edition. *American Journal of Occupational Therapy, 68*(Supp. no. 1), S1–S48. https://doi.org/10.5014/ajot.2014.682006

Bagley, H. J, Short, H., Harman, N. L., Hickey, H. R., Gamble, C. L., Woolfall, K., Young, B., & Williamson, P. R. (2016). A patient and public involvement (PPI) toolkit for meaningful and flexible involvement in clinical trials—a work in progress. *Research Involvement and Engagement, 2*, 15. https://doi.org/10.1186/s40900-016-0029-8

Brown, T. (2012). Assessment, measurement, and evaluation/Why can't I do what everyone expects me to do? In S. J. Lane & A. C. Bundy (Eds.), *Kids can be kids: A childhood occupations approach* (pp. 320–348). F. A. Davis Co.

Campbell, L., Novak, I., McIntyre, S., & Lord, S. (2013). A KT intervention including the evidence alert system to improve clinician's evidence-based practice behaviour: A cluster randomised controlled trial. *Implementation Science, 8*, 132–138. https://doi.org/10.1186/1748-5908-8-132

Cheah, S., & Presnell, S. (2011). Older people's experiences of acute hospitalisation: An investigation of how occupations are affected. *Australian Occupational Therapy Journal, 58*(2), 120–128. https://doi.org/10.1111/j.1440-1630.2010.00878.x

Cox, D. R., & Reid, N. (2000). *The theory of the design of experiments.* CRC Press.

Craig, P., Dieppe, P., Macintyre, S., Michie, S., Nazareth, I., & Petticrew, M. (2008). Developing and evaluating complex interventions: The new Medical Research Council guidance. *British Medical Journal, 337*, a1655. https://doi.org/10.1136/bmj.a1655

Craig, P, Dieppe, P., Macintyre, S., Michie, S., Nazareth, I., & Petticrew, M. (2019). *Developing and evaluating complex interventions*. Medical Research Council. https://mrc.ukri.org/documents/pdf/complex-interventions-guidance/

Creswell, J. L., & Plano Clark, V. (2011). *Designing and conducting mixed methods research*. Sage Publications.

Creswell, J. W. (2014). *Research design: Qualitative, quantitative and mixed methods approaches* (4th edn). Sage Publications.

Cusick, A., & Kielhofner, G. (2006). Professional responsibility and roles in research. In G. Kielhofner (Ed.), *Research in occupational therapy: Methods of inquiry for enhancing practice* (pp. 46–57). F. A. Davis Co.

Evans, J. J., Gast, D. L., Perdices, M., & Manolov, R. (2014). Single case experimental designs: Introduction to a special issue of Neuropsychological Rehabilitation. *Neuropsychological Rehabilitation, 24*(3–4), 305–314. https://doi.org/10.1080/09602011.2014.903198

Fossey, E., Harvey, C., Mcdermott, F., & Davidson, L. (2002). Understanding and evaluating qualitative research. *Australian and New Zealand Journal of Psychiatry, 36*, 717–732. https://doi.org/10.1046/j.1440-1614.2002.01100.x

Gustafsson, L., Molineux, M., & Bennett, S. (2014). Contemporary occupational therapy practice: The challenges of being evidence based and philosophically congruent. *Australian Occupational Therapy Journal, 61*(2), 121–123. https://doi.org/10.1111/1440-1630.12110

Hoffman, T., Bennett, S., & Del Mar, C. (2010). *Evidence-based practice across the health professions*. Churchill Livingstone.

Lannin, N. A., Cusick, A., McClusky, A., & Herbert, R. D. (2007). Effects of splinting on wrist contracture after stroke: A randomized controlled trial. *Stroke, 38*, 111–116. https://doi.org/10.1161/01.STR.0000251722.77088.12

Miller, M. L., & Kirk, J. (1986). *Reliability and validity in qualitative research*. Sage Publications.

Mokkink, L. B., Terwee, C. B., Patrick, D. L., Alonso, J., Stratford, P. W., Knol, D. L., Bouter, L. M., & de Wet, H. C. W. (2010). The COSMIN Study reached international consensus on taxonomy, terminology, and definitions of measurement properties for health-related patient-reported outcomes. *Journal of Clinical Epidemiology, 63*(7), 737–745. https://doi.org.10.1016/j.jclinepi.2010.02.006

Mokkink, L. B., de Wet, H. C. W., Prinsen, C. A. C., Patrick, D. L., Alonso, J., Bouter, L. M., & Terwee, C. B. (2018a). COSMIN risk of bias checklist for systematic reviews of patient-reported outcome measures. *Quality of Life Research, 27*(5), 1171–1179. https://doi.org/10.1007/s11136-017-1765-4

Mokkink, L. B., Prinsen, C. A. C., Patrick, D. L., Alonso, J., Bouter, L. M., de Wet, H. C. W, & Terwee, C. B. (2018b). *COSMIN methodology for systematic reviews of patient-reported outcome measures (PROMs)—User manual (version 1.0)*. https://www.cosmin.nl/wp-content/uploads/COSMIN-syst-review-for-PROMs-manual_version-1_feb-2018.pdf

Moyers, P. A. (2010). Competence and professional development. In K. Sladyk, K. Jacobs, & N. MacRae (Eds.), *Occupational therapy essentials for clinical competence* (pp. 749–764). SLACK Inc.

Mulligan, S. (2003). *Occupational therapy evaluation for children: A pocket guide*. Lippincott Williams & Wilkins.

Occupational Therapy Australia. (2010). *Australian Minimum Competency Standards for New Graduate Occupational Therapists*. https://www.otaus.com.au/sitebuilder/aboutus/knowledge/asset/files/16/australian_minimum_competency_standards_for_new_grad_occupational_therapists.pdf>

Pizzo, E., Doyle, C., Matthews, R., & Barlow, J. (2015). Patient and public involvement: How much do we spend and what are the benefits? *Health Expectations, 18*(6), 1918–1926. https://doi.org/10.1111/hex.12204

Rosenbaum, P. R. (2002). *Observational studies*. Springer.

Sackett, D. L., Rosenberg, W. M., Gray, J. A., Haynes, R. B., & Richardson, W. S. (1996). Evidence-based medicine: What it is and what it isn't. *British Medical Journal, 312*, 71–72. https://doi.org/10.1136/bmj.312.7023.71

15 Evidence-based practice in occupational therapy

Reinie Cordier and Sarah Wilkes-Gillan

Chapter objectives

Upon completion of this chapter, the reader will be able to:

*   Define the concept of evidence-based practice and its importance to occupational therapy practice.
*   Explain the three-step process of locating, analysing and applying evidence.
*   Differentiate between tools to appraise the quality of the evidence.
*   Discuss current and future direction of evidence-based practice in the clinical context.
*   Identify areas of research waste and discuss solutions to avoid research waste.
*   Explain the importance of knowledge translation.

Key terms

evidence-based practice; level of evidence; methodological quality, knowledge translation

Introduction

Evidence-based practice (EBP) is fundamental to occupational therapy practice. EBP has been defined as: 'the conscientious, explicit, and judicious use of current best evidence in making decisions about the care of individual patients' (Sackett et al., 1996, p. 71). EBP combines the concepts of scientific research-based knowledge and individual practitioner knowledge to provide the most effective, client-centred health care to our clients. As occupational therapists we assist clients with complex health care needs. As such we often have clinical questions such as: 'Has the intervention that I plan on using with my client been shown to be effective for people with similar health conditions?'; 'How many intervention sessions does my client need before I can expect to see some observable improvements?'; and 'Is the intervention I'm seeing delivered while on clinical placement effective for the client?' or 'Will this intervention be as effective for my client once they are discharged from the hospital and are at home?' Using an EBP approach ensures we are seeking to answer these clinical questions and results in our clients receiving the best and most up-to-date treatment. EBP also facilitates client-centred decision-making and assists us to manage rapid changes in knowledge and to manage the information available to us (Bennett & Bennett, 2000).

It is worth noting at this point that reference is made to both EBP and evidence-informed practice in literature, two related constructs. EBP means that research is conducted through validated scientific processes that can be extensive and complex. This process is what most people think of when thinking about research, as in creating an answerable question, searching for evidence, evaluating for validity, integrating what has been found, and then evaluating outcomes (Woodbury & Kuhnke, 2014). Most often evidence-based research is seen in clinical settings, as studies can be controlled and evaluated more effectively. Evidence-informed practice means various practice settings use research that is already available and has been tested and applied. This evidence is then combined with the experiences and expertise of the practice setting to best fit the population served (Woodbury & Kuhnke, 2014). For the purpose of this chapter we will refer to EBP, whilst acknowledging the importance of co-production in research and evaluating the appropriateness of interventions and services by incorporating the perspectives of service users.

On an applied level, EBP assists our clinical reasoning and decision-making process, therefore influencing 'what we do' and 'why we do it'. As shown in Figure 15.1, EBP integrates the concepts of scientific knowledge (e.g., *research evidence that is currently available*), clinical expertise and experience (e.g., *what we, or our colleagues, know has or has not worked in the past with similar clients*), the client's individual circumstances (e.g., *the client's preferences, values, resources available to them*) and our practice context and resources available to us as occupational therapists (e.g., *our work setting, assessment tools and equipment used, funding, training*). When using an EBP approach, our clinical reasoning becomes more apparent and serves to reinforce our accountability to our clients, our funders and our profession. EBP also informs decision-making regarding where best to direct health resources and funding, such as whether or not to invest in a particular piece of equipment or to dedicate time to conducting a particular intervention (Hoffmann et al., 2017). This raises the importance of shared decision-making. Shared decision-making involves occupational therapists and clients collaboratively making a health-related decision after having discussed the options, the likely benefits and harms of each option, and considered the client's values, preferences and circumstances.

Once we have a clinical question, we can phrase this question into an answerable research question (refer to Chapter 13). After formulating our research question, we can use the following three-step EBP process: Step 1—locating the best available evidence; Step 2—analysing and appraising the evidence we find; and Step 3—applying the research-proven scientific evidence to our interventions for our clients. This process supports health professionals in their decision-making to eliminate ineffective, inappropriate, unnecessarily expensive and potentially harmful practices (Hamer & Collinson, 2014). It is well worth keeping in mind that as both a student and future occupational therapist you will come across some issues and research questions with limited evidence to draw from. In these situations, it is important to consider and integrate all aspects of EBP as outlined in Figure 15.1 to inform decision-making.

Step 1: Locating the evidence

This step answers the question: *How do I find good evidence?* The purpose of reviewing research and taking an EBP approach is to find the best available evidence that is specific to both the practice context in which you work and the individual needs of the client. Is there evidence that can support my decision? Is there evidence that supports the

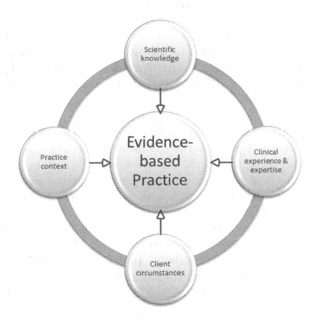

Figure 15.1 Concept of evidence-based practice.

recommendations I make to my client? Considering the accessibility to health information for clients due to the internet and an exponentially growing body of information and evidence is important. Clinicians must be able to decipher the available information and navigate the questions and concerns their clients may have based on the best possible evidence available (Hoffmann et al., 2017). Clients are likely to share information relating to their health challenge that they located from the internet and various other sources. As a clinician you need to have the skills to evaluate and interpret the findings for the client in terms of the quality of the information they provided. You also need to help them interpret often contradictory findings with varying levels of quality. This provides the client with the choice to select the most appropriate care options that are relevant to their condition or treatment.

To determine if occupational therapy students understood and valued the importance of EBP and if they planned on using it in practice, a study was conducted by Stronge and Cahill (2012) involving final-year students from four universities in Ireland in 2008. A Knowledge, Attitude and Behaviour Questionnaire was used to survey the students. All students reported that they had a clear understanding of EBP and were willing to practice EBP in the future. The majority (85 per cent) reported accessing evidence weekly or more often. The internet (28 per cent) and textbooks (27 per cent) were the most popular sources of evidence. The students listed a number of important barriers to EBP, including: difficulty in finding evidence (55 per cent), lack of time in finding evidence (31 per cent), and fieldwork educators not practising EBP (27 per cent) (Stronge & Cahill, 2012).

Similarly, most practising occupational therapists recognise the importance of EBP to guide their clinical decision-making. However, they report workload pressures and lack of time for reading as difficulties in applying this to practice. Another challenge for occupational therapists to adopt an EBP approach is the skill of literature searching and appraising, as well as interpreting the research with regard to their practice in relation to their own context and their client groups (Bennett et al., 2017). To meet the needs of those seeking to identify the best available evidence, a number of resources are available. These resources can be categorised into those that have already been appraised by experts in the area and those where the located information still needs to be appraised. Appraisal is a process where the information presented is critiqued to determine its quality.

Locating appraised evidence

Cochrane Reviews are *systematic reviews* of primary research in human health care and health policy, and are internationally recognised as the highest standard in *evidence-based health care*. They investigate the effects of interventions for prevention, treatment and rehabilitation. You can read more about Cochrane Reviews on their website (http://www.cochrane.org/what-is-cochrane-evidence).

OTseeker is a database that contains abstracts of systematic reviews, randomised controlled trials and other resources relevant to occupational therapy interventions. Most trials have been critically appraised for their validity and interpretability. In one database, OTseeker provides fast and easy access to information from a wide range of sources to inform occupational therapy. You can find more information via the web link http://www.otseeker.com.

Until 2019, the Critically Appraised Papers (CAPs) department of the *Australian Occupational Therapy Journal* published critically appraised summaries of qualitative and quantitative research relevant to occupational therapy. The main aim of this department is to keep occupational therapists up to date with recent advances relevant to their profession. This is achieved by summarising and appraising original research studies or reviews of research, which are of sound methodological quality. In June 2019, the *Australian Occupational Therapy Journal* introduced the Cochrane Corner, a knowledge translation initiative where within-discipline experts present and frame evidence from Cochrane resources in a way that will help make the awareness, accessibility and uptake of evidence relevant to professionals in the field.

Clinical practice guidelines provide a critical review of specific assessments and interventions detailing best practice and are designed to overcome the primary barrier to EBP reported by therapists: lack of time to identify the information. Clinical guidelines are usually created for a particular population group and are used within the context of practice (Heiwe et al., 2011). These guidelines involve grading systems to help you understand the quality of evidence and apply the information to your own practice. Clinical practice guidelines support clinicians when implementing a new approach and organisational approaches. Guidelines can help occupational therapists to consider the context within which the intervention is performed or interventions for other health professionals when working in an interdisciplinary team (Bayley et al., 2012; Van't Leven et al., 2012). An important component of guidelines is to consider the lack of evidence and to report the most important findings from the scientific evidence base as a set of implementable actions (Kelly & Bonnefoy, 2007). Clinical guidelines can also provide support for occupational therapy programs.

Locating evidence that still requires appraisal

Using library database searches, you can also find peer-reviewed journal articles about research. There are a number of databases available, each with a specific focus.

The Cumulative Index to Nursing and Allied Health Literature (CINAHL), PsycINFO, ERIC, Proquest, Embase, SCOPUS, PubMed, Medline and Web of Science are databases commonly used by occupational therapists. If you are a student or practitioner, access to these databases will be provided via your university or local health service library. These databases will give you access to research evidence, which you will then need to analyse and appraise so that you can implement this information into practice. Most university librarians are helpful in teaching students how to develop and conduct a comprehensive search strategy.

Step 2: Analysing and appraising the evidence

This step involves answering the question: 'How do I interpret the evidence I've found?' and 'What is the quality of the evidence I've found?' When seeking to understand the evidence you have located, it is important to understand that the quality of all types of information is not considered equal. Some study designs have relatively more weighting when making decisions (e.g., systematic reviews of randomised controlled trials vs single case design). Similarly, some data sources are more trustworthy then others (Cochrane Reviews vs websites that do not report peer-reviewed articles). As such, when you are searching for evidence, you need to keep in mind the level of study design, methodological quality and purpose of the research.

Level of design

Evidence has different *levels* of design (e.g., systematic reviews, randomised controlled trials, case studies). It is important to note that there are multiple guidelines pertaining to hierarchies of evidence that can be used, depending on the type of research question you aim to address (e.g., prevalence, prognosis, long-term outcomes) (Bennett, 2015). Hierarchies of evidence take into account different study designs in hierarchies based on their ability to address different types of questions and to control for bias. Thus, hierarchies of evidence match study designs to address different types of questions in a type of matrix. In this chapter we use evidence levels of intervention research as an example. When considering the level of evidence, the more robust the study design (e.g., a systematic review of randomised controlled trials [RCTs]), the more we can trust the findings of the study.

The National Health and Medical Research Council (NHMRC) provides levels of study designs. As shown in the first column of Table 14.1, systematic reviews of randomised controlled trials provide the most robust evidence, with case study design with a low number of participants providing weaker evidence. However, it is still important to consider all levels of evidence when trying to find answers to clinical questions. It is also important to consider the evidence from qualitative studies as well, since not all occupational therapy practices readily lend themselves to be evaluated via randomised controlled trials methodologies.

Methodological quality

As shown in Table 15.1 in the second column, these studies will also vary in their *methodological quality* (e.g., how well has the systematic review been designed?). There are multiple information sources that can tell us how well the study was designed.

Table 15.1 Tools for understanding the quality of scientific evidence

The National Health and Medical Research Council (NHMRC)			The Evidence Alert Traffic Light Grading System	
Levels of Evidence	Grades of Recom.*	Description of Recommendation	Traffic light grade	Examples
I = Systematic Review	A—Excellent	Body of evidence can be trusted to guide practice. Several supporting studies with low risk of bias.	Green—GO	High-quality systematic reviews and meta-analyses that demonstrate clinically significant positive effects for the intervention; a number of RCTs demonstrate effectiveness across different setting; no dispute of effectiveness from high-quality studies. For example: Self-management programs for chronic musculoskeletal pain conditions: a systematic review and meta-analysis (Du et al., 2011). The evidence from this study indicates that it is recommended to provide self-management programs to adult patients with arthritis. Self-management is a safe, community-based and effective way for patients with arthritis to manage pain and disability (GO).
II = RCT	B—Good	Evidence can be trusted to guide practice in most instances. Population studied is similar to target population. Most studies consistent with low risk of bias or inconsistent findings between studies can be explained.	Green-Yellow—MEASURE	High quality RCTs but with a limited range, may show a small effect of the intervention, or a variation of the intervention was investigated and because it is based in sound theory and practice could be applied to your setting. For example: Assessing an internet-based parenting intervention for mothers with a serious mental illness: a randomised controlled trial (Kaplan et al., 2014). The study found that participation in an online parenting intervention for mothers with a serious mental illness enhanced parenting and coping skills, and decreased parental stress. This RCT establishes that mothers with a SMI are interested in and capable of receiving online parenting education and support (MEASURE).
III = Quasi-experimental studies IV = Non Experimental	C—Satisfactory	Evidence provides some support and may be applicable to practise with consideration. Population in studies differ from target population, but may be able to apply findings. Some inconsistency around findings with a moderate risk of bias.	Yellow—MEASURE	The findings from the studies might be compromised because of the quality of the design or bias. May have smaller numbers involved in the experiment. For example: Feasibility of a home-based program to improve handwriting after stroke: a pilot study (Simpson et al., 2016). The quasi-experimental study found that delivery of a four-week handwriting intervention with eight supervised sessions in the community was feasible; however, recruitment of an adequate sample size is required to determine effectiveness (MEASURE).

| V = case report/ program evaluation VI = opinion pieces | D—Poor | Weak evidence, not applicable to practice context. Different population investigated and findings not transferable. Inconsistent evidence with high risk of bias. | Red—STOP | Single case studies and opinion pieces that report small positive effects which are not generalisable to your setting. The intervention may have been investigated by the company or people responsible for selling the product, or may have funded the investigation. For example: Occupational therapy using sensory integration to improve participation of a child with autism: a case report (Schaaf et al., 2012). Even though the study reported improvement in sensory processing and enhanced participation in home, school and family activities, the case study by itself is too weak to support use (STOP). |
| | | | Red—STOP | High-quality evidence, such as a systematic review or RCT, suggests this approach is not effective or may have negative effects. Also consider the risk of the intervention when compared to the potential benefits. For example: Does EEG-neurofeedback improve neurocognitive functioning in children with ADHD? (Vollebregt et al., 2014). A systematic review and a double-blind placebo-controlled study. The systematic review found no significant treatment effect on any of the neurocognitive variables. Existing literature fails to support any benefit of neurofeedback on neurocognitive functioning in ADHD (STOP). |

Note: *Recom. = Recommendations
Source: Adapted from NHMRC (2009) and Novak (2012)

These include the 'limitations section' of the journal article, as well as a number of checklist points such as: sample size/number of participants in the study, blinding (of the participants or researchers conducting the study), randomisation (to the intervention or waitlist group), bias, and controlling for confounding variables. (Did boys receive more benefits than girls from the intervention? Did patients taking medication get more benefits than those who did not take medication?) A description of different types of biases is provided in Figure 15.2.

There are a number of critical appraisal tools that can assist you in locating and understanding these checklist points, including: McMaster Critical Appraisal Tool, Kmet, A Measurement Tool to Assess Systematic Reviews (AMSTAR), PEDro scale, Critical Appraisal Skills Programme (CASP) Checklists, Joanna Briggs Institute Model of Evidence-Based Healthcare and COnsensus-based Standards for the selection of Health Measurement INstruments (COSMIN).

Using the NHMRC grade system of recommendation, the number of studies (e.g., more than two), the level of the studies design (e.g., RCTs) and the methodological quality of the studies (e.g., low risk of bias) can be combined to guide practice based on the findings of the studies (e.g., Grade A, Excellent, Body of evidence from the studies can be trusted to guide practice). More information on the NHMRC can be accessed via their website at https://www.nhmrc.gov.au/.

Studies that demonstrate: i) consistency/similar findings; ii) a robust methodological design; iii) large/observable client benefits/outcomes; iv) generalisability beyond participants in the study to the relevant client population; and v) directly applicable findings to occupational therapy practice would be considered excellent evidence to guide practice. This is where systematic reviews and meta-analysis of treatment, assessments and general investigations are helpful as they gather and interpret the evidence. Compare this to studies with a high risk of bias (e.g., small sample size, no randomisation of participants), inconsistent evidence found between studies (e.g., some studies report the

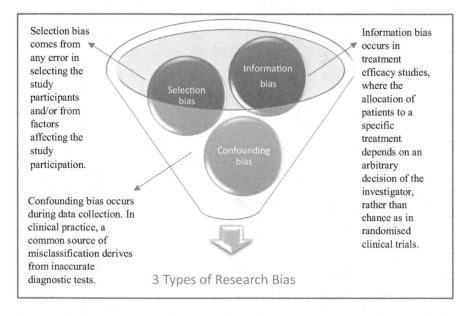

Figure 15.2 Types of research bias.

intervention to be effective and others ineffective), restricted clinical impact (e.g., only boys improved as a result of the intervention) and findings not generalisable or applicable to your context.

Purpose/type of evidence

The evidence you locate will vary in *purpose* (e.g., to investigate effectiveness, feasibility, appropriateness). Once a study has been found effective, it is also important to consider if it is a feasible and appropriate approach. Evans (2003) argued that for health care interventions to achieve a *gold standard*, evidence must be demonstrated in three areas: *effectiveness* (Does the intervention work as intended?), *feasibility* (Are adequate resources available for implementation?) and *appropriateness* (What is the impact of the intervention from the participants' perspective?).

Integrating the aspects of the evidence in context

A *systematic review* (i.e., systematic methods to collect secondary data, critically appraise research studies, and synthesize findings) and *meta-analysis* (i.e., to systematically merge findings of single, independent studies, using statistical methods to calculate an overall or 'absolute' effect) represent high-level evidence. A systematic review and meta-analysis may show an intervention is very *beneficial* (highly effective) at improving children's handwriting. However, the intervention may require six months of intervention twice a week, making it very *costly* (less feasible) for families. Further, children may *dislike* going, need to leave school early, and may also need to do hours of home activities every week, having a *stressful* impact on parents (decreased appropriateness). Therefore, it is important to consider the information presented with a discerning eye and determine if the information is reliable and trustworthy for you to be able to make an informed decision.

Step 3: Applying the evidence to practice

In this step of the EBP process, you are seeking to answer the question, 'How do I apply the evidence?' Once you have identified the level, quality and purpose of the evidence you have located, you need to make an informed decision of how best to apply this information to your practice. The Evidence Alert Traffic Light Grading System (Novak, 2012) presented in Table 14.1 provides you with actions to take based on the evidence you have located. In your plans to apply the evidence you have found it is also important to reconsider your practice setting, what other supports will be needed to provide this intervention for your clients and your client's goals, preferences, values and circumstances. You need to ask the questions: 'What additional support, costs and logistics are needed before you can begin the intervention? (*feasibility*)', 'Will the intervention be *appropriate* from my client's perspective? 'Does the evidence suggest this approach will be *effective* in improving outcomes for my client?'

The action for *green* light evidence is, where applicable, to use this approach (GO). The action for *yellow* light evidence is to apply this approach with caution, as there may be insufficient or conflicting evidence. In this instance, best practice is to use outcome measures and attainment of client goals to evaluate if this approach has been effective for your client (MEASURE). The action for *red* light evidence is not to use this approach or to discontinue this approach if it is already being used (STOP).

The application of evidence-based practice in Australia

Occupational therapists' perceptions of barriers to implementing evidence-based practice and educational needs were examined by surveying 649 members of the national professional association—Occupational Therapy Australia. The majority of the respondents were positive about EBP, with 96 per cent agreeing that EBP is important (Bennett et al., 2003). However, only 56 per cent reported using research to make clinical decisions. The vast majority of occupational therapists reported relying on clinical experience (96 per cent), and information from continuing education (82 per cent) and colleagues (80 per cent). Lack of time, not having enough evidence in occupational therapy (63.4 per cent) and skills in locating the evidence (54.7 per cent) were identified as the main barriers to the implementation of EBP. Over half (52 per cent) expressed strong interest in further developing their EBP skills, and most (80 per cent) expressed an interest in the availability of brief summaries of evidence (Bennett et al., 2003). Because of these barriers, occupational therapists may be more likely to rely on their clinical experience rather than on published research findings when making clinical decisions (McKenna et al., 2005).

Implementing the above steps

The case study below provides an example of the process involved in locating the evidence, how the occupational therapist can analyse and appraise the evidence, and how this information can be applied when planning interventions.

Case study

Case study: Jack

Claire is an occupational therapist with three years of clinical experience. She provides intervention to children with various conditions and occupational challenges at their homes and schools. One of Claire's clients is Jack, a seven-year-old boy diagnosed with Attention Deficit Hyperactivity Disorder (ADHD). Jack is currently taking medication for his ADHD symptoms and to support his learning at school. His mother and teacher have identified that he has difficulty interacting with other children. Jack does not have any friends. Jack's mother and teacher have asked Claire to provide an intervention to address Jack's social difficulties.

Step 1: Locating the evidence

Claire uses her professional network by calling her colleagues who are occupational therapists working in schools to ask if they have implemented any social skills interventions. She then conducts a library database search using the terms 'ADHD' and 'social skills training' to find peer-reviewed journal articles. While Claire couldn't find any Australian guidelines for the treatment of ADHD, she found some recent guidelines written by the American Psychiatric Association. Claire also phoned her mentor as her mentor has over 20 years of clinical experience in this area and has connections with university researchers who are occupational therapists.

Step 2: Analysing and appraising the evidence

Claire informs her mentor that her colleagues who work in schools have run social skills training groups in the library at lunch time with a group of children with different diagnoses, all of whom have social difficulties. They describe the group as difficult to run, as all of the children in the group have social difficulties, with multiple children often being disruptive, thus making it hard to run the group. Claire also shows her mentor an article she found in her database search by Storebø et al. (2011). The article is a systematic review of 11 randomised controlled trials (RCTs). The article concluded that there was little evidence that social skills training improves the social skills of school-aged children with ADHD. Most of the RCTs included in the review reported using social skills training interventions which were conducted with groups of children with ADHD in clinic settings, away from the child's everyday environment and peers. The ADHD guidelines Claire found recommend a combined approach, where children take medication and engage in other interventions at the same time. When synthesising all the collected evidence, Claire and her mentor decide not to implement a social skills training intervention the way it is most commonly implemented, as there is strong evidence to suggest this approach will not be effective (STOP). After further reading, Claire and her mentor decide they will include typically developing peers and video-modelling in the social intervention for Jack. In systematic reviews, these components were found to be effective for improving the social skills of children diagnosed with autism. They also find some emerging evidence (e.g., NHMRC level II and IV studies) for using these approaches with children with ADHD (Wilkes–Gillan et al., 2016; Wilkes et al., 2011).

Step 3: Using the evidence

Claire recommends that Jack continue taking his medication (ADHD guidelines) during the intervention which will be conducted at Jack's school. The intervention will involve Jack and two typically developing peers (clinical experience and quality of evidence). Claire will support the three children as they play in the playground together. She will also video-record them playing, so she can play the footage back to them at the start of their next session (video–modelling and quality of evidence). As Claire has based her intervention on research that is strong in children with autism and emerging in children with ADHD, the intervention will last for one school term. Claire's mentor advised that she use a social skills assessment before and after the intervention (MEASURE) to investigate if the intervention is effective for Jack (clinical experience and quality of evidence).

The future of evidence-based practice

Considering the recurring theme of clinicians identifying the need for EBP, but reporting barriers in the practical application, both internationally and in Australia, a multifaceted approach to address EBP in occupational therapy is needed. Systems to reduce the time involved in identifying appropriate and high-quality evidence, as well as education and training of how to understand and apply evidence, are necessary (Bennett et al., 2003).

In recognition of the importance of EBP, occupational therapy students must be able to demonstrate the ability to locate, analyse and appraise, and implement evidence upon completion of their degree prior to registering as an occupational therapist. EBP is taught in occupational therapy courses around the world and health professionals attend EBP workshops as part of continuing professional development to ensure the practice recommendations resulting from evidence are shared and translated into practice. There is still a need to develop practice guidelines in many areas, especially in areas of inter-disciplinary care (Newhouse & Spring, 2010).

While best practice guidelines are becoming more readily available to clinicians, ro-bust, evidence-based guidance regarding the most effective treatment approaches may not currently be available, with more research needed in many areas. Until guidelines applicable to your practice context become available, less formal approaches are neces-sary for gathering evidence and information (Kelly & Bonnefoy, 2007). Examples of less formal approaches include: gathering evidence from different stakeholders (includ-ing clients, clinicians and managers), reviewing existing practices, combining existing practices with EBP to develop specific guidelines for your context, and examining the evidence available in similar conditions and contexts.

If you are a student, you may notice that some experienced practitioners do not prac-tise rigorous EBP, instead relying on previous experience and findings to guide their decision-making process and recommendations. While some practitioners are still over-coming the barriers to implementing an EBP, as reflected by data from the Cochrane Library, many are ensuring an evidence-based approach.

Increasing the value of research and reducing research waste

The Lancet (one of the world's most highly ranked peer-reviewed medical journals). published a series of papers that, collectively, recommend how to increase the value of research and reduce waste in research. The papers covered the following topics: (1) decisions about which research to fund based on issues relevant to users of research (Chalmers et al., 2014); (2) improvements in the appropriateness of research design, methods and analysis (Ioannidis et al., 2014); (3) issues of efficient research regulation and management (Salman et al., 2014); (4) the role of fully accessible research informa-tion (Chan et al., 2014); and (5) the importance of unbiased and usable research reports (Glasziou et al., 2014). This information is important for occupational therapy students to be aware of as they begin to understand and implement research. This can apply to tasks and assessments in units of study, clinical placements and students who will con-sider completing honours programs as part of their undergraduate degree.

(1) Funding and research value

Annual global investment into biomedical research continue to rise, which has led to an increase in health research and outcomes for the public. However, the increase in research has also led to research waste. Examples of research waste include, over replication of research topics and data, conducting too many small studies in under-researched areas, and untargeted research (see Figure 15.3). Chalmers et al. (2014) suggested the following recommendations for research funders with the aim to reduce waste and increase the value of research (see Figure 15.3):

- insisting proposals are justified by systematic review evidence synthesising research about what is known and not known;
- strengthening the sharing of information about research that is in progress to encourage collaboration and reduce duplication; and
- engaging research users to decide which research to support and prioritise.

(2) Research design, conduct and analysis

Avoidable weakness in research design, conduct and analysis are all reasons studies can potentially produce misleading results – this wastes valuable resources. Some common weaknesses in research design that can lead to waste are distinguishing small effect sizes from bias, lack of detail in written protocols, poor documentation of research, power calculations for sample size that are too low and lack of involvement of experienced statisticians (see Figure 15.3). Ioannidis et al. (2014) put forth the following recommendations with the aim to address these problems:

- making full research protocols publicly available;
- improving research methodology and design by continuing to train researchers, through reporting standards, and by ensuring no conflict of interest in stakeholders; and
- rewarding methodological rigour and well conducted research.

(3) Regulation and management

Even after important research has been identified and the study design is appropriate and robust, waste can occur from the regulation and management of research (Salman et al., 2014). Poor management can lead to poor recruitment and retention of participants. In order to reduce research waste:

- Regulators should work and partner with researchers, patients, and health professionals to streamline research guidelines and processes;
- Researchers and research managers should increase efficiency of recruitment, retention and data monitoring; and
- All involved should promote the integration of research into everyday clinical practice (see Figure 15.3).

(4) Fully accessible research information

Health research is commonly documented in study protocols, research reports and journal articles. However, full study reports and datasets containing participant-level information are rarely made available. This lack of information about studies can result in wasted investment and bias, which can ultimately impact the care of health care

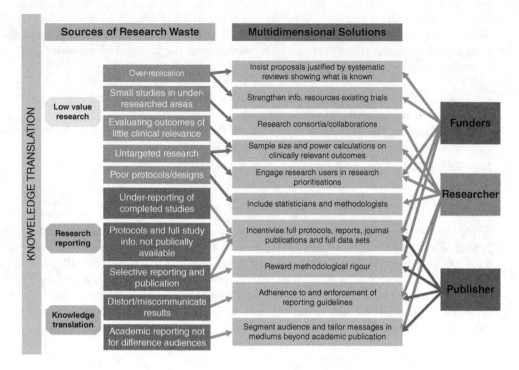

Figure 15.3 Sources of research waste and multidimensional solutions.

consumers as well as the furthering of research. Chan et al. (2014) suggest three actions to take when attempting to address this issue:

- For institutions and funders to recognise full dissemination of research;
- For investigators, funders, sponsors and regulators to adopt standards for sharing full study reports and data sharing; and
- Enforcing study registration policies and sharing of participant-level data (see Figure 15.3).

(5) Incomplete or unusable research reports

Adequate reporting of research is important to ensure resources invested in the research are not wasted. There are reporting guidelines (e.g., CONSORT, STARD, PRISMA and ARRIVE) that aim to help researchers improve the quality of their reporting. However, these guidelines are often not readily adopted or adhered to—with many studies providing insufficient information on interventions to be replicable or omitting key information (Glasziou et al., 2014). In order to address these issues, the following actions should be taken:

- Funders, institutions and publishers should move towards infrastructure to support and enforce good and complete reporting; and
- Improving the capacity of both authors and reviewers to provide high-quality complete reporting of research (see Figure 15.2).

Knowledge translation

Research waste can also impact knowledge translation (see Figure 15.3). Knowledge translation is the end goal of research—it involves the implementation of research into the everyday health care practices and organisations. Knowledge translation is about the usefulness of research and involves all aspects, from the design of the research through to dissemination of results and implementation (Wensing & Grol, 2019). Although there have been recent advances in research, the uptake and implementation of research in everyday health care settings and practices is still lacking (Wensing & Grol, 2019). Wensing and Grol (2019) outline some of the main reasons for slow development in this field, as well as practical strategies for advancing knowledge translation.

The main reasons for slowed development are:

- A lack of alignment or match between the problem and approaches to implementation;
- Concepts, frameworks and theories to help support implementation of research;
- Stakeholder involvement to co-design research and support the successful implementation of research in practice—this aims to bridge the gap from translation to service provider uptake;
- Evaluation of outcomes and implementation programs; and
- Measurement of outcomes of improvement, transfer and implementation.

The following are recommended strategies when aiming to successfully implement research into practice:

- Researchers and advisors are encouraged to work in multidisciplinary teams and partner with organisations where the research would be implemented;
- Increasing recognition of published work and funding;
- Adopting structured approaches regarding stakeholder involvement;
- Improving the quality of evaluation processes between health care professionals, mangers and policy makers; and
- Developing and evaluating new outcome measures with robust psychometric qualities.

Conclusion

Evidence-based practice is fundamental to occupational therapy practice. It informs our clinical reasoning and decision-making process in determining best-practice for our clients. The ability to be skilled consumers of research is therefore a critical skill for occupational therapy practitioners and students alike. This chapter provided an overview of the concept of evidence-based practice and how it encompassed scientific knowledge as well as clinical expertise, client preference and context. The three-step process of evidence-based practice was described: Step 1—locate, Step 2—analyse and appraise, and Step 3—apply evidence to our own clinical practice. Tools that were useful in understanding quality of evidence were presented, as well as a vignette of this process in action. Current and future directions in evidence-based practice were discussed, including barriers to implementation, research waste and translating research into practice.

Summary

- EBP involves integrating scientific knowledge, clinical experience and expertise, client circumstance and the practice context.
- EBP involves a process of locating, analysing, appraising and implementing the evidence.
- As occupational therapists, we must use an EBP approach to ensure our knowledge is up to date and that our clients receive the best available treatment.
- Occupational therapists should ensure research isn't wasted and consider how the research we read can be implemented in our everyday work settings and practices.

Review questions

1. What is evidence-based practice and why is it important to occupational therapy practice?
2. Describe the three-step process of evidence-based practice.
3. Clinicians have identified a number of barriers to incorporating evidence-based practice in everyday practice—what are these barriers and how may they be overcome?
4. What are three areas that contribute to research waste and how does this impact knowledge translation?

References

Bayley, M. T., Hurdowar, A., Richards, C. L., Korner-Bitensky, N., Wood-Dauphinee, S., Eng, J. J., McKay-Lyons, M., Harrison, E., Teasell, R., Harrison, M., & Graham, I. D. (2012). Barriers to implementation of stroke rehabilitation evidence: Findings from a multi-site pilot project. *Disability and Rehabilitation*, *34*(19), 1633–1638. https://doi.org/doi:10.3109/09638288.2012.656790

Bennett, S. (2015). Using evidence to guide practice. In C. Baum, C. Christiansen, & J. Bass (Eds.), *Occupational Therapy: Performance, participation and well-being* (4th edn, pp. 93–109). SLACK Inc.

Bennett, S., & Bennett, J. W. (2000). The process of evidence-based practice in occupational therapy: Informing clinical decisions. *Australian Occupational Therapy Journal*, *47*(4), 171–180. https://doi.org/10.1046/j.1440-1630.2000.00237.x

Bennett, S., Hannes, K., & O'Connor, D. (2017). Appraising and interpreting systematic reviews. In T. Hoffmann, S. Bennett, & C. Del Mar (Eds.), *Evidence-based practice across the health professions* (3rd edn, pp. 292–322). Elsevier Australia.

Bennett, S., Tooth, L., McKenna, K., Rodger, S., Strong, J., Ziviani, J., Mickan, S., & Gibson, L. (2003). Perceptions of evidence-based practice: A survey of Australian occupational therapists. *Australian Occupational Therapy Journal*, *50*(1), 13–22. https://doi.org/10.1046/j.1440-1630.2003.00341.x

Chalmers, I., Bracken, M. B., Djulbegovic, B., Garattini, S., Grant, J., Gülmezoglu, A. M., Howells, D. W., Ioannidis, J. P. A., & Oliver, S. (2014). How to increase value and reduce waste when research priorities are set. *The Lancet*, *383*, 156–165. https://doi.org/10.1016/S0140-6736(13)62229-1

Chan, A.-W., Song, F., Vickers, A., Jefferson, T., Dickersin, K., Gøtzsche, P. C., Krumholz, H. M., Ghersi, D., & van der Worp, H. B. (2014). Increasing value and reducing waste: Addressing inaccessible research. *The Lancet*, *383*, 257–266. https://doi.org/10.1016/S0140-6736(13)62296-5

Du, S., Yuan, C., Xiao, X., Chu, J., Qiu, Y., & Qian, H. (2011). Self-management programs for chronic musculoskeletal pain conditions: A systematic review and meta-analysis. *Patient Education & Counseling*, *85*(3), e299–310. https://doi.org/10.1016/j.pec.2011.02.021

Evans, D. (2003). Hierarchy of evidence: A framework for ranking evidence evaluating healthcare interventions. *Journal of Clinical Nursing*, *12*(1), 77–84. https://doi.org/10.1046/j.1365-2702.2003.00662.x

Glasziou, P., Altman, D. G., Bossuyt, I., Clarke, M., Julious, S., Michie, S., Moher, D., & Wager, E. (2014). Reducing waste from incomplete or unusable reports of biomedical research. *The Lancet*, *383*, 267–276. https://doi.org/10.1016/S0140-6736(13)62228-X

Hamer, S., & Collinson, G. (2014). *Achieving evidence-based practice: A handbook for practitioners.* Elsevier Health Sciences.

Heiwe, S., Kajermo, K. N., Tyni-Lenné, R., Guidetti, S., Samuelsson, M., Andersson, I.-L., & Wengström, Y. (2011). Evidence-based practice. Attitudes, knowledge and behaviour among allied health care professionals. *International Journal for Quality in Health Care*, *23*(2), 198–209. https://doi.org/10.1093/intqhc/mzq083

Hoffmann, T., Bennett, S., & Del Mar, C. (Eds.). (2017). *Evidence-based practice across the health professions* (3rd edn). Elsevier Australia.

Ioannidis, J. P. A., Greenland, S., Hlatky, M. A., Khoury, M. J., Macleod, M. R., Moher, D., Schulz, K. F., & Tibshirani, R. (2014). Increasing value and reducing waste in research design, conduct and analysis. *The Lancet*, *383*, 166–175. https://doi.org/10.1016/S0140-6736(13)62227-8

Kaplan, K., Solomon, P., Salzer, M. S., & Brusilovskiy, E. (2014). Assessing an internet-based parenting intervention for mothers with a serious mental illness: A randomized controlled trial. *Psychiatric Rehabilitation Journal*, *37*(3), 222–231. https://doi.org/10.1037/prj0000080

Kelly, M. P., & Bonnefoy, J. (2007). *The social determinants of health: Developing an evidence base for political action.* Universidad del Desarrollo, Chile and National Institute for Health and Clinical Excellence.

McKenna, K., Bennett, S., Dierselhuis, Z., Hoffmann, T., Tooth, L., & McCluskey, A. (2005). Australian occupational therapists' use of an online evidence-based practice database (OTseeker). *Health Information & Libraries Journal*, *22*(3), 205–214. https://doi.org/10.1111/j.1471-1842.2005.00597.x

Newhouse, R. P., & Spring, B. (2010). Interdisciplinary evidence-based practice: Moving from silos to synergy. *Nursing Outlook*, *58*(6), 309–317. https://doi.org/10.1016/j.outlook.2010.09.001

NHMRC. (2009). *NHMRC additional levels of evidence and grades for recommendation for developers of guidelines.* NHMRC. https://www.mja.com.au/sites/default/files/NHMRC.levels.of.evidence.2008-09.pdf

Novak, I. (2012). Evidence to practice commentary: The evidence alert traffic light grading system. *Physical and Occupational Therapy in Paediatrics*, *32*, 256–259. https://doi.org/10.3109/01942638.2012.698148

Sackett, D. L., Rosenberg, W. M., Gray, J. A., Haynes, R. B., & Richardson, W. S. (1996). Evidence based medicine: What it is and what it isn't. *British Medical Journal*, *312*, 71–72. https://doi.org/10.1136/bmj.312.7023.71

Salman, R. A.-S., Beller, E., Kagan, J., Hemminki, E., Phillips, R. S., Savulescu, J., Macleod, M. R., Wisely, J., & Chalmers, I. (2014). Increasing value and reducing waste in biomedical research regulation and management. *The Lancet*, *383*, 176–185. https://doi.org/10.1016/S0140-6736(13)62297-7

Schaaf, R. C., Hunt, J., & Benevides, T. (2012). Occupational therapy using sensory integration to improve participation of a child with autism: A case report. *American Journal of Occupational Therapy*, *66*(5), 547–555. https://doi.org/10.5014/ajot.2012.004473

Simpson, B., McCluskey, A., Lannin, N., & Cordier, R. (2016). Feasibility of a home-based program to improve handwriting after stroke: A pilot study. *Disability and Rehabilitation*, *38*(7), 673–682. https//doi.org/10.3109/09638288.2015.1059495

Storebø, O., Skoog, M., Damm, D., Thomsen, P., Simonsen, E., & Gluud, C. (2011). Social skills training for attention deficit hyperactivity disorder (ADHD) in children aged 5 to 18 years. *Cochrane Database of Systematic Reviews*, December 7(12), CD008223. https//.doi.org/10.1002/14651858.CD008223.pub2

Stronge, M., & Cahill, M. (2012). Self-reported knowledge, attitudes and behaviour towards evidence-based practice of occupational therapy students in Ireland. *Occupational Therapy International*, *19*(1), 7–16. https://doi.org/10.1002/oti.328

Van't Leven, N., Graff, M. J. L., Kaijen, M., de Swart, B. J. M., Olde Rikkert, M. G. M., & Vernooij-Dassen, M. J. M. (2012). Barriers to and facilitators for the use of an evidence-based occupational therapy guideline for older people with dementia and their carers. *International Journal of Geriatric Psychiatry*, *27*(7), 742–748. https://doi.org/10.1002/gps.2782

Vollebregt, M. A., van Dongen-Boomsma, M., Buitelaar, J. K., & Slaats-Willemse, D. (2014). Does EEG-neurofeedback improve neurocognitive functioning in children with attention-deficit/hyperactivity disorder? A systematic review and a double-blind placebo-controlled study. *Journal of Child Psychology & Psychiatry*, *55*(5), 460–472. https://doi.org/10.1111/jcpp.12143

Wensing, M., & Grol, R. (2019). Knowledge translation in health: How implementation science could contribute more. *BMC Medicine*, *17*(88). https://doi.org/10.1186/s129616-019-1322-9

Wilkes-Gillan, S., Bundy, A., Cordier, R., Lincoln, M., & Chen, Y.-W. (2016). A randomised controlled trial of a play-based intervention to improve the social play skills of children with attention deficit hyperactivity disorder (ADHD). *PLoS One*, *11*(8), e0160558. https//doi.org/10.1371/journal.pone.0160558

Wilkes, S., Cordier, R., Bundy, A., Docking, K., & Munro, N. (2011). A play-based intervention for children with ADHD: A pilot study. *Australian Occupational Therapy Journal*, *58*(4), 231–240. https://doi.org/10.1111/j.1440-1630.2011.00928.x

Woodbury, M. G., & Kuhnke, J. L. (2014). Evidence-based practice vs. evidence-informed practice: What's the difference? *Wound Care Canada*, *12*(1), 18–21. https://www.woundscanada.ca/docman/public/wound-care-canada-magazine/2014-vol-12-no-1/584-vol12no1full/file

16 Clinical reasoning in occupational therapy practice

Justin Scanlan, Jennie Brentnall and Carolyn Unsworth

Chapter objectives

Upon completion of this chapter, the reader will be able to:

- Describe the process of clinical reasoning in occupational therapy practice.
- Identify six aspects of clinical reasoning in occupational therapy, and three influences on clinical reasoning.
- Describe how these aspects of and influences on clinical reasoning can be applied in different stages of the occupational therapy process.
- Present a framework to support the development of clinical reasoning skills in novice occupational therapists.

Key terms

clinical reasoning; professional reasoning; decision-making; client-centred practice; novice and expert practitioner; reflection; intuition; worldview

Introduction

Clinical reasoning in occupational therapy is a complex process. Although it is often described as a 'tacit' process (understood without necessarily being able to be expressed), this chapter presents a framework for clinical reasoning to support novice occupational therapists to develop skills in collaborative service planning and decision-making. The framework incorporates six aspects of clinical reasoning (narrative reasoning, interactive reasoning, procedural reasoning, conditional reasoning, pragmatic reasoning and ethical reasoning) and three influences on clinical reasoning (worldview, intuition and reflection), and describes how these different aspects of and influences on reasoning can be applied at different stages of the occupational therapy process (formulating an impression, information gathering and planning, and monitoring). Applying this framework, novice occupational therapists are supported to consider a range of factors essential to supporting clients' attainment of optimal occupational performance and participation. Over time, with practice and critical self-reflection, the novice occupational therapist will develop more expert clinical reasoning and these processes will become tacit and therefore will be more flexible, integrated and efficient.

Clinical reasoning in occupational therapy practice

The aim of occupational therapy is to assist clients (e.g., individuals, families, groups and communities) to move towards the occupational futures they want. This can be achieved through facilitating changes to people, environments, occupations, or combinations of all three. The various settings in which occupational therapists work also influence the focus and duration of therapy. Therefore, occupational therapists must simultaneously consider what their clients wish to achieve, barriers and facilitators to achieving these outcomes, the types of services that are likely to be most effective, the current body of empirical evidence that supports or endorses the intervention methods proposed, and the expectations of service settings.

Many novice occupational therapists seek to find an 'instruction manual' to guide decision-making. As appealing as this idea is, the nature of occupational therapy practice means that such an instruction manual would be impossible to write. Each client has a unique set of skills, values, interests, roles, habits, routines, strengths and difficulties, and each functions in a unique context (Taylor & Kielhofner, 2017). Since occupational therapists must consider the complex interplay between people, their environments and their occupations, there are an infinite number of possible interventions. Although some occupational therapy interventions will be similar to others, no two plans will ever be exactly the same due to the unique situation of each client.

The process undertaken by occupational therapists to consider and weigh all the relevant factors when developing, implementing and reviewing collaborative intervention plans has been referred to as *clinical reasoning* (Mattingly & Fleming, 1994a; Rogers & Masagatani, 1982; Unsworth & Baker, 2016) or *professional reasoning* (Schell & Schell, 2018; Schell, 2019). Researchers investigating clinical reasoning in occupational therapy have often described it as a *tacit* process: one that is understood, but is difficult to describe (e.g., Fleming, 1991a; Mattingly, 1991a; Neistadt, 1996; Schell & Cervero, 1993). While this is true, such conceptualisations are not particularly helpful in assisting novice occupational therapists develop sound clinical reasoning skills.

In this chapter, six key aspects of clinical reasoning and three influences on clinical reasoning are presented, as well as a framework linking these to support the reasoning process. With practice and critical reflection, the process of clinical reasoning becomes more flexible, integrated and efficient. Occupational therapy practice occurs in a vast array of *clinical* and *non-clinical* settings, and with a variety of *clients* (e.g., individuals, families, groups or communities) who have a diverse range of factors that might hinder optimal occupational performance and participation. For simplicity, in this chapter, the term *clients* is used to refer to individuals, families, groups or communities with whom occupational therapists might work, and the term *conditions* is used to refer to impairments, situations or other factors that reduce clients' abilities to achieve optimal occupational performance and participation.

Aspects of clinical reasoning

Narrative reasoning

Narrative reasoning focuses on clients' occupational stories (Bonsall, 2012; Mattingly, 1991b). What have been their valued and meaningful roles and occupations in the past? How are those valued and meaningful roles and occupations enacted in their current situations (e.g., have their current conditions impacted on their ability to engage in these roles and occupations)? What do clients want for their occupational futures (e.g., do they want to return to previous occupations; do they wish to engage in new, more meaningful occupations; or have they lost hope so they can no longer see useful future occupations)?

The occupational focus of narrative reasoning supports occupational therapists to focus on the most important aspect of practice: occupational performance and participation (Bonsall, 2012; Mattingly, 1991b; Mattingly, 1998; Neistadt, 1996). This focus also allows the exploration and understanding of clients' values, their beliefs in their abilities, and the types of things that are important to them. All of these factors are critical in making decisions that are the most supportive of clients achieving their desired occupational futures.

The process of occupational *story making* (creating a picture of clients' desired occupational futures) can support clients and therapists to take action in the therapeutic process (Bonsall, 2012). Additionally, narrative reasoning allows the exploration of how clients have *made sense* of their situations and how their conditions impact on their daily lives. This process of making sense of experiences (Christiansen, 1999; Levine & Reicher, 1996) is important to consider in planning assessment, goal-setting and interventions.

Interactive reasoning

Interactive reasoning (Mattingly & Fleming, 1994b) considers clients in the context of their relationships with their occupational therapists, health care and support services, and informal supports (e.g., friends and family). This aspect of reasoning prompts occupational therapists to focus on maximising the quality of therapeutic relationships, identify how clients' current and previous interactions with health or social services may influence their current therapeutic interactions, and consider how much and what type of informal supports they receive (Schwartzberg, 2001). This aspect of reasoning therefore guides the therapist in adjusting their interactions with clients.

Interactive reasoning helps occupational therapists to understand potential barriers or enablers to optimal engagement with the therapeutic process and what supports might be available to clients. Consider the difference in approach that would be necessary for an individual client with good family and community supports and a positive, trusting relationship with health services, compared with a community that has previously had negative interactions with health services, that might not recognise and prioritise occupational needs for support, or that may lack access to services and family or community supports. Interactive reasoning guides the understanding of these issues and allows occupational therapists to design plans that takes these issues into account.

Procedural reasoning

Procedural reasoning (Fleming, 1991a) is the process whereby occupational therapists consider 'for this specific condition, what are the most suitable services to achieve the desired outcomes?' In other disciplines, procedural reasoning might be referred to as *diagnostic reasoning, scientific reasoning* or *hypothetico-deductive reasoning*. Procedural reasoning supports occupational therapists to engage with clients to consider a variety of different intervention options to develop a 'short list' of potentially effective approaches.

Evidence-based practice is central in this aspect of clinical reasoning. Developing a PICO question (**P**articipants, **I**ntervention, **C**omparison, **O**utcome) (Del Mar et al., 2017) can be very useful in guiding this search.

Procedural reasoning is arguably the most concrete aspect of clinical reasoning. For this reason, it is often the first aspect considered by novice occupational therapists. While this process is important, it is critical for occupational therapists to avoid a *one size fits all* approach. The six aspects of and three influences on clinical reasoning presented in this chapter together enable occupational therapists to consider the variety of factors important to clients' situations, avoiding an exclusive focus on diagnoses or impairments.

Conditional reasoning

The fourth aspect of reasoning, conditional reasoning (Fleming, 1991a), considers, 'what is the best intervention approach for this specific client, with these specific values, needs, desires and hopes for the future, in this specific context?' It includes consideration of clients' current condition, their potential future condition and the importance of clients engaging fully in the intervention process to support optimal outcomes. Using this aspect of reasoning guides occupational therapists to consider potential future outcomes for their clients. At this point, occupational therapists should consider what interventions or approaches are most suitable for their clients 'in a perfect world', rather than considering what is *practical* or *feasible* (Scanlan & Hancock, 2010). While the consideration practicality and feasibility is important (and is considered in pragmatic reasoning), if consideration is not first given to what would be optimal, important intervention options may be overlooked.

Pragmatic reasoning

Pragmatic reasoning is concerned with what is possible to achieve given the practical constraints and opportunities in the therapy environment or context (Unsworth, 2004; Unsworth & Baker, 2016). Pragmatic reasoning includes the thinking the therapist undertakes when considering the local practice culture, funding and reimbursement issues, access to equipment and resources, and issues around time such as the number of clients to see, client length of stay and needing to treat individual clients simultaneously (Schell & Cervero, 1993; Unsworth, 2004). When reasoning pragmatically, it is important that the therapist holds the client's best interests uppermost in their mind and guards against making decisions based only on 'what is easiest' or 'what is always done here'.

Pragmatic reasoning supports occupational therapists to consider the *best fit* intervention approaches for their clients, given the limitations of the systems in which their services are offered (Cohn et al., 2010). These limitations might include the availability of funding, access to community supports or accommodation, or the length of time available for therapeutic interventions. While all of these factors exert a significant influence on the clinical reasoning process, ethical reasoning as described next ensures that occupational therapists take an ethical approach to clinical reasoning that does not rule out essential interventions just because they are difficult to achieve. Pragmatic and ethical reasoning sometimes necessitate that occupational therapists take on advocacy roles to support their clients to access necessary resources.

Ethical reasoning

The final aspect of clinical reasoning is ethical reasoning. Ethical reasoning considers what is necessary for the individual and moral outcomes. It accompanies the analysis of moral dilemmas when one moral conviction or action may conflict with another (Barnitt, 1993; Kanny & Slater, 2018). For example, a therapist will rely on their ethical reasoning to help determine the most successful ways to work with a client whose primary goal is to be able to independently take drugs, which is illegal, and may also temporarily reduce the client's cognitive capacity, thus making them vulnerable to negative events. Ethical reasoning ensures all clients receive services in a fair and equitable manner and relies heavily on the therapists' worldview.

Influences on clinical reasoning

Worldview

In a seminal review, Wolters (1989) described 'worldview' as encompassing individuals' assumptions about life and reality. It includes values, beliefs and attitudes, motivation, ability to read the culture, faith and spirituality, and personal style (Unsworth, 2004). Worldview thereby shapes all thinking, including the clinical reasoning processes of therapists. Our worldview gives us a global outlook and is shaped by our personal-cultural-historic context. Every person's worldview is unique, and although an individual may be aware of their worldview, a therapist is generally not able to 'reason' with it. Rather, worldview is an influence on clinical reasoning.

Intuition

Intuition may be defined as immediate and 'whole' (as opposed to fragmented) knowledge, that is, without conscious reasoning (Chaffey et al., 2012; Unsworth, 2017; 2020). Intuition informs knowledge and is in turn supported by the individual's understanding of their emotions. More experienced therapists appear to be more comfortable with trusting and acting upon their intuition, which some therapists call their 'gut instinct'. Novice therapists can benefit from discussing intuition in different therapeutic environments with experienced therapists to try to access, understand and begin to build their own intuition.

Reflection

Reflection involves spending time thinking critically about events and encounters, and responses to these. This may be about past experiences (reflection on action), in the present (reflection in action), or looking forward in anticipation (reflection for action). In his seminal work, Schön (1983) described reflection as a bridge to link theory and practice. It is thereby a key enabler of clinical reasoning as thinking about therapeutic encounters and their success, as well as how they could be improved, assists novice therapists to hone practice and attain expert status faster. Hence, reflective practice is embedded in occupational therapy practice guidelines and standards internationally (Occupational Therapy Board of Australia, 2018; World Federation of Occupational Therapists, 2016), and most occupational therapy students learn about reflective practice in their education program and have time for reflective journal writing embedded in their fieldwork education placements (Craig-Duchesne et al., 2018; Wong et al., 2016). While there is a high level of interest and engagement across the profession in reflective practice, a key barrier is a lack of time (Knightbridge, 2019). Students are therefore encouraged to routinely build time into their schedule to create opportunities for both group and individual reflection.

Bringing it all together

An overview of the different elements of clinical reasoning is presented in Figure 16.1. The first four types of reasoning (narrative, interactive, procedural and conditional) are combined to determine *optimal* intervention approaches. These options are constantly reviewed and analysed using pragmatic and ethical reasoning to determine the *best fit* approach to interventions which is then used to develop intervention plans and goals. The worldview, intuition and reflections of therapists all influence how clinical reasoning plays out in each therapeutic encounter.

Given the holistic approach of occupational therapy, this overall process of clinical reasoning is perhaps more complex than may be observed in the clinical reasoning processes undertaken by other health professionals (Fleming, 1991b; Unsworth, 2017; Unsworth & Baker, 2016). Specifically, clinical reasoning in occupational therapy requires the consideration of clients' current and future occupational functioning, and how they engage and relate to others and their environments. Without this broad focus, occupational therapy intervention plans are likely to be misaligned with clients' needs and goals and may not optimise the contribution of support systems.

Throughout the intervention process, there should be regular monitoring. Results of ongoing monitoring provide feedback into the clinical reasoning process and may result in changes to plans and goals. It is therefore useful to conceptualise the process of clinical reasoning as a spiral. With each successive loop of continuing assessment and

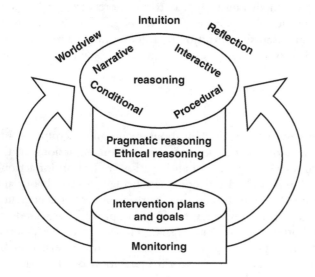

Figure 16.1 A framework for clinical reasoning in occupational therapy.

evaluation, the understanding of clients' unique situations becomes more comprehensive and the overall quality of clinical reasoning is improved (Higgs & Jones, 2000).

Using clinical reasoning at different stages of the occupational therapy process

Occupational therapists use clinical reasoning in all aspects of their work, but in general this process can be broken into three stages. These stages are: formulating an impression; information gathering and planning; and monitoring. Key considerations for occupational therapists at each stage of the process are summarised in Table 16.1.

Developing from a novice to an expert practitioner

Over time and with experience, reasoning processes become more embedded in occupational therapists' everyday thinking and go from very conscious processes to more *tacit* (semi-automatic) processes (Fleming, 1991a; Gibson et al., 2000; Mattingly & Fleming, 1994a; Unsworth, 2001). Although often not easily distinguished, the phases of development of expertise have been described as Novice, Advanced beginner, Competent, Proficient and Expert (Unsworth, 2001). It is also important to consider that not all therapists will reach expert status in their career, and that time and experience, while supporting expert practice, are not synonymous with being an expert occupational therapist. Students and novice occupational therapists often experience clinical reasoning as time-consuming and effortful (Gibson et al., 2000). It can be disconcerting to watch more experienced therapists articulate well-reasoned intervention plans very quickly, and difficult to see and explain the process of determining those plans. Often experts appear to make inexplicable leaps in their reasoning. This reflects the increased efficiency of the clinical reasoning process as expertise emerges.

The process of development from a novice practitioner to a more expert practitioner takes experience and well-developed reflective skills (Craig-Duchesne et al., 2018; Gibson et al., 2000; Harries, 2007; Wong et al., 2016). Students can benefit from working with peers to review each other's clinical reasoning processes and challenge one another to ensure important factors are recognised and considered in order to create plans that are best aligned to clients' needs and desires. Critical reflection on clinical reasoning with supervisors, peers and senior clinicians, particularly during fieldwork placements and in practice after graduation, assists in the refinement of these skills.

With ongoing, careful consideration and reflection, expertise in clinical reasoning develops over time. Even expert practitioners need to continue reflecting on their practice and clinical reasoning processes (Creek, 2007). Without this process of reflection, clinical decisions can become too automated and may fail to consider the unique situations and needs of each client. Other factors also influence the development of clinical reasoning skills. These include organisational factors such as how much employers value continuing professional development and support the provision of high-quality supervision; the service setting; and individual therapists' cognitive skills and commitment to ongoing development.

Table 16.1 Overview of considerations at different stages of the clinical reasoning process

	Narrative	Interactive	Procedural	Conditional	Pragmatic and ethical
Overall aim	To understand clients' roles and occupational functioning, the impacts of their situations on occupational functioning and their desired occupational functioning for their futures (Bonsall, 2012; Mattingly, 1991b)	To maximise the quality of therapeutic relationships by understanding clients' supports and engagement with service systems (Mattingly & Fleming, 1994b)	To understand clients' conditions, likely prognoses and evidence–based interventions that are likely to support optimal outcomes (Fleming, 1991a)	To consider the current and future impact of the condition and establish intervention approaches that will engage clients in therapy and support optimal outcomes for the future (Fleming, 1991a)	To consider the limitations on potential interventions/supports alongside what is necessary for clients (Edwards et al., 2004; Unsworth, 2004)
Considerations: *Formulating an impression*	• Roles and occupations typical for clients with given characteristics (e.g., age) • History and duration of clients' conditions • The likelihood that clients are still adjusting to their conditions • The potential that clients have developed coping strategies for managing the impact of their conditions on their day-to-day functioning	• Clients' living arrangements • Clients' current support services • Whether clients have previously received occupational therapy services • Information about how clients have engaged with services previously • Limitations imposed by the setting on how clients are engaged	• The potential functional impact of clients' conditions on their daily functioning • The likely trajectory of clients' conditions (improving, remaining stable, deteriorating) • Whether clients are likely to require short-term or ongoing supports • Evidence–based approaches to support optimal outcomes for the challenges that clients experience	• What do clients want for their futures? • How is their condition likely to impact on their lives now and into the future? • What approaches will engage clients in therapy?	• Limitations imposed by the service setting in terms of what clients can be offered • The kinds of services that are and will be available to clients • Other services that can be engaged to ensure that clients' needs are met, collectively

Considerations: *Information gathering and planning*	• Clients' occupational histories • Clients' most valued roles and occupations • The impact of clients' conditions on their abilities to engage in their roles and occupations • Clients' wishes for their occupational futures (e.g. return to previous roles/occupations; explore new opportunities)	• Understanding of how clients have engaged with services in the past, and whether they are likely to have difficulties engaging with services in the future • Understanding of how clients are engaging in the current therapeutic relationship • Supports that clients currently have access to and that might be required • What clients need from services, and how differing needs such as encouragement and support, practical assistance to achieve goals, and hope to set goals for the future can be met • The limitations on current services and in the current setting	• Approaches with the best evidence for supporting clients to achieve their desired occupational goals • The advantages and disadvantages of potential approaches, and the acceptability of each to clients Note: advice from senior colleagues and peers can be very helpful in this process.	• The optimal approaches for clients • The most acceptable approach to clients, considering their abilities to complete the required activities or achieve changes in environments • The approaches clients believe will be most successful • All things considered, the approaches likely to be most suited to assist clients to meet their desired occupational futures	• Considering the 'optimal' and 'most appropriate' approaches, the pragmatic limitations to implementation • Limitations on funding and service structures that limit how interventions can be delivered • Given these limitations, the interventions that can be delivered that will still support good outcomes for clients • 'Trade-offs' clients are willing to make • With the limitations imposed, whether clients are still receiving appropriate services or if advocacy is required

Considerations: *Monitoring*
• The specific outcomes that can be expected to be achieved and how these can be measured
• If, on balance, outcomes are less than expected, further consideration of:
  • clients' current difficulties or their desired occupational futures (narrative reasoning);
  • clients' understanding of their conditions and their relationships with support networks (interactive reasoning); and
  • the most effective interventions for clients' specific situations to achieve desired goals (procedural and conditional reasoning).

Conclusion

Clinical reasoning is an important skill that therapists develop as they gain experience in practice settings. It provides the basis for professional decision-making and day-to-day problem-solving. Different types of clinical reasoning are used depending on the contextual requirements and practice requirements of the client, family and others around them. It is important for students to be cognisant of the different types of clinical reasoning, and factors that may influence reasoning such as the therapist's worldview, intuition and ability to reflect, so that they can start to implement them during their practice education placements.

Summary

- Clinical reasoning in occupational therapy requires the simultaneous consideration of a range of factors to support optimal collaborative decision-making with clients.
- In this chapter, six aspects of clinical reasoning have been presented as essential in the occupational therapy process: narrative reasoning, interactive reasoning, procedural reasoning, conditional reasoning, pragmatic reasoning and ethical reasoning.
- In an optimal clinical reasoning process, narrative, interactive, procedural and conditional reasoning are all considered, and then a selection of intervention options are identified and reviewed in terms of what is practical and feasible given the limitations of the situation (pragmatic reasoning), as well as what is just and fair for the individual (ethical reasoning).
- Clinical reasoning is influenced by a therapist's worldview, capacity for reflection and growth, and intuition.
- Although initially complex and time-consuming, with practice and reflection the clinical reasoning of novice occupational therapists becomes more flexible, integrated and efficient.

Review questions

1. Describe the six aspects of clinical reasoning and how each of these supports the development of optimal intervention plans.
2. How can pragmatic and ethical reasoning influence (both positively and negatively) an overall intervention plan?
3. Describe considerations in your clinical reasoning when working with a client who has had previously negative interactions with health services, does not recognise or prioritise the need for support to meet occupational needs, and has limited or no family or community supports (particularly consider your interactive, conditional, pragmatic and ethical reasoning)?
4. Using narrative and conditional reasoning, describe how working with a client to identify a 'desired occupational future' can help to drive therapeutic action.
5. In occupational therapy, it is not possible to determine an intervention plan based only on the client's diagnosis or current limitations. Provide some of your clinical reasoning to explain why this isn't possible.
6. As individuals, we often don't spend much time thinking about our worldview, until it is challenged or it becomes apparent that this is the underlying reason for a conflict. Reflect on your worldview of the concept of education: is education a right or a privilege? Should you have to pay for your primary, secondary and tertiary education? Is education the key to knowledge and therefore power?

References

Barnitt, R. E. (1993). 'Deeply troubling questions': The teaching of ethics in undergraduate courses. *British Journal of Occupational Therapy*, *56*(11), 401–406. https://doi.org/10.1177/030802226930560104

Bonsall, A. (2012). An examination of the pairing between narrative and occupational science. *Scandinavian Journal of Occupational Therapy*, *19*(1), 92–103. https://doi.org/10.3109/11038128.2011.552119

Chaffey, L., Unsworth, C., & Fossey, E. (2012). The relationship of intuition and emotional intelligence among occupational therapists in mental health practice. *American Journal of Occupational Therapy*, *66*(1), 88–96. https://doi.org/10.5014/ajot.2012.001693

Christiansen, C. H. (1999). Defining lives: Occupation as identity: an essay on competence, coherence, and the creation of meaning. *American Journal of Occupational Therapy*, *53*(6), 547–558. https://doi.org/10.5014/ajot.53.6.547

Cohn E. S., Schell, B. A. B., & Crepaeu, E. B. (2010). Occupational therapy as a reflective practice. In N. Lyons (Ed.), *Handbook of reflection and reflective inquiry*. Springer.

Craig-Duchesne, C., Rochette, A., Scurti, S., Beaulieu, J., & Vachon, B. (2018). Occupational therapy students' experience with using a journal in fieldwork and factors influencing its use. *Reflective Practice*, *19*(5), 609–622. https://doi.org/10.1080/14623943.2018.1538953

Creek, J. (2007). The thinking therapist. In J. Creek & A. Lawson-Porter (Eds.), *Contemporary issues in occupational therapy: Reasoning and reflection* (pp. 1–22). John Wiley & Sons.

Del Mar, C., Hoffmann, T., & Glasziou, P. (2017). Information needs, asking questions, and some basics of research studies. In T. Hoffmann, S. Bennett, & C. Del Mar (Eds.), *Evidence-based practice across health professions* (3rd edn, pp. 16–40). Elsevier.

Edwards, I., Jones, M., Carr, J., Braunack-Mayer, A., & Jensen, G. M. (2004) Clinical reasoning strategies in physical therapy. *Physical Therapy*, *84*(4), 312–335. https//doi.org/10.1093/ptj/84.4.312

Fleming, M. H. (1991a). The therapist with the three-track mind. *American Journal of Occupational Therapy*, *45*(11), 1007–1014. https://doi.org/10.5014/ajot.45.11.1007

Fleming, M. H. (1991b). Clinical reasoning in medicine compared with clinical reasoning in occupational therapy. *American Journal of Occupational Therapy*, *45*(11), 988–996. https://doi.org/10.5014/ajot.45.11.988

Gibson, D., Velde, B., Hoff, T., Kvashay, D., Manross, P. L., & Moreau, V. (2000). Clinical reasoning of a novice versus an experienced occupational therapist: A qualitative study. *Occupational Therapy in Health Care*, *12*(4), 15–31. https://doi.org/10.1080/J003v12n04_02

Harries, P. A. (2007). Knowing more than we can say. In J. Creek & A. Lawson-Porter (Eds.), *Contemporary issues in occupational therapy: Reasoning and reflection* (pp. 161–188). John Wiley & Sons.

Higgs, J., & Jones, M. (2000). *Clinical reasoning in the health professions*. Butterworth-Heinemann.

Kanny, E. M., & Slater, D. Y. (2018). Ethical reasoning. In B. A. Schell & J. W. Schell (Eds.), *Clinical and professional reasoning in occupational therapy* (pp. 188–208). Lippincott Williams & Wilkins.

Knightbridge, L. (2019). Reflection-in-practice: A survey of Australian occupational therapists. *Australian Occupational Therapy Journal*, *66*(3), 337–346. https://doi.org/10.1111/1440-1630.12559

Levine, R. M., & Reicher, S. D. (1996). Making sense of symptoms: Self-categorization and the meaning of illness and injury. *British Journal of Social Psychology*, *35*(2), 245–256. https://doi.org/10.1111/j.2044-8309.1996.tb01095.x

Mattingly, C. (1991a). What is clinical reasoning. *American Journal of Occupational Therapy*, *45*(11), 979–986. https://doi.org/10.5014/ajot.45.11.979

Mattingly, C. (1991b). The narrative nature of clinical reasoning. *American Journal of Occupational Therapy*, *45*(11), 998–1005. https://doi.org/10.5014/ajot.45.11.998

Mattingly, C. (1998). In search of the good: Narrative reasoning in clinical practice. *Medical Anthropology Quarterly*, *12*(3), 273–297. https://doi.org/10.1525/maq.1998.12.3.273

Mattingly, C., & Fleming, M. H. (1994a). *Clinical reasoning: Forms of inquiry in therapeutic practice.* F. A. Davis Co.

Mattingly, C., & Fleming, M. H. (1994b). Interactive reasoning: Collaborating with the person. In C. Mattingly & M. H. Fleming (Eds.), *Clinical reasoning: Forms of inquiry in therapeutic practice* (pp. 178–196). F. A. Davis Co.

Neistadt, M. E. (1996). Teaching strategies for the development of clinical reasoning. *American Journal of Occupational Therapy, 50*(8), 676–684. https://doi.org/10.5014/ajot.50.8.676

Occupational Therapy Board of Australia. (2018). *Australian occupational therapy competency standards 2018.* https://www.occupationaltherapyboard.gov.au/Codes-Guidelines/Competencies.aspx

Rogers, J. C., & Masagatani, G. (1982). Clinical reasoning of occupational therapists during initial assessment of physically disabled patients. *Occupational Therapy Journal of Research, 2*(4), 195–219. https://doi.org/10.1177/153944928200200401

Scanlan, J. N., & Hancock, N. (2010). Online discussions develop students' clinical reasoning skills during fieldwork. *Australian Occupational Therapy Journal, 57*(6), 401–408. https://doi.org/10.1111/j.1440-1630.2010.00883.x

Schell, B. A. B. (2019). Professional reasoning in practice. In B. A. Boyt Schell & G. Gillen (Eds.), *Willard & Spackman's occupational therapy* (13th edn, pp. 482–497). Wolters Kluwer.

Schell, B. A. B., & Cervero, R. M. (1993). Clinical reasoning in occupational therapy: An integrative review. *American Journal of Occupational Therapy, 47*(7), 605–610. https://doi.org/10.5014/ajot.47.7.605

Schell, B. A. B., & Schell, J. W. (2018). *Clinical and professional reasoning in occupational therapy* (2nd edn). Lippincott Williams & Wilkins.

Schön, D. A. (1983). *The reflective practitioner: How professionals think in action.* Basic.

Schwartzberg, S. (2001). *Interactive reasoning in the practice of occupational therapy.* Pearson.

Taylor, R. R., & Kielhofner, G. (2017). *Kielhofner's model of human occupation: Theory and application* (5th edn). Lippincott Williams & Wilkins.

Unsworth, C. A. (2001). The clinical reasoning of novice and expert occupational therapists. *Scandinavian Journal of Occupational Therapy, 8*(4), 163–173. https://doi.org/10.1080/110381201317166522

Unsworth, C. A. (2004). Clinical reasoning: How do pragmatic reasoning, worldview and client-centredness fit? *British Journal of Occupational Therapy, 67*(7), 10–19. https://doi.org/10.1177/030802260406700103

Unsworth, C. A. (2017). An overview of professional reasoning within occupational therapy practice. In M. Curtin, M. Egan, & J. Adams (Eds.), *Occupational therapy for people experiencing illness, injury or impairment* (7th edn, pp. 90–104). Elsevier.

Unsworth, C. A. (2020). The evolving theory of clinical reasoning. In E. A. S. Duncan (Ed.), *Foundations for practice in occupational therapy* (6th edn). Elsevier.

Unsworth, C. A., & Baker, A. (2016) A systematic review of professional reasoning literature in occupational therapy. *British Journal of Occupational Therapy, 79*(1), 5–16. https://doi.org/10.1177/0308022615599994

Wolters, A. M. (1989). On the idea of worldview and its relationship to philosophy. In P. A. Marshall, S. Griffioen, & R. Mouw (Eds.), *Stained glass: Worldviews and social science* (pp. 14–25). University Press of America.

Wong, K. Y., Whitcombe, S., & Boniface, G. (2016). Teaching and learning the esoteric: An insight into how reflection may be internalised with reference to the occupational therapy profession. *Reflective Practice, 17*(4), 472–482. https://doi.org/10.1080/14623943.2016.1175341

World Federation of Occupational Therapists. (2016). *Minimum standards for the education of occupational therapists (Revised 2016).* https://www.wfot.org/assets/resources/COPYRIGHTED-World-Federation-of-Occupational-Therapists-Minimum-Standards-for-the-Education-of-Occupational-Therapists-2016a.pdf#:~:text=The%20World%20Federation%20of%20Occupational%20Therapists%20%28WFOT%29%20Minimum,quality%20assurance%20for%20development%20beyond%20the%20levels%20specified

17 Occupational therapy models of practice

Merrill Turpin and Jenniffer García

Chapter objectives

Upon completion of this chapter, the reader will be able to:

- Understand the importance of theory in guiding occupational therapy practice.
- Briefly overview six occupational therapy models of practice.
- Understand different ways occupational therapy currently presents the relationship between person, environment and occupation.

Key terms

human occupation; theory and practice; occupational therapy models of practice

Introduction

In any given practice situation, occupational therapists have to make decisions about action, that is, they need to decide what to *do* with a specific client. This is a complex process, in part due to the diversity of individual needs and circumstances. Occupational therapists have to deal with disparate information, sometimes contradictory, and connect it in a meaningful way that helps them to formulate a plan of action. They have to combine knowing and doing.

Knowing and doing are generally referred to as theory and practice, respectively. Both inform each other. Without theory, practitioners are akin to technicians. Without practice, theory has no grounding in the world. Combining the two is crucial to occupational therapy. Over time and through a process of integrating professional knowledge and skills with their personal values, beliefs and commitments, occupational therapists will develop a professional framework to guide their thinking. This combines propositional knowledge (generalised, knowing *that*) with professional craft knowledge (specific, knowing *how*) and personal knowledge (knowing oneself) (Higgs et al., 2001).

Models of practice provide guidance for combining knowledge and action. Occupational therapy has a well-developed collection of discipline-specific models of practice. These aim to guide practice by: i) making explicit the assumptions of the profession; ii) providing a framework for organising knowledge (both generalised knowledge and that pertaining to a particular client such as assessment results and narrative information); and iii) outlining a process to use when addressing issues relevant to occupational therapy practice (Turpin & Iwama, 2011).

This chapter provides a brief overview of six occupational therapy models of practice—Occupational Performance Model (Australia) (OPMA) (Chapparo & Ranka, 1997), Model of Human Occupation (MOHO) (Kielhofner, 2008), Person–Environment–Occupation (PEO) model (Law et al., 1996), Canadian Model of Occupational Performance and Engagement (CMOP-E) (Townsend & Polatajko, 2007), Person–Environment–Occupation-Performance (PEOP) model (Baum et al., 2015) and Kawa model (Iwama, 2006). To illustrate combining theory and practice, these models of practice are used to discuss the case study of Maria.

Case study

Maria is a 60-year-old woman who has had mental health issues since she was 20. Throughout her life she has abused prescription medication, leaving her with reduced cognitive function. She suffered from severe depressive episodes and has made three suicide attempts. She was recently diagnosed with bipolar disorder, after receiving a litany of misdiagnoses and being prescribed various psychotropic medications. Adverse side-effects of her medications include dry mouth, dizziness and tremor.

Maria did not finish high school nor pursue further education. She has three adult daughters, three grandchildren and divorced five years ago. When married, she was a stay-at-home mother. After her divorce, economically, she needed to work and started full time as a sales assistant. She faces ongoing challenges within the work environment, because she forgets clients' requests, has limited endurance for standing for long periods of time and is bullied by her boss and workmates. Her social network is limited to one friend and she is both dependant on and aggressive towards her daughters. She receives some financial support from her ex-husband but manages money very poorly.

Occupational Performance Model (Australia) (OPMA)

The OPMA is widely used in Australia, although it does not represent an official position of Occupational Therapy Australia. It was first published as a monograph in 1997 (Chapparo & Ranka, 1997) and has a comprehensive website (http://www.occupationalperformance.com). We have placed OPMA first, because its structure follows the tradition of occupational performance models, the dominant occupational therapy models in the 1970s. While it represents the biopsychosocial shift in thinking in occupational therapy of the 1990s, it includes performance areas and performance components (major features of the occupational performance models, see Turpin & Iwama, 2011). The OPMA focuses on occupational performance, defined as 'the ability to perceive, desire, recall, plan and carry out roles, routines, tasks and subtasks for the purpose of self-maintenance, productivity, leisure and rest in response to demands of the internal and/or external environment' (Chapparo & Ranka, 1997, p. 4). It centres on the person in context, referring to internal (within the person) and external (outside of the person) environments.

The *internal environment* has four levels: occupational roles, performance areas, performance components and the core elements of body, mind and spirit. The primary concern is the performance of *occupational roles*, and all occupational therapy

interventions should work towards this. Occupational roles are influenced by expectations of what is required (i.e. a person's own expectations as well as those of others—
significant others and society) and they change over time as abilities and circumstances
alter. Occupational roles have three dimensions—knowing, doing and being. Knowing refers to understanding desired or expected occupational roles; doing refers to
carrying out those roles; and being refers to the satisfaction or fulfilment a person
might obtain from them. Occupational roles form the intersection of the internal and
external environments.

Performance areas and *performance components* are classic dimensions of occupational performance models. In the OPMA, the *performance areas* are self-maintenance, rest, leisure
and productivity. The model emphasises that particular occupations should be classified
into these areas by the performer (e.g., an occupation might be work for one person and
leisure for another). The five *performance components* are biomechanical, sensory-motor,
cognitive, intrapersonal and interpersonal. Each is presented from the perspective of
the performer and the demands of the task (e.g., respectively, a person's strength and
range of motion and an object's weight and size). The final internal level consists of the
core element—the interaction of body, mind and spirit. As Chapparo and Ranka (1997)
explained, 'Relative to occupational performance, the body-mind-spirit core element
of this model translates into the 'doing-knowing-being' dimensions of performance'
(p. 13). That is, the body provides the means of doing, the mind enables knowing and
the spirit is the foundation for being.

The *external environment* is the context surrounding the internal environment and has
four interconnected dimensions—physical, sensory, cultural and social. The physical
environment includes both the natural and constructed surroundings and determines
the skills and abilities required to perform occupation in a particular location and position. The sensory environment provides sensory cues. The cultural environment includes the values, beliefs, ideals and customs that are shared among social groups and
influences what people choose to do and believe they are expected to do. The social
environment is created by the patterns of relationships between people.

In addition to the four dimensions of the environment, *space* and *time* influence occupational performance. Both have *physical* and *felt* dimensions. Physical space includes the
wider physical world, objects and body structures. Felt space is the subjective experience of space. For example, the same space might feel safe to some people and unsafe to
others, or claustrophobic to some and comfortable to others. Regarding time, physical
time refers to chronological time, while felt time is the subjective experience of time,
with highly personal meaning.

Case study: OPMA perspective

In terms of the *internal environment*, Maria's main occupational roles are as mother,
grandmother and worker. Her main performance component problems lie in the *cognitive, interpersonal* and *intrapersonal performance components*, manifesting as poor planning
and problem solving, paranoid ideation, severely reduced memory and lack of initiative
(cognitive); misunderstanding of other people's intentions and lack of empathy (interpersonal); and poor emotional regulation (intrapersonal). An example of a performance
area that is affected is self-maintenance. She needs supervision with medication and
financial management and her daughters are key to providing this. In terms of the *external environment*, she is socially isolated and bullied at work (social environment), and has

experienced these challenges all her adult life (time). A full OPMA analysis would show how the four internal levels affect each other and how they are shaped by the external environment.

Model of Human Occupation (MOHO)

The MOHO has been published for over four decades and in five book editions (1985, 1995, 2003, 2008, 2017), and is the most widely used occupational therapy model (Forsyth et al., 2019). It was first published when the major alternatives were the occupational performance models, and it represented a major departure from that way of thinking. MOHO addresses how occupation is a) chosen, b) patterned, and c) performed in the contexts in which people live and act. It assumes a close association between person and environment and outlines three interacting elements of the person—volition, habituation and performance capacity.

First, *volition* is the motivation for choosing occupation and has the following three components. *Personal causation* refers to a person's thoughts and feelings about his or her ability to perform everyday activities effectively (sense of agency). *Values* are 'beliefs and commitments about what is good, right and important to do' (Forsyth et al., 2019, p. 603). *Interests* develop over time according to what a person finds enjoyable and satisfying. Whether or not particular occupations remain in a person's occupational repertoire depends on his or her experiences.

Second, *habituation* relates to the patterns and routines into which people organise their occupations, and habits and roles are its main components. *Habits* develop when familiar things are done in familiar environments and can involve learned ways of undertaking tasks and the enactment of regular routines. *Roles* have social expectations and responsibilities, as well as implications for identity. People internalise role expectations through their interactions with others and people develop an identity associated with these roles.

Third, *Performance capacity* is 'a person's underlying mental and physical abilities and how those abilities are used and experienced in occupational performance' (Forsyth et al., 2019, p. 604). It has both objective and subjective components. Objective capacities can be observed, measured and modified using a range of different frameworks such as motor control, cognitive and sensory approaches. The subjective experience of performance capacity includes how people experience abilities and impairments and how they perceive the world.

The *environment* is the context in which human occupation occurs and has physical, social, cultural, economic and political features. The physical environment includes spaces and objects. The social environment includes both social groups and tasks. Along with the cultural environment, it contributes to the expectations of and opportunities available to people and shapes their views regarding valuable and worthwhile occupations. The economic and political environments determine the resources and occupational roles available.

MOHO identifies three 'levels' of human occupation, referred to as *dimensions of doing*, with each embedded within the broader one above and all being influenced by volition, habituation, personal capacity and environmental conditions. The broadest level is *occupational participation* or taking part in society. This occurs through work, play and activities of daily living. Performance capacities, habituation, volition and environmental conditions all influence occupational participation. Next is *occupational performance*, the actual performing of occupation. The final dimension of doing is *skill*. Skills are grouped into motor skills (those relating to moving self and objects); process skills (those required to logically sequence actions over time); and communication and interaction skills (those required for conveying need and intentions, and acting with others).

Finally, human occupation results in occupational identity, competence and adaptation. Over the course of people's lives, they build *occupational identities*, that is, a sense of themselves as occupational beings. People's occupational identities are shaped by their awareness of what they are good at and capable of, what they find interesting and satisfying to do, the roles they have, what they feel obliged to do, and their perceptions of the demands and supports of the environment. People have *occupational competence* when they are able to sustain a pattern of occupational participation that reflects their occupational identity. While occupational identity relates to subjective experience, occupational competence is about creating action from that identity. Both contribute to a person's *occupational adaptation* over time.

The complex interaction between people and their environment shapes human occupation. When the capacities of people correspond to the demands of the environment and available resources, occupational performance is facilitated. When people perform well, they are likely to feel good about themselves and their abilities and pursue opportunities for repeating such experiences. When the fit is poor and occupational performance is reduced, a change in either performance capacity or the environment, or both, may be required in order to increase the fit. Reduced access to resources from the political and economic environment can limit opportunities to increase the fit between the environmental demands and the person's abilities.

Case study: MOHO perspective—worker role

In terms of *volition*, Maria has limited interest in working but does so because she needs to earn more money to afford her medications. She has a reduced sense of self-efficacy, shaped by continued criticism from her mother and ex-husband about being lazy and disorganised, as well as negative interactions with co-workers. In contrast, winning an award at work made her feel good about herself for the first time in her life.

Regarding *habituation*, she puts a lot of effort into strategies to support her worker role, such as noting due dates, setting alarms and using memory aids. However, this effort causes her stress and she feels exhausted all the time. As a result, she sleeps whenever she is at home. Her lack of time and exhaustion reduces her ability to engage in her other roles of mother, grandmother and friend and keeps her socially isolated.

Her *performance capacity* is limited by objective components: her cognitive decline and reduced physical capacity (associated with her age, passive lifestyle, and the side effects of the medications). The subjective experience of a menacing work environment reinforces her feelings of incompetence and dependence.

The *environment* of work is physically and cognitively demanding and includes bullying from co-workers and her boss. Consequently, there is a poor fit between her and her environment, but she needs to keep working to earn the money she needs.

Person–Environment–Occupation (PEO) model

The PEO model was published in 1996 (Law et al., 1996) and no further editions have been undertaken. The model is concerned with the relationship among person, environment and occupation and its contribution to occupational performance through the *'person–environment–occupation fit'* (PEO fit) (Law et al., 1996, p. 17). Greater or lesser PEO fit leads to enhanced or reduced occupational performance.

The model differs from many other models at the time, in that it uses an ecological framework and describes a 'transactive' (as distinct from interactive) relationship between people and their environments. In an interactive approach, person and environment are conceived as separate entities that interact and can be studied separately. In a transactive approach, a person's occupational performance cannot be separated from the context in which it occurs. Therefore, occupational performance is context-, person- and occupation-specific. It results from particular people doing particular things in particular places in particular circumstances.

In a transactive relationship, a change in any of person, environment and occupation will change the others in ways that cannot be controlled or predicted. Therefore, the unit of study and analysis is an *event*, rather than the separate components of person, environment and occupation. By exploring the event as a whole, attention centres on the way PEO fit changes with a change to any components. Changes in PEO fit are also evident when taking a lifespan perspective, in that PEO fit is assumed to change over time and with different circumstances. This lifespan perspective is presented diagrammatically using a cylinder that can be transected at different places to represent the PEO fit at different times in a person's life.

The PEO model also discusses each component. The *person* is 'a dynamic, motivated and ever-developing being, constantly interacting with the environment' (Law et al., 1996, p. 17). It takes a lifespan perspective, whereby people change over time, as they grow and develop and move through their life stages. However, they also change in response to alterations in the environment surrounding them. Their attributes, characteristics, abilities and skills change, as well as how they think and feel about themselves, their sense of identity and their sense of what they are capable of doing and achieving. As occupational performance can be measured both objectively and subjectively, the model advocates that people's capacities should be measured (e.g., through objective assessment) and their experiences and perceptions also should be explored (e.g., through self-report).

The *environment* is inseparable from the person. It is defined broadly, understood as shaping and being shaped by people, and has five aspects: cultural, socio-economic, institutional, physical and social. Some or all of these five aspects will combine to shape occupational performance. Environments also change over the course of people's lives. People might relocate geographically, find themselves in altered circumstances, or their environments might change because they have changed their roles, routines and habits. Changes in environments rarely relate to only one environmental aspect. For example, a change in physical environment might have implications for the social environment. To illustrate how people and environments are intertwined, internalised cultural views shape what people want and need to do and socio-economic circumstances will shape what they have the opportunities to do and the resources available to them.

Finally, *occupation* is what people do in their contexts. Occupation is considered in terms of three aspects of human action—activity, task and occupation, which are considered 'nested within each other' (Law et al., 1996, p. 16). These three aspects of human action might appear dated in the light of more recent taxonomies of occupation (see Townsend & Polatajko (2007) in which task is nested within activity, rather than activity being the basic unit of a task).

Case study: PEO perspective—visiting her daughter

Maria received plane tickets to visit one of her daughters, who was living abroad. Although feeling excited, she was concerned about travelling by herself to a country in which people speak a different language. Her other two daughters dropped her off at the airport and an assistant took her to the first plane. However, during the stopover, she missed her connecting flight because she became disoriented and lost in the airport. She was distressed and unable to plan what to do. Because she did not arrive on the correct plane, her daughter realised that she must still be at the transit airport and made phone calls to the airline. After getting help from the airline, Maria arrived at her daughter's home many hours later than expected. She was quite shaken by the experience. During her visit, she became withdrawn and was completely dependent on her daughter for every decision, because everything was so different.

The PEO fit changes if any one or more components change. In Maria's situation, the primary changes were the occupation (she hadn't flown very much) and the environment (being in a very different place). These changes had a dramatic effect on the PEO fit and also led to altered behaviour (person). When compared with how she manages in her daily life at home, even though it is difficult and exhausting, she still manages to work. In contrast, during the visit, she became incapable of making decisions.

Canadian Model of Occupational Performance and Engagement (CMOP-E)

CMOP-E was published in *Enabling Occupation II: Advancing an Occupational Therapy Vision for Health, Well-being and Justice through Occupation* (Townsend & Polatajko, 2013) by the Canadian Association of Occupational Therapists (CAOT) (along with the Canadian Practice Process Framework [CPPF] and the Canadian Model of Client-Centred Enablement [CMCE]). The three main components of the model are person, occupation and environment.

CMOP-E still retains the essential structure of the original CMOP, published in 1997. Like OPMA, the influence of the occupational performance models is evident in its inclusion of both performance components and performance areas. The person is presented as having three performance components—affective, cognitive and physical—as well as a central core of spirituality. The performance areas of ADL/self-maintenance, work/productive activities, and play/leisure provide the framework for categorising occupation.

Occupation is the core domain of occupational therapy and the 'bridge' that connects person and environment (Townsend & Polatajko, 2007, p. 23). It is defined as:

> groups of activities and tasks of everyday life, named, organised, and given value and meaning by individuals and a culture. Occupation is everything people do to occupy themselves, including looking after themselves (self-care), enjoying life (leisure), and contributing to the social and economic fabric of their communities (productivity).
> (definition of occupation retained from the first edition of *Enabling Occupation*—CAOT 1997, cited in Townsend & Polatajko (2007, p. 17)).

The environment has four aspects—physical, institutional, cultural and social—and surrounds the person, emphasising that each person lives in a specific environmental context that affords (and constrains) possibilities for occupation.

Enablement through occupation is conceptualised as the core of occupational therapy. While occupational performance is an enduring component of the model, the concept of engagement was added to the second edition to emphasise that people can engage in occupation without necessarily performing it. As an exemplar, Townsend and Polatajko (2007) described a father and his severely disabled son who undertook extreme sporting events together such as marathons, triathlons and ironman events. The son engaged in these (but did not perform them), while being pushed in a wheelchair, pulled in a dinghy or pulled behind his father's bicycle.

Occupational therapy *enables* the following: i) engagement in everyday life; ii) performance of occupation; and iii) the creation of a just society in which people are able to participate. Therefore, occupational therapy practice can target both individual and societal levels. Accordingly, CMOP-E identifies six categories of client—individuals, families, groups, communities, organisations (e.g., government, non-government and corporate agencies; clubs and associations) and populations.

Client-centred practice is also considered fundamental to occupational therapy. It involves collaboration and power sharing, working *with* people rather than doing to or for them, and prioritising client goals and outcomes. Townsend and Polatajko (2007) explained that both client-centred practice and engagement can be encountered at the level of the client and therapist or at the broader systems surrounding them. For example, factors influencing the personal level might include the client's culture and level of education, the therapist's capacity to recognise the client's expertise and to share power. Factors influencing the broader level could include management policy and practice or government philosophy and the equity of resource distribution.

Case study: CMOP-E perspective—the pandemic

In 2020, the world was consumed by the COVID-19 pandemic. Being in the 'at risk' category because of her age and health condition, government policy forced Maria to stay at home (i.e., the institutional environment disrupted her physical, social and cultural environments). While she continued to receive money from her employer, and, therefore, was able to afford her medications, she was unable to go to work or see her children and grandchildren (her main occupational roles). At a personal level, she began to feel fragile, sad and irritable (affective components). She felt that her memory and ability to stay focused had deteriorated because of constantly worrying that she would catch the virus and become a burden on her daughters (cognitive components). All of this made her feel worthless (spiritual core). Because of this disconnection between her and her environment, her occupation became quite disrupted and she was unable to do her usual activities. She felt 'all at sea'.

Through an online consultation with the occupational therapist who had worked with her the last time she was hospitalized in a mental health unit, Maria was able to identify and participate in meaningful activity. Together they organized a routine in which she participated in an online knitting group with the goal of knitting a scarf for each of her grandchildren. The occupational therapist coordinated with a community group to deliver a box of wool to her. This enabled Maria's occupational engagement and social participation, and enabled her to fulfil her occupational roles (restoring occupation as a bridge between person and environment).

Person–Environment–Occupation–Performance (PEOP) model

The PEOP is in its fourth edition (1991, 1997, 2005, 2015). The model has undergone significant conceptual development and each version of the model differs substantially than previous ones. Baum et al. (2015) referred to it as 'an ecological-transactional systems model' (p. 49), meaning that it centres on people in the environmental systems in which they live. In understanding and facilitating human occupational performance, the model draws upon a wide base of knowledge, including 'healthcare, disability studies, social policy, technology, rehabilitation science, and public health' (Baum et al., 2015, p. 50).

The model is based on the following four assumptions:

1. It values collaboration. Because clients know what is valued by and meaningful to them, intervention planning should be a collaborative process. Clients could be individuals and families (receiving direct intervention) or other health care providers, professionals in other sectors such as architects, or whole communities (intervention through consultation).
2. It focuses on occupational performance, which is defined as 'the doing of meaningful activities, tasks and roles through complex interactions between the person and environment' (Baum et al., 2015, p. 52). Occupational performance supports *participation* (active engagement and involvement in social life) and *well-being*, and connects the individual to his or her socio-cultural environment through roles.
3. It emphasises a systems perspective. In systems theory, the components of the system influence each other and the system as a whole. In occupational performance, the components are the activity, task or role being performed, the environment influencing them and the person performing them. The primary interaction occurs between person and environment, and the meaningfulness of occupation is dependent on this interaction. The mutual influence of components is seen when, through occupational performance, the person both changes the environment and is also changed (e.g., his or her self-perception and actual skills).
4. It supports client-centred practice. Ultimately, occupational therapists aim to enable people to perform the activities, tasks and roles that are meaningful for them and serve a purpose in their daily lives. Forming partnerships with those people is central to achieving this aim. The fourth edition of the PEOP model comprises four interacting elements—person, environment, occupation and the narrative. Occupational performance, leading to participation and well-being, results when there is an optimal person–environment fit. The narrative and occupational performance interact dynamically. The narrative refers to 'the past, current and future perceptions, choices, interests, goals and needs that are unique to the Person, Organization or Population' (Baum et al., 2015, p. 54), these last three being categories of the client. The personal narrative includes perception and meaning, choices and responsibilities, attitudes and motivation, and needs and goals. An organisational narrative comprises mission and history, focus and priorities, stakeholders and values, and needs and goals. A population narrative will include environments and behaviours, demographics and disparities, incidence and prevalence, and needs and goals.

The PEOP model provides detailed elements of person and environment. The elements related to the person are cognitive, psychological, physiological, sensory, motor and spiritual. In discussing the psychological elements of the person, Baum et al. (2015) emphasised the importance of understanding 'the roles, activities and goals of the client' (p. 53), as these provide the motivation for occupational performance. The environment includes culture, social determinants, social support and social capital, education and policy, the physical and natural environment, and assistive technology. Occupation comprises activities, tasks and roles (Baum et al., 2015).

Case study: PEOP perspective

Maria has been admitted to the acute mental health ward. Given her history of severe suicide attempts, upon reporting having recurrent suicidal ideation, she was immediately hospitalised. She has been feeling very anxious, irritable, and depressed lately. In addition to the stress of being socially isolated during the pandemic, her ex-husband wants to decrease the pension he provides. Maria feels worthless and incapable of returning to work.

The occupational therapist on the ward found it easy to build rapport with Maria and engage her in attending occupational therapy sessions. Maria is well known on this ward and feels 'at home', valued and protected. After a couple of sessions together, Maria indicated that she would like to work toward a post-discharge goal of initiating retirement and finding something to return meaning to her life. By listening to her narrative, the occupational therapist understood that Maria had never enjoyed her current work. She had a childhood dream of being a midwife and working with babies. When she was married, the economic situation and lack of support from her husband (environmental factors), as well as her own learning difficulties and the mental health issues she faced through her life (personal factors), had combined to prevent her achieving these dreams. By working collaboratively, Maria and her occupational therapist discovered that the hospital near her home was seeking *cuddle carers* who could volunteer at least twice a week at the neonatology unit. This seemed the perfect opportunity for Maria. The prospect of undertaking this role, has made Maria feel excited and optimistic about her life. The occupational therapist has met with Maria's family and contacted the hospital to ensure that she is supported to perform this role. Maria describes this occupation as the most meaningful work she will have done in her life and is really looking forward to it.

Kawa model

'The Kawa model: Culturally relevant occupational therapy' was published in 2006 (Iwama, 2006). It was developed because the existing occupational therapy models were not appropriate to Japanese culture, and a substantial portion of the Kawa model book was devoted to explaining aspects of that culture. At the time, Iwama claimed that the degree to which occupational therapy was culturally bound was largely unrecognised. More recently, Nelson et al. (2017) stated that recognition of 'occupation and health as culturally bound constructs' in occupational therapy had increased in focus over the previous decade (p. 73). The model explores the notion of occupation from a collectivist perspective, in which a 'decentralised self' requires reordering of the doing, being and becoming framework (Wilcock, 1998) to belonging, being and then doing. Iwama (2006) challenged occupational therapy 'to make its ideas, ideology, theory and the practices that follow, relevant to many, many groups of people' (p. 50). The work of Nelson et al. provides an example of the model being used for another collectivist culture, Australian Aboriginals and Torres Strait Islanders.

Kawa is the Japanese word for river. Just as a river flows from its source to the ocean, metaphorically, a person's life 'flows' from birth to death. The water flowing through the river represents the life energy, or life flow. In the model, the *life flow* could be that of a person or family, or the life of an organisation.

The river metaphor aptly represents the aim in collectivist cultures of creating harmony with one's surroundings. A river is shaped by the unique geography over which it courses, following valleys, flowing over and around rocks and falling in waterfalls. Similarly, the flow of the water itself can etch into the landscape, creating new channels. As Iwama (2006) explained, 'collectively oriented people tend to place enormous value on the *self* embedded in relationships. There is greater value in 'belonging' and 'interdependence', than a unilateral agency and in individual determinism. In such experience, the interdependent self is deeply influenced and even determined by the surrounding social context, at a given time and place' (p. 145).

Cross-sections depicting river elements can reveal the state of a person's river (life flow) at different times in their life. The elements are as follows:

Water (*misu*) represents life flow. As a fluid, water will easily take on the shape of a container and fill the spaces completely. However, the power of its flow gives it the capacity to carve new channels. So, too, people can conform to the demands of their surroundings, while also influencing them.

The surroundings (social and physical environments) are represented by the *river walls and floor* (*Kawa no soku-heki* and *Kawa no Zoko*, respectively). In collectivist cultures, these are important factors in determining a person's life flow because the environmental culture is instrumental in determining how people experience 'self' in the meanings they ascribe to their actions.

Rocks (*iwa,* large rocks or crags) represent circumstances that impede the life flow and are considered by the person as problematic and difficult to remove. Potential rocks include impairments to body structures and functions, difficulties with activities of daily living, lack of money and difficult social relations.

Driftwood (*ryuboku*) represents personal attributes and resources, which could relate to personal characteristics and abilities (e.g., values, personality, skills) as well as material assets (e.g., wealth, special equipment) and living situation (e.g., rural and urban, shared accommodation). These can affect circumstances and life flow in positive and negative ways. Compared to rocks, driftwood is less permanent and more amenable to the flow of the river. The *spaces* between obstructions (*sukima*) represent places in a person's life where life energy and life flow are still occurring (Kawa model uses a strengths-based approach, seeking to identify strengths rather than problems). Identification of *sukima* enables an occupational therapist to work by strategically building on opportunities to maximise life flow. The *Orang Tang* fish and *sparkles* have been added since the original publication and represent things that are going well in a person's life. The spaces, fish and sparkles prompt identification of personal and situational strengths that could be built upon to increase life flow.

Case study: Kawa model perspective—Maria's life flow

Looking at the *river walls and floor*, it is clear that Maria has had a hard life. Her river has been 'blocked' for much of her life. In her younger days, her life flow was restricted by the mental health issues experienced by her own mother, her complex social circumstances and the learning difficulties that made schooling challenging. As an adult, she has had a long history of emotional and mental struggles, lack of proper diagnosis, medication abuse and being neglected by her former husband. There are many *rocks* that have obstructed her life flow.

The Kawa model uses a strengths-based approach through the concepts of *driftwood*, *Orange Tang* and *sparkles*, and *sukima* (spaces between obstructions). She is provided with substantial support from her daughters (helping to optimise the spaces between obstructions); she has a long-term belief in engaging in volunteer activities with vulnerable groups in her community, and is looking forward to her planned volunteer work at the hospital; and she is motivated to be part of a group of retired women. These are aspects of her life that can be built on to improve her life flow and shape the course of her river for the next phase of her life.

Issues evident in the models

Comparison of occupational therapy practice models highlights that occupational therapy is primarily concerned with occupation, which includes people's action (doing) in specific contexts at specific times, as well as the meaning of that action in the context of their everyday lives. Central to the occupational therapy notion of occupation is the relationship between person, environment and occupation (Joosten, 2015). The nature of this relationship varies across models. It is presented as transactive, interactive or with occupation serving as a bridge between person and environment. A deeply contextualised understanding of occupation is common throughout the practice models.

Although the outcome of this relationship is commonly presented as occupational performance, more recently a concern for participation in everyday life and in society has been made explicit. For example, in the CMOP-E, the scope of occupational therapy includes enabling a just society. This is consistent with the way the 'client' is conceptualised. While the client was conceived as an individual for most of occupational therapy's history, contemporary models make explicit that the client could be an individual, family or other group, an organisation, or a population.

Conclusion

Both theory and practice (knowing and doing, respectively) are important for occupational therapy. Models of practice are frameworks to support using theory to inform practice. They provide guidance for organising knowledge in a way that enables decision making about action. Six occupational therapy models of practice have been presented and used to discuss the case of Maria. These case vignettes only provide a 'snapshot' of how each model could be used to understand the case. In practice, a full analysis with a chosen model of practice would need to be undertaken.

Summary

- Theory and practice are both important for professional practice.
- Occupational therapy has a well-developed collection of models of practice, which aim to guide occupational therapists in combining theory and practice.

- Comparing occupational therapy models of practice emphasises that the core concern for occupational therapy is occupation embedded in a multi-dimensional environmental context. The main differences between the models of practice pertain to the nature of the relationship among person, environment and occupation.
- Current occupational therapy models of practice conceptualise 'client' broadly as including individuals, families and groups, organisations, and populations.

Review questions

1. How do the different occupational therapy models of practice conceptualise the relationship between person, environment and occupation?
2. How has conceptualisation of the 'client' in occupation changed?
3. What are the main components of each model of practice?

References

Baum, C. M., Christiansen, C. H., & Bass, J. D. (2015). The Person–Environment–Occupation–Performance (PEOP) model. In C. H. Christiansen, C. M. Baum, & J. D. Bass (Eds.), *Occupational therapy: Performance, participation, and well-being* (pp. 49–56). SLACK Inc.

Chapparo, C., & Ranka, J. (1997). *OPM: Occupational Performance Model (Australia).* Occupational Performance Network.

Forsyth, K., Taylor, R. R., Kramer, J. M., Prior, S., Ritchie, L., & Melton, J. (2019). The Model of Human Occupation. In B. A. Boyt Schell & G. Gillen (Eds.), *Willard & Spackman's occupational therapy* (13th edn, pp. 601–621). Lippincott Williams & Wilkins.

Higgs, J., Tichen, A., & Neville, V. (2001). Professional practice and knowledge. In J. Higgs & A. Titchen (Eds.), *Practice knowledge and expertise in the health professions* (pp. 3–9). Butterworth Heinemann.

Iwama, M. K. (2006). *The Kawa model: Culturally relevant occupational therapy.* Churchill Livingstone.

Joosten, A. V. (2015). Contemporary occupational therapy: Our occupational therapy models are essential to occupation centred practice. *Australian Occupational Therapy Journal, 62*(1), 219–222. https://doi.org/10.1111/1440-1630.12186

Kielhofner, G. (2008). *Model of Human Occupation: Theory and application* (4th edn) Lippincott Williams & Wilkins.

Law, M., Cooper, B., Strong, S., Stewart, D., Rigby P., & Letts, L. (1996). The Person–Environment–Occupation model: A transactive approach to occupational performance. *Canadian Journal of Occupational Therapy, 63*(1), 9–23. https://doi.org/10.1177/000841749606300103

Nelson, A., McLaren, C., Lewis, T., & Iwama, M. (2017). Cultural influences and occupation-centred practice with children and families. In S. Rodger & A. Kennedy-Behr (Eds.), *Occupation-centred practice with children: A practical guide for occupational therapists* (pp. 73–90). John Wiley & Sons.

Townsend, E., & Polatajko, H. (2007). *Enabling occupation II: Advancing an occupational therapy vision for health, well-being, & justice through occupation.* CAOT Publications ACE.

Townsend, E. A, & Polatajko, H. J. (2013). *Enabling occupation II: Advancing an occupational therapy vision for health, well-being, and justice through occupation* (2nd edn). CAOT Publications ACE.

Turpin, M. J., & Iwama, M. K. (2011). *Using occupational therapy models in practice: A fieldguide.* Churchill Livingstone.

Wilcock, A. A. (1998). Reflections on doing, being and becoming. *Canadian Journal of Occupational Therapy, 65*(5), 248–256. https://doi.org/10.1177/000841749806500501

Part III

Practice issues

18 Fundamentals of occupational therapy

Understanding the environment

Tammy Aplin, Emma Crawford and Desleigh de Jonge

Learning objectives

Upon completion of this chapter, the reader will be able to:

1. Understand the importance of the environment in occupational therapy practice and in shaping people's lives overall.
2. Be familiar with the terminology and frameworks used to describe the environment.
3. Be able to explain the transactional nature of person, environment and occupation, and the enabling and constraining impact of the environment on occupational performance, participation and life chances.
4. Be able to consider and understand the environment, with reference to the eight dimensions.
5. Be able to describe the influence of the eight dimensions of the environment on people's everyday occupations.

Key terms

environment; micro-, meso-, exo- and macrosystem; bioecological model of human development; press competence model; physical environment; personal environment; temporal environment; social environment; cultural environment; institutional environment; socio-economic environment; virtual environment

Introduction

The role of the environment in promoting health and well-being has been acknowledged in occupational therapy since the early days of the profession. Occupational therapy viewed people as active beings operating in, and interacting with, the world around them. One of the profession's founders highlighted the need for people to actively engage with the environment, stating: 'Our conception of man is that of an organism that maintains and balances itself in the world of reality and actuality by being in active life and active use' (Meyer, 1922, p. 5).

This understanding shaped the profession's response to the sterile, unstimulating hospital and institutional environments of the time. In these environments, returning soldiers, people with infectious diseases and the 'mentally ill' experienced extended periods of isolation from the community. With little to do, they could become disruptive or despondent (Parent, 1978). Chapter 3 provides more information about the history of the profession over this period in Australia. Early occupational therapy practitioners recognised that by acting on these environments they could be agents of change (Laurence & Banks, 1978). They worked to improve people's recovery and well-being by creating comfortable real-world environments with regular routines to promote occupational engagement and mastery.

Occupational therapy has built a unique and comprehensive understanding of the environment's role in promoting occupational performance, participation, ongoing well-being and life chances, reflected in our models. The first recognition of environment in occupational therapy models was in the 1980s (Reed & Sanderson, 1999). Since this time occupational therapy interventions have focused on changing the environment such as sensory rooms, accessible and enriching play environments, restructuring and modifying educational, workplace and home environments, providing caregiver and community education, advocacy, and policy work. A rich understanding of the environment has also enabled occupational therapists to understand how the environment influences uptake and outcomes of interventions. The range of environmental assessments and interventions provided by occupational therapists is vast and reflective of the central role the environment plays in occupational therapy. While these cannot be considered in depth in this chapter, a brief overview is provided in Table 1 of common environmental assessments and interventions addressing the environment.

Table 18.1 Examples of occupational therapy assessments and interventions addresing the environment

Assessments	*Interventions*
• Occupational analysis • Interview with client about different dimensions of the environment and their impact on life • Gathering narrative interviews, observation notes and/or surveys (e.g., to understand impact of new funding model, to understand a practice context, to inform a quality improvement project, or to identify systemic disadvantage) • Home, school, worksite visit • Ergonomic assessment of workplace • Access assessment of public buildings • Human rights assessment • Community consultation • Needs analysis • Standardised measures of the environment broadly which include multiple dimensions • Standardised measures of the community • Standardised measures of home and residential environments • Standardised measures of school environment • Standardised measures of social support • Standardised measures of the workplace • Standardised measures of social determinants of health	• Redesign/modification of workplaces • Home modifications • Sensory rooms • Design of workplaces, school, play, residential and institutional housing environments • Assistive and mainstream technology (e.g., wheelchairs, pressure relieving devices, hoists, bathroom/toilet aids, communication aids, switches, tablets and smartphones) • Context therapy • Caregiver, family and community education • Facilitate formal or informal support • Individual advocacy • Systems advocacy for institutional change or education/social attitude change • Social inclusion initiatives • Government and organisational policy development and change • Changing service and organisation structures (e.g., governance, policy, processes) • Working towards changing funding structures • Service re-design to ensure services are physically, culturally and socially accessible such as service co-design (e.g., intake procedures, bookings, reception areas, community worker support) • Community development work • Participatory Occupational Justice Framework projects (Whiteford et al., 2018). • Cultural responsiveness training • Cultural responsiveness initiatives based on formal frameworks including IAHA Cultural Responsiveness in Action Framework (2020) or Making Connections Framework (Nelson et al., 2017) or other approaches • Quality improvement projects

The environment is a complex concept, described variously within and outside the discipline of occupational therapy. To provide a deep understanding of the environment, this chapter will overview a number of influential models/frameworks, whose key concepts informed contemporary occupational therapy models, described in Chapter 17. Before considering how we as occupational therapists may change the environment to enhance occupational performance, it is important that these key concepts are understood as they describe the environment and its impact on people's lives. With this knowledge we are better able to partner with people and provide more tailored assessments and interventions. The chapter therefore presents, firstly, how the environment is conceived as having constraining or enabling impact on daily activities. Secondly, the multiple layers of the environment are discussed. Thirdly, the influence of the environment on people's ongoing health/well-being and life chances are considered. Fourthly, how we shape, and are shaped by, the environment is then presented in a discussion of the transactive nature of the environment. The chapter concludes with a detailed discussion of the dimensions of the environment, namely, the physical, personal, social, temporal, cultural, institutional, socio-economic and virtual dimensions, with particular reference to the case study of Sarah.

Case study: Sarah's story—understanding the environment

Red-faced, too warm and slightly frazzled, Sarah bumped into a desk that was too close to the front door of the classroom when she rolled in ten minutes late. She could not sneak through the back door like other late students because of the steps. In their guidance session before class, the very reason she was late, the councillor had encouraged Sarah to, 'think about how lucky you are to have your new wheelchair funded by the National Disability Insurance Scheme'. Sarah wondered what was lucky about having spina bifida, standing out, being stuck at the front of the classroom and unable to fit between the desks, being teased. Tina got it. Tina wasn't in a wheelchair: kids made unkind remarks because of her skin colour. Tina whispered across her desk, 'did you watch "Outta school" last night?' Sarah remembered the pangs of envy she felt as she watched the stories of adolescents leaving school after year ten to work and travel. 'I was thinking, we should get out of school!'

In a bustle of excitement, Tina rushed to the newsagency where Sarah had been working for the past six years since they finished school. She held up an official-looking letter. 'I'm going back to school at the age of 21! Mum says she's proud of the strong Aboriginal woman I've grown up to be.' Sarah lifted her eyebrows and widened her eyes to show that she was looking at Tina's acceptance letter. 'Sorry, I was daydreaming about the day we decided to leave school because of that TV show. It was a bit rash, but I'm glad. You've helped your family so much with your little brothers and they're doing so well at school because of everything you and your parents do. You've got great experience working at the real-estate agency. I know my mum and dad appreciate me working here. It made sense for our family, financially, but I'm so much more confident now... All people see is my chair. They don't know that I'm a go-getter who is smart with my money and loves book-keeping for my parent's shop. And if there's a desk in my way now, I just convince someone that the whole room needs rearranging. At least, that's what I'll do when I get into business admin at TAFE.' Sarah noticed she was rambling nervously. Congratulating Tina on the great news, she hastily said goodbye. Red-faced, too warm and slightly frazzled, she rolled out the door ten minutes before her shift ended so she could stop at her apartment before visiting the family she volunteered with in an English tutoring program for refugees. Tina wondered why Sarah was in such a hurried fluster. Sarah wondered if she too would find an acceptance letter to TAFE in her mailbox today.

The environment: Key concepts from an occupational perspective (environment enables and constrains)

The environment in which we live can enable or restrict us in our daily lives. The way in which the environment might constrain our lives is known as environmental press. Environmental press, demonstrated in Figure 18.1 on the x-axis, was proposed by Lawton and Nahemow (1973) in their *Press-Competence Model*. This model shows how the environment interacts with the person to result in behaviour and effect, i.e. the things we do and feel. If the environment has too much press or places too many demands on the person's level of competence (abilities residing within the individual) negative behaviour or affect results (Lawton & Nahemov, 1973; Lawton, 1982). For example, excessive environmental press contributed to Sarah's choice to leave school before completing year 12 despite her aspirations for further study.

Figure: Press-competence model. Adapted from Lawton, M. P. (1982). Competence, environmental press, and the adaptation of older people. In M. P. Lawton, P. G. Windley & T. O. Byerts (Eds.), Aging and the environment: Theoretical approaches (pp. 33-59). New York: Springer, p. 44. Sourced from original : Lawton, M. P., & Nahemow, L. (1973). Ecology and the ageing process. In C. Eisdorfer., & M. P., Lawton (Eds.), The psychology of adult development and aging (pp. 619-674). Washington, DC: American Psychological Association

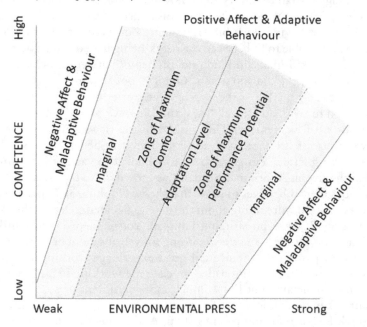

Figure 18.1 Press competence model from Lawton and Nahemov's Ecological Model of Ageing. Source: Lawton & Nahemow (1973, pp. 619–674)

Layers of the environment

There are many aspects to the environment. Some aspects are in the person's immediate environment whilst others are in the broader community. Bronfenbrenner describes four layers, the micro-, meso-, exo- and macrosystem as shown in Figure 18.2—the Bi-oecological Model of Human Development (Bronfenbrenner, 1979; Bronfenbrenner & Morris, 2006). The inner layer is the immediate or microsystem, which includes the person's family, friends, school, neighbourhood and home, and represents the people and organisations that the person interacts with most. For Sarah, this would be her parents, Tina, her workplace and where she volunteers. The next layer is the mesosystem, which describes the interconnections between microsystems. For Sarah, this layer would include the interactions between her parents' shop and her local community. The next layer is the exosystem. This includes aspects of the community which impact indirectly on the person. For example, the local council where Sarah lives would fund and organise local community events and supports such as support groups for youth. Finally, in the outer layer is the macrosystem. This includes the overarching culture, ideology and structures of the society in which the person lives (Bronfenbrenner, 1979; Bronfenbrenner & Morris, 2006). For Sarah, this would include Australian culture and norms within and for groups that she identifies with, such as the norms and expectations for women and people with a disability. National policies such as the National Disability Insurance Scheme would also fit in the macrosystem as they determine what resources are available to support Sarah.

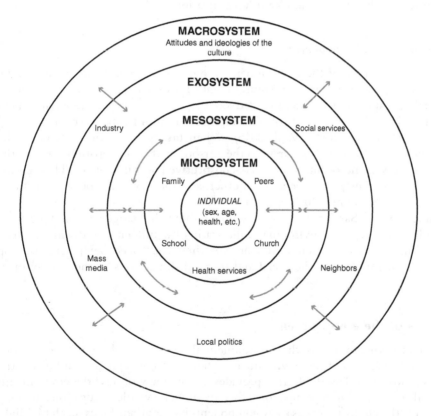

Figure 18.2 Bronfenbrenner's Bioecological Model of Human Development.
Source: Velez-Agosto et al. (2017, pp. 900–910)

The environment influences life chances and health

When the impacts of the environment are considered over time, it is recognised as influencing our life chances and health. This can be illustrated by Sarah and Tina's story. Both Sarah and Tina grew up in the same area, went to the same school and have parents who loved and cared for them. Yet their life chances and health will be different due to their environment. For example, while going through high school Tina had a lot of friends and exercised frequently through sporting groups. In contrast, these opportunities did not exist for Sarah as there were no wheelchair sports offered in her school or community. Tina was offered a job by her Mum's friend in real-estate. Since starting the job Tina has moved into higher positions and is now selling property. She has just bought her first home. Sarah in contrast may not have been considered for a similar role because of access issues to workplaces or local business owners not understanding her abilities. As a result of her environment, Sarah has not had as many opportunities for physical fitness, social connection or economic participation as Tina, which may impact her health and well-being in the future. This comparison highlights the importance of a sociological perspective of health, where health is understood to be impacted by an accumulation of social factors, and not simply a result of immediate biological or psychological factors (Germov, 2019). These social factors (i.e., 'the conditions in which people are born, grow, work, live and age, and the wider set of forces and systems sharing the conditions of daily life') are described as the social determinants of health (World Health Organization, 2020) and are considered to be the most important factors in determining our health (World Health Organization, 2020).

Transactional nature of environment

The transactional nature of the environment recognises that while we are shaped by the environment, we also shape the environment. This concept, which is evident in occupational therapy models, was founded on the concept of person–environment transaction described in the work of philosophers, environmental psychologists and gerontologists (Bunting, 2016; Wahl, 2015). When taking a transactional view, the environment cannot be seen as separate to the person (or their occupations); rather the environment, person and occupation are co-constitutive (Bunting, 2016). They are intertwined, and constantly influencing each other, and therefore cannot be understood in isolation (Aplin & Tanner, 2019; Bunting, 2016).

For example, when Sarah was young she learnt about the dangers of smoking from teachers in her kindergarten environment, illustrating the influence of the institutional and social dimensions of her environment. She then convinced her parents to stop smoking, in turn influencing the social and physical dimensions of the environment around her.

Dimensions of the environment

The above conceptualisations of the environment allow us to understand the relationship between ourselves and the environment. These key concepts have informed the profession's guiding models. Table 18.2 provides an overview of how the environment is conceptualised in common occupational therapy models. While occupational therapy models include the environment as a key component, it is not their focus. Each highlight

Table 18.2 Common occupational therapy models' conceptualisation of the environment

Occupational therapy model	Conceptualisation of the environment	
	Aspects of environment	Influence of environment
Model of Human Occupation (MOHO) (Kielhofner, 2008)	Physical, social, cultural, economic and political considerations.	The environment supports, constrains and gives meaning to individual's occupations. Environment seen as influencing and being influenced by the person. Culture, political and economic conditions are considered broader aspects which influence the person, spaces, objects, social groups and occupational forms/tasks.
Canadian Model of Occupational Performance and Engagement (CMOP-E) (Canadian Association of Occupational Therapists, 1997; Townsend & Polatajko, 2007)	Cultural, institutional, physical and social aspects.	Environment affords occupational possibilities and is unique for each individual. Interactions between the person, environment and occupation are dynamic. Interactions between person and environment are bi-directional.
The Person–Environment–Occupation Model (PEO) (Law et al., 1996)	Cultural, socio-economic, institutional, physical and social considerations. Consideration of environmental domains from the perspective of person, household, neighbourhood or community. The temporal aspect of the environment is identified as an important consideration, with reference to time points across the lifespan.	Environment dictates behaviour and is influenced by the person. This two-way influence of person and environment is considered as 'transaction' The environment is the context within which occupational performance occurs and is considered to have constraining and enabling effects on occupational performance
The Kawa model (Iwama, 2006)	The environment is the river bed (river walls and floor) representing the physical and social context of the person that influences life flow. Rocks represent circumstances that block life flow and cause dysfunction. This may include personal circumstances but may also include external, environmental circumstances. The temporal aspect of the environment (past, present and future) is considered in terms of the river's make-up at different points along the river's path.	A metaphorical model using a river to represent life flow—the river bed (environment) and rocks (circumstances) can impede the flow of the water (life flow) or create room for the water to flow freely (life flow which may include occupational engagement). The Kawa river metaphor can be applied at an individual, family, group or organisational level; thus the influence of environment on life flow can be considered for individuals, groups, communities and organisations.
The Person–Environment–Occupation-Performance (PEOP) model (Baum & Christiansen, 2005)	Natural environment, social support, economic systems, culture and values, and the built environment and technology.	The environment is extrinsic to the person and can be enabling, supporting or restrictive to the performance and participation of individuals, organisations or communities.

different aspects of the environment and acknowledge the concepts described above variably. Therefore, to further understand the environment, and its elements, eight dimensions of the environment are presented below. These dimensions are drawn from literature which broadly examines the environment, along with occupational therapy models and literature, to provide a comprehensive understanding of the environment.

Physical environment

The physical environment includes things that we can touch, see, smell and hear. This includes the natural and built environment, structures, objects, layout, space, location and ambient conditions (American Occupational Therapy Association, 2014; Aplin & Tanner, 2019; Law et al., 1996; Townsend & Polatajko, 2007). The natural environment includes everything living and non-living in our natural world, for example the trees, grass and animals (American Occupational Therapy Association, 2014; Townsend & Polatajko, 2013). The built environment describes built structures and objects that we live around and within (Townsend & Polatajko, 2007). Objects include furniture, products, equipment such as Sarah's wheelchair, and items that we use day to day. How the structures and objects are placed or arranged creates the layout of our environments and influences our space (Sanford & Bruce, 2010).

The space in our environment can be understood as the areas in between the natural and built environment, for example, how much space there is in a living room, parking space or personal space. These elements of the physical environment can impact widely on people's lives. For example, the limited space and layout of the desks at Sarah's school meant she was forced to always sit at the front of the class.

Another important aspect to the physical environment is location. This considers elements relevant to the home or where the person lives, such as family and friends, schools, shops, and other services or facilities, such as transport (Aplin & Tanner, 2019). Location also includes the topography or lay of the land, which refers to how steep or flat the land is (Aplin & Tanner, 2019). For Sarah, a steep road or pathway makes it difficult for her to get to where she wants to go in her wheelchair. The ambient conditions are also important to consider, including the lighting, airflow, breezes, shade, the weather and temperature, along with noise and odour (Aplin & Tanner, 2019).

Personal environment

The personal environment refers to emotions associated with the environment, including our sense of privacy, freedom, control and independence, safety and security, identity and connectedness with places (Aplin et al., 2013; 2015; Aplin & Tanner, 2019).

Privacy is defined as being alone and free from disturbance or intrusion from others (Oxford English Dictionary, 2019). Our sense of privacy and how much control we have over our privacy varies throughout the day, across our lives, and depends on the space and place. For example, at home we often have more privacy than in public places such as work or school (Aplin & Tanner, 2019). For privacy to occur in our homes, we also need to have control and freedom in our homes.

Our sense of control, freedom and independence is an important aspect of how we experience environments. For example, at work or at school we have little control over the spaces we use, whereas at home we have a greater sense of control, freedom and independence. Our sense of safety and security at home is both physical and emotional

(Aplin & Tanner, 2019). For example, Sarah may feel safe at home because she has good security features, but it may also come from being in a familiar and known environment, living with her parents who make her feel safe. In comparison, Sarah may feel unsafe or at risk when making her way home alone along quiet streets at night.

Our deepest feelings associated with the environment are in relation to identity and connection (Aplin & Tanner, 2019). There are places in our lives that are linked to our sense of self. For example, our homes as personal places, which we have decorated and organised in our own way, reflect our identities and are linked to our sense of self (Despres, 1991; Sixsmith, 1986). At a deeper level, we can have a strong sense of connection or belonging to a place, a home, or home town (Aplin & Tanner, 2019; Rowles, 2000). This deep connection to place comes from living in and being in a place over time, where memories are formed (Aplin & Tanner 2019; Rowles, 2000).

Social environment

The social environment describes the complexities of our relationships, connections and influence of others in our world. It includes our relationships with others, the attitudes and expectations of others, along with social events (Law et al., 1996; Townsend & Polatajko, 2007; World Health Organization, 2001). Relationships incorporate our connections with those closest to us, such as our family, friends and pets, as well as our involvement with community, neighbours, workplace and school colleagues. Our relationships impact our lives in every way, both positively and negatively. For example, Sarah's best friend Tina provides a positive impact through friendship. In contrast, some peers at school who teased Sarah had a negative impact as they contributed to her leaving school early.

The widely held expectations and attitudes within the social environment influence our participation and life chances strongly. These attitudes and social expectations or norms,\ come from all levels of society, from those close to us at the microsystem, from our communities (exosystem), and from society broadly (macrosystem) (Townsend & Polatajko, 2007; World Health Organization, 2001). For example, Sarah's parents and teachers may have held low expectations for her about her future, i.e. the type of job she may have as an adult, where she might live or how independent she would be. Sarah's parents, teachers and peers were likely influenced by wider societal expectations and norms of people with disability.

Social events also influence our day-to-day lives and participation (American Occupational Therapy Association, 2014). Social events include events such as a family get-together or dinners, parties, and traditional events and celebrations, along with more community or societal events like a market, exhibition, cultural festival or national holiday. When thinking about social events, the social and physical environment are intertwined and create environments which are supportive or restrictive for people. For example, the volume of people at a sports arena may make it difficult for Sarah to mobilise through the crowds whilst a small community sports event in an open field would be more manageable.

Temporal environment

The temporal environment acknowledges that our lives and the world we live in are not static. There are two main elements of the temporal environment, cyclical and linear time (Werner et al., 1985).

Cyclical time refers to the routines and patterns of our lives, those daily, weekly and yearly occurrences in our lives (Law et al., 1996; Werner et al., 1985). We all have routines and patterns in life. Sarah, for example, works five days a week eight to four, volunteers to teach a family of refugees English on Wednesday evenings, and takes her dog for a walk every morning. These routines provide structure and predictability to Sarah's life and allow her to plan ahead and make appropriate arrangements.

Linear time refers to the past, present and future, thinking about the influence of history and our lifespan (Law et al., 1996; Werner et al., 1985). For instance, Sarah and Tina are thinking about their future a lot at the moment and making plans to return to study. Considering the past, Tina (Sarah's friend) is an Aboriginal woman and has been adversely affected by discriminatory policies and attitudes towards her ancestors and possibly towards herself since the British colonisation in Australia. In the present, she is able to access some additional support for her studies as an Aboriginal woman through an Indigenous student support program. Tina has strong ideas about being a role model for her younger family members when she is older by gaining a higher level qualification and being engaged in a successful career.

Cultural environment

Culture is the confluence of beliefs, values, knowledge, perspectives, attitudes, norms and customs that stem from people belonging to a society or group (Hammell, 2013). All groups have their own unique culture, including groups based on ethnicity, gender, religion, sexuality, age, profession, ability and socio-economic status. Behaviours and beliefs can seem to be common sense or 'right', when in fact they are reflections of culture (Hammell, 2013) and may not be the most appropriate, effective or meaningful ways for people from other groups. For example, the way Sarah might dress, talk or eat her breakfast each day might seem inconsequential to her, and may be different from the clothing, food, language and customs of the migrant families that she volunteers with or the ways her friend Tina, who is an Aboriginal woman, understands and goes about her everyday activities. Nonetheless, these are reflective of her own cultural background and provide her a reference point for understanding her own and other people's cultural norms, beliefs, behaviours and traditions.

When considering the culture as a dimension of the environment that influences day-to-day lives, it is important to first be aware of our own culture as it shapes our perspective (Hammell, 2013). Connecting and listening to people's stories can reveal the ways in which culture shapes what is important to us, the things we do and how we do them (Nelson et al., 2017).

In the Australian context, the health of Aboriginal and Torres Strait Islander people is of particular importance for achieving overall well-being and health equality, and therefore, culturally responsive practice is paramount (Australian Government, 2015; Indigenous Allied Health Australia, 2020). A gap in many health outcomes between Aboriginal and Torres Strait Islander people and non-Indigenous Australians (Close the Gap Campaign Steering Committee, 2019) highlights the need for health services and health professionals to reflect on their own practice, along with the services they work for, to consider how they might best work in ways that are responsive and collaborative. Therefore, being culturally responsive is critical (Indigenous Allied Health Australia, 2020; Nelson et al., 2017). Chapter 11 describes a strengths-based approach when engaging with people from an Aboriginal and Torres Strait Islander background.

Institutional environment

People's lives occur within a web of services, systems, organisations and policies. This web is the institutional context that they interact with as they go about their lives. Institutions contribute to the structure of society, such as how and when health and therapy services might be accessed, and the distribution of power and resources, including funding for services, equipment and support (Townsend & Polatajko, 2013). However, the institutional environment goes beyond health and therapy services and relates to all aspects of life. The institutional aspect of the macro environment includes housing services and organisations, utilities, telephone and internet communications platforms and providers, consumer goods, architectural and building services, transport, civil and legal protection, associations, organisations, businesses, media, welfare, health, education, employment and political activity (World Health Organization, 2001).

Some of the institutions that Sarah interacts with include her parents' newsagency business; government policy, organisation and funding associated with the National Disability Insurance Scheme; her previous school; architectural services and policies (such as the Building Code) that influence accessibility; the TV show that she watched on government-subsidised free-to-air television; TAFE; and the non-profit volunteer organisation. While a lack of school accessibility and a television show discouraged Sarah from pursuing education beyond year ten, TAFE and government funding have subsequently enabled her to extend her education.

For Sarah, and all of us, it is important to understand that our actions are influenced, but not completely determined, by the expectations and requirements of institutions (Kantartzis & Molineux, 2011). Sarah's personal characteristics of being highly motivated, being financially responsible and listening to her parents were also influential in her decision making. The institutional structures and personal characteristics interact to determine occupational engagement (Crawford et al., 2016). Institutions shape and can often challenge, but do not always determine, the ways in which people carry out their occupations.

Socio-economic environment

The socio-economic macro environment refers to whether a person lives in poverty, wealth or somewhere in between. It is, therefore, a matter of equity, access and occupational justice (Galvaan, 2012; Sofo & Wicks, 2017). What someone chooses to do in their life is influenced by their external environment, including resource availability (Galvaan, 2012). For Sarah, her socio-economic context contributed to her choice to finish school at year ten because it was financially beneficial to her family. If Sarah's family's financial situation had been different, then her choices might have also been different. For example, her family might not have seen value in Sarah working in their business if they had increased wealth and therefore encouraged her to continue to complete year 12. If she had lived in poverty with parents who had not had educational opportunities due to financial constraints within their own families, they might have wanted her to continue to complete her full high school education to take advantage of an opportunity that they did not have. Socio-economic context can influence people's participation and life in many ways, in combination with personal and other environmental factors (Sofo & Wicks, 2017).

Virtual environment

The virtual environment has become increasingly important since the digital revolution. The recent global pandemic has amplified this, with a rapid increase in the use of technology to create and maintain connections as well as access and sustain services, employment and education. Once considered a convenient adjunct to life, being able to access and effectively navigate through the virtual environment is now considered a necessity. Computers and smart devices, connected to the internet, provide access to education, health and government services; shopping; banking; entertainment; information systems; social networks; and storage of personal documents, photos, audio and video recordings (Jaeger, 2011). These technologies also provide enormous benefits as services can be offered remotely using video consultation technologies.

In addition, these modalities improve access to expertise that may not be available locally and reduce the travel costs associated with accessing, and providing, services (Rogers 2010). However, the digital divide can make it difficult for many older people and people with disabilities to access these online services, due to lack of awareness and access to the virtual world as well as the cost of these technologies (Jaeger, 2011). For Sarah, the virtual environment enabled her to apply for TAFE to multiple cities using her smartphone. However, the cost of a new laptop and internet services may be difficult on her minimum wage. Sarah was able to access health services via telehealth using her smartphone during the COVID-19 lockdown and plans to access advice on suitable technologies for her return to study from the disability support officer at her new institution.

Conclusion

This chapter has discussed the history and conceptualisations of the environment in occupational therapy. Eight dimensions of the environment were presented with reference to the case study of Sarah to provide an understanding of the multiple aspects and complexities of the environment and how it influences day-to-day life and occupational engagement for all of us. This in-depth and nuanced understanding of the environment and its transactional nature is critical to occupational therapy practice.

Summary

- Occupational therapy's history is founded on a deep understanding of the environment and how it can be acted on to create change.
- The environment can enable or constrain our day-to-day lives and over time influences our life chances and health.
- The transactional nature of the environment means that we are shaped by the environment and we can shape the environment.
- To conceptualise and understand the environment more deeply, eight dimensions of the environment can be considered: the physical, personal, social, temporal, cultural, institutional, socio-economic and virtual.

Review questions

1. Identify one activity in your life where you are bored or stressed doing the activity. Locate the activity in Figure 18.1 on the Press Competence Model. Where would

you rate your competence and the environmental press? And describe what aspects of the person (you) and your environment are contributing to the press.

2. To understand how the environment influences life chances and health, choose two dimensions of the environment and describe aspects of these dimensions that have influenced your life chances and health in a positive or negative way.

3. For each of the eight dimensions of the environment name one facilitator and one barrier that impacts your role as a student.

References

American Occupational Therapy Association. (2014). Occupational Therapy Practice Framework: Domain and Process, 3rd edition. *American Journal of Occupational Therapy, 68*(Supp. 1), S1–S48. https://doi.org/10.5014/ajot.2014.682006

Aplin, T., de Jonge, D., & Gustafsson, L. (2013). Understanding the dimensions of home that impact on home modification decision making. *Australian Occupational Therapy Journal, 60*(2), 101–109. https://doi.org/10.1111/1440-1630.12022

Aplin, T., de Jonge, D., & Gustafsson, L. (2015). Understanding home modifications impact on clients and their family's experience of home: A qualitative study. *Australian Occupational Therapy Journal, 62*(2), 123–131. https://doi.org/10.1111/1440-1630.12156

Aplin, T., & Tanner, B. (2019). The home environment. In E. Ainsworth & D. de Jonge (Eds.), *An occupational therapists guide to home modification practice* (2nd edn, pp. 1–16). SLACK Inc.

Australian Government. (2015). *Implementation plan for the National Aboriginal and Torres Strait Islander Health Plan 2013–2023.* Commonwealth of Australia. https://www1.health.gov.au/internet/main/publishing.nsf/Content/AC51639D3C8CD4ECCA257E8B00007AC5/$File/DOH_ImplementationPlan_v3.pdf

Baum, C. M., & Christiansen, C. H. (2005). The Person–Environment–Occupation–Performance: An occupation-based framework for practice. In C. H. Christiansen, C. M. Baum, & J. D. Bass (Eds.), *Occupational therapy: Performance, participation, and well-being* (pp. 243–266). SLACK Inc.

Bronfenbrenner, U. (1979). *The ecology of human development.* Harvard University Press.

Bronfenbrenner, U., & Morris, P. A. (2006). The Bioecological Model of Human Development. In W. Damon & R. M. Lerner (Eds.), *Handbook of child psychology volume 1: Theoretical models of human development* (6th edn, pp. 794–828). Wiley & Sons.

Bunting, K. L. (2016). A transactional perspective on occupation: A critical reflection. *Scandinavian Journal of Occupational Therapy, 23*(5), 327–336. https://doi.org/10.3109/11038128.2016.1174294

Canadian Association of Occupational Therapists. (1997). *Enabling occupation: An occupational therapy perspective.* CAOT Publications ACE.

Close the Gap Campaign Steering Committee. (2019). *Close the Gap report—'Our Choices, Our Voices'.* https://www.humanrights.gov.au/our-work/aboriginal-and-torres-strait-islander-social-justice/publications/close-gap-report-our

Crawford, E., Turpin, M., Nayar, S., Steel, E., & Durand, J. (2016). The structural-personal interaction: Occupational deprivation and asylum seekers in Australia. *Journal of Occupational Science, 23*(3), 321–338. https://doi.org/10.1080/14427591.2016.1153510

Despres, C. (1991). The meaning of home: Literature review and directions for future research and theoretical development. *Journal of Architectural and Planning Research, 8*(2), 96–115. https://www.jstor.org/stable/43029026

Galvaan, R. (2012). Occupational choice: The significance of socio-economic and political factors. In G. Whiteford & C. Hocking (Eds.), *Occupational science: Society, inclusion, participation* (pp. 152–162). Wiley-Blackwell.

Germov, J. (2019). *Second opinion: An introduction to health sociology* (6th edn). Oxford University Press.

Hammell, K. (2013). Occupation, well-being, and culture: Theory and cultural humility. *Canadian Journal of Occupational Therapy, 80*(4), 222–234. https://doi.org/10.1177/0008417413500465

Indigenous Allied Health Australia. (2020). *Cultural responsiveness in action framework*. https://iaha.com.au/workforce-support/training-and-development/cultural-responsiveness-in-action-training/

Iwama, M. K. (2006). *The Kawa model: Culturally relevant occupational therapy*. Elsevier Health Sciences.

Jaeger, P. T. (2011). *Disability and the Internet: Confronting a digital divide*. Lynne Rienner Publishers

Kantartzis, S., & Molineux, M. (2011). The influence of western society's construction of a healthy daily life on the conceptualisation of occupation. *Journal of Occupational Science, 18*(1), 62–80. https://doi.org/10.1080/14427591.2011.566917

Kielhofner, G. (2008). *Model of Human Occupation: Theory and application* (4th edn). Lippincott Williams & Wilkins.

Laurence, M. K., & Banks, S. I. (1978). Milieu therapy and the elderly: A role for the occupational therapist consultant. *Canadian Journal of Occupational Therapy, 45*(4), 171–173. https://doi.org/10.1177/000841747804500407

Law, M., Cooper, B., Strong, S., Stewart, D., Rigby, P., & Letts, L. (1996). The Person–Environment–Occupation model: A transactive approach to occupational performance. *Canadian Journal of Occupational Therapy, 63*(1), 9–23. https://doi.org/10.1177/000841749606300103

Lawton, M. P. (1982). Competence, environmental press, and the adaptation of older people. In M. P. Lawton., P.G. Windley, & T. O. Byerts (Eds.), *Aging and the environment* (pp. 33–59). Springer.

Lawton, M. P., & Nahemow, L. (1973). Ecology and the ageing process. In C. Eisdorfer & M. P. Lawton (Eds.), *The psychology of adult development and aging* (pp. 619–674). American Psychological Association.

Meyer, A. (1922). The philosophy of occupation therapy. *Archives of Occupational Therapy, 1*, 1–10.

Nelson, A., McLaren, C., Lewis, T., & Iwama, M. (2017). Cultural influences and occupation-centred practice with children and families. In S. Rodger & A. Kennedy-Behr (Eds.), *Occupation-centred practice with children: A practical guide for occupational therapists* (pp. 73–90). Wiley.

Oxford English Dictionary. (2019). *privacy, n.* Oxford University Press. https://www.oed.com/view/Entry/151596?redirectedFrom=privacy

Parent, L. H. (1978). Effects of a low-stimulus environment on behavior. *American Journal of Occupational Therapy, 32*(1), 19–25.

Reed, K. L., & Sanderson, S. N. (1999). *Concepts of occupational therapy* (4th edn). Lippincott Williams & Wilkins.

Rogers, L. (2010). Developing simulations in multi-user virtual environments to enhance healthcare education. *British Journal of Educational Technology, 42*(4), 608–615. https://doi.org/10.1111/j.1467-8535.2010.01057.x

Rowles, G. (2000). Habituation and being in place. *Occupational Therapy Journal of Research, 20*(Suppl 1), 52S–67S. https://doi.org/10.1177/15394492000200S105

Sanford, J. A., & Bruce, C. (2010). Measuring the physical environment. In E. Mpofu & T. Oakland (Eds.), *Rehabilitation and health assessment: Applying ICF guidelines* (pp. 207–228). Springer.

Sixsmith, J. (1986). The meaning of home: An exploratory study of environmental experience. *Journal of Environmental Psychology, 6*(4), 281–298. https://doi.org/10.1016/S0272-4944(86)80002-0

Sofo, F., & Wicks, A. (2017). An occupational perspective of poverty and poverty reduction. *Journal of Occupational Science, 24*(2), 244–249. https://doi.org/10.1080/14427591.2017.1314223

Townsend, E. A., & Polatajko., H. J. (2007). *Enabling occupation II: Advancing an occupational therapy vision of health, well-being and justice through occupation*. CAOT Publications ACE.

Townsend, E., & Polatajko, H. (2013). *Enabling occupation II: Advancing an occupational therapy vision for health, well-being and justice through occupation* (2nd edn). CAOT Publications ACE.

Wahl, H-W. (2015). Theories of environmental influences on aging and behaviour. In N. Pachana (Ed.), *Encyclopedia of geropsychology* (pp. 1–9). Springer.

Werner, C. M., Altman, I., & Oxley, D. (1985). Temporal aspects of home: A transactional perspective. In I. Altman & C. M. Werner (Eds.), *Home environments* (Vol. 8, pp. 1–32). Plenum.

Whiteford, G., Jones, K., Rahal, C., & Suleman, A. (2018). The Participatory Occupational Justice Framework as a tool for change: Three contrasting case narratives. *Journal of Occupational Science, 25*(4), 497–508. https://doi.org/10.1080/14427591.2018.1504607

World Health Organization. (2001). *International Classification of Functioning, Disability and Health.* World Health Organization.

World Health Organization. (2020). *Social determinants of health.* https://www.who.int/social_determinants/sdh_definition/en/

Velez-Agosto, N. M., Soto-Crespo, J. G., Vizcarrondo-Oppenheimer, M., Vega-Molina, S., & Garcia Coll, C. (2017). Bronfenbrenner's Bioecological Theory revision: Moving culture from the macro into the micro. *Perspectives on Psychological Science, 12*(5), 900–910. https://doi.org/10.1177/1745691617704397

19 The occupational therapy practice process

Louise Gustafsson, Stephen Isbel and Alexandra Logan

Chapter objectives

Upon completion of this chapter, the reader will be able to:

- Articulate the importance of using an occupation-focused practice process.
- Describe the main features of the Canadian Practice Process Framework, the Occupational Therapy Intervention Process Model and the MOHO-Therapeutic Reasoning Process.
- Understand how to apply three occupational therapy processes.

Key terms

occupational therapy process; Canadian Practice Process Framework; Occupational Therapy Intervention Process Model; MOHO-Therapeutic Reasoning Process

Introduction

The occupational therapy process is a framework that occupational therapists can apply to support occupation-centred thinking and action when interacting with individuals, groups, communities or populations. The occupational therapy process is not a formula that can be used in all situations, but is driven by theory and is client-centred. As all individuals, groups, communities and populations differ, so can the process used to engage, assess and intervene in occupational therapy. This chapter will describe three occupational therapy processes and apply each to a case study to illustrate how it can be used in practice.

The Canadian Practice Process Framework

The Canadian Practice Process Framework (CPPF) is an occupation-focused, client-centred framework where the client can be an individual, group, community or population (Polatajko et al., 2007). It contains the core process elements of assessment, intervention and evaluation, while accounting for societal and practice influences on both the client and the therapist. The CPPF comprises four elements: the societal context, the practice context, frames of references and the eight process-based action points. The CPPF is organised in this way to acknowledge that what occurs when delivering occupational therapy is influenced by the physical, cultural, social and institutional context in which the process takes place. The CPPF also acknowledges that personal and

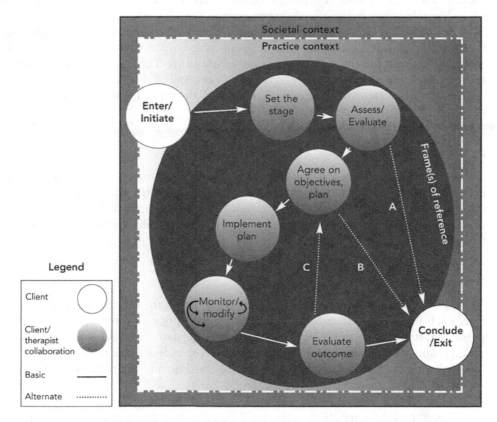

Polatajko, H. J., Craik, J., Davis, J., & Townsend, E. A. (2007). Canadian Practice Process Framework. In E. A. Townsend & H. J. Polatajko, *Enabling occupation II: Advancing an occupational therapy vision for health, well-being, & justice through occupation* (p. 233). Ottawa, ON: CAOT Publications ACE.

Figure 19.1 Canadian Practice Process Framework (CPPF).

environmental factors will influence the occupational therapy process. Figure 19.1 is a diagrammatical representation of the CPPF and each element will be described.

Societal context

The occupational therapy process takes place 'within a broad societal context comprised of cultural, institutional, physical and social environmental elements' (Craik et al., 2013, p. 235). This can include aspects of the natural and built environment (physical context) or family support (social context), or ethnicity, race and gender (cultural context), or political and economic considerations (institutional context).

Practice context

The practice context is embedded with the societal context and takes place when the therapist meets their client to start the therapeutic relationship. The practice context includes how the therapist is expected to behave and to elicit the client's perception of his or her role in the occupational therapy process (Craik et al., 2013, p. 236).

When working with individuals or groups of people, it is important to understand that the therapist and the individual or group will have different values, beliefs and attitudes that will influence the therapeutic relationship. These are known as personal factors which acknowledges that people and groups will differ around what interventions they will accept, who they will see if they become unwell, and explanation of their health and well-being (Helman, 2007).

Frame of reference

A frame of reference is used to explain and understand a situation and to guide practice reasoning. In occupational therapy practice and specifically in relation to the CPPF, a frame of reference helps the therapist to frame their thinking in relation to their own skills and knowledge, their client and the context in which the therapeutic relationship takes place.

Action points

The CPPF contains eight action points embedded within the societal and practice context. Each point requires an action to be completed prior to moving on to the next point. It is important to remember that there are alternate pathways through the eight action points, such as when the evaluation of outcome indicates the need for new objectives to be formulated and a therapy plan can be continued or the process can conclude.

1. Enter/initiate
    This is the time when the occupational therapist first meets the client, based upon a referral or other request to see the client. A focus is on identifying occupational challenges and establishing a collaborative relationship to support enablement. The occupational therapist explains their role and a mutual decision is made to continue or discontinue with the process.

2. Set the stage
    This is a point where the client and therapist collaborate to establish common ground and mutual expectations. In doing this, values, beliefs and assumptions can be explored and clarified along with identifying occupational issues and possible goals.

3. Assess/evaluate
    An occupation-focused assessment is required to establish the occupational status of the client and identify influencing personal, environmental and occupational factors. Results from the initial top-down, occupation-focused assessment may inform the need for further body structure/function (bottom-up) assessment, depending on the occupational issues identified and the practice area.

4. Agree on objectives and plan
    This is the stage when the client identifies priority occupational issues and occupational goals are established. The occupational therapist and the client then agree on a plan to meet the stated goals. The plan may include a range of approaches from underpinning frames of reference.

5. Implement the plan

    Implementation of the plan is a collaborative process between the client and the occupational therapist. The occupational therapist facilitates the plan by using enabling skills so that the client has a sense of empowerment throughout the process.

6. Monitor and modify

    The plan should be a flexible and dynamic process. Changes in the societal and practice contexts, as well as personal and environmental factors, will mean that plans need to be reviewed.

7. Evaluate outcome

    The occupational therapy process involves assessing a client and establishing goals and objectives. An essential part of the process is to determine if these goals have been met and modifying the intervention if they have not been met.

8. Conclude/exit

    In most cases the occupational therapy process will conclude once the goals have been met. In some cases, not all goals can be met and referral to other services may be appropriate. In most cases, a written summary of the occupational therapy process is made available to the client, as well as options for re-entry if required.

Occupational Therapy Intervention Process Model (OTIPM)

The Occupational Therapy Intervention Process Model (OTIPM) (Fisher & Maraterella, 2019) outlines the steps required to implement occupation-centred reasoning throughout all phases of the occupational therapy process. Like other practice processes, the OTIPM supports occupation-centred reasoning that is client-centred. Unlike other practice processes, greater detail is provided to support planning and implementation of occupation centred-evaluation and approaches to intervention, which in turn supports reasoning that is truly top-down. The OTIPM characterises occupational therapy practice in three stages: 1) evaluation and goal setting; 2) intervention; and 3) re-evaluation (Figure 19.2) and can be applied when working with individuals through to communities.

The Transactional Model of Occupation describes the complexity of occupation, which includes occupational performance, occupational experience and participation, and guides this understanding within the OTIPM. The transactional perspective reinforces that people do not produce occupation and cannot be separated from their situational contexts. In this model, the *geopolitical*, *sociocultural* and *temporal* elements are the broadest, overarching elements including, for example, geographic and economic influences; rules, regulations and norms; and patterns, sequences and rhythms. Examples of elements in the *social* and *physical* environment include spaces, tangible objects and people, whether they are present or not. The *task* and *client* elements describe what is expected during occupation (e.g., structure, tools, purpose and outcome) and the influences that are internal to the client (e.g., age, gender and life stage; habits, routines, rituals and roles; attitudes, beliefs and values; and body functions). The occupational therapist must be aware of all elements and how changes in one will result in changes within other situational elements and occupation, as well as how occupation influences the situational elements. This is a dynamic and ongoing transactional process.

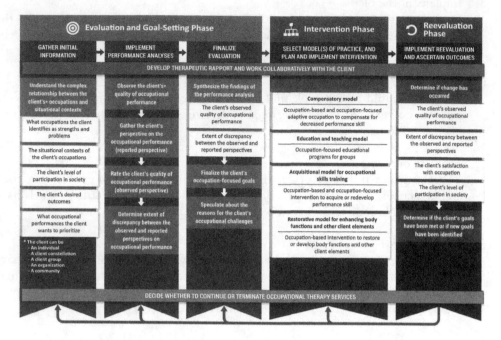

Figure 19.2 Occupational Therapy Intervention Process Model.
Source: Maraterella and Fisher (2019). Used with permission

Evaluation and goal setting

This stage commences after an initial referral or request for occupational therapy service has been received. In this stage, the occupational therapist gathers information needed to understand the client's occupations and the situational contexts of those occupations. Developing therapeutic rapport and a collaborative relationship with the client begins in this phase but continues throughout the entire process. Once the occupational therapist understands what occupations the client wants to prioritise, a performance analysis, for example, Assessment of Motor and Process Skills (Fisher & Bray-Jones, 2011) is conducted to determine the quality of the client's occupational performance at the level of performance skills performed or not performed effectively. The occupational therapist and client then collaborate in the development of the client's occupation–focused goals. Finally, the occupational therapist considers possible reasons for the observed problems of occupational performance.

Intervention

In this stage, the intervention model is selected, and interventions are planned and implemented to address the client's problems of occupational performance. This may include a compensatory, acquisitional, restorative, or education and teaching approach. The compensatory approach involves introducing adaptive equipment or assistive technology, alternative or compensatory strategies, and/or modifying external elements influencing occupation. The acquisitional approach involves the development of occupational performance through engagement in occupation. The restorative approach focusses on developing underlying body functions or other client elements through engagement in occupation. While all approaches include an educational component, the education and teaching approach is chosen to share occupation-focused knowledge with individuals or groups using lectures or workshops. The chosen approaches are collaboratively planned and implemented with the client.

Re-evaluate

Progress and the outcomes of the occupational therapy intervention are re-evaluated through various methods, including performance analyses and a review of the client's goals. At the end of each phase, the occupational therapist determines whether to continue or terminate services. In the re-evaluation phase, this may lead to the identification of new goals and re-entry into the most appropriate step in the OTIPM.

Model of Human Occupation (MOHO)—Therapeutic Reasoning Process

The Therapeutic Reasoning Process (TRP) (Forsyth, 2017) is an occupation focused, client-centered practice model that embeds the four elements of the Model of Human Occupation (MOHO) (Figure 19.3) at each step of occupational therapy—in other words, the TRP is a method of putting the MOHO into practice for therapists.

The MOHO 'lens' is used to understand the dynamic and reciprocal interaction between a person's 'open' systems of volition, habituation and performance capacity. As depicted in Figure 19.3, the TRP involves seven 'steps'.

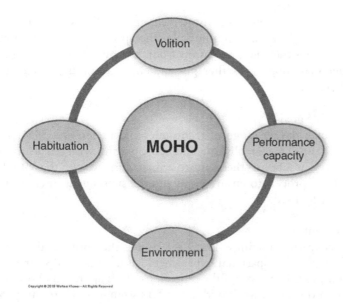

Figure 19.3 The four elements of the Model of Human Occupation.

Step 1: Theory-driven questions

Theory-driven questions guide therapists to consider how these internal processes are impacted by the external social and physical environment. This initial step is crucial in getting to know the person, and their unique circumstances and the ways they 'do' their chosen occupations (occupational skills, performance and participation). Information gathered on these concepts often raise broader questions relating to occupational identity, competence and adaptation.

Step 2: Administering standardised assessment(s)

The TRP is a form of procedural reasoning with MOHO guiding the therapist's thinking at each step in the process. Therefore, the selection of standardised assessments will be based on information needed to answer the theory-driven questions from Step 1. There are numerous standardised assessments that align with the MOHO, which allow therapists to respond to their theory-driven questions; however, subscribing to the TRP does not mean therapists need to restrict their selection to only MOHO assessments. An example of a MOHO-aligned assessment tool is the Model of Human Occupation Screening Tool (MOHOST).

Step 3: Occupational formulation

Occupational formulation draws the assessment strands together to provide a uniquely occupational perspective to the client's life circumstance. The purpose of the formulation is to highlight personal and environmental strengths and attributes that can act as mechanisms for change. The formulation may also highlight functional limitations and environmental demands for consideration when setting goals and doing intervention planning. Wherever possible it is important to collaborate with the client to create an occupational formulation; this aids client-centered practices and creates genuine partnership needed in the following steps.

Step 4: Identifying occupational changes

Despite humans being innately occupationally driven, many clients find framing goals for the future a challenge. This step prompts the therapist to explore with the client what occupational changes the client may want from therapy. Understanding the subjective nature of change may support the therapist and client to solidify the desired goals and outcomes for therapy.

Step 5: Developing measurable goals

Occupational therapists may have a range of techniques and preferences (SMART goals or Goal Attainment Scaling) for establishing and collaborating with clients to develop measurable goals. This step supports therapists to remain aligned with the MOHO theory during the goal setting process to ensure goals and the subsequent intervention planning stay occupationally focused.

Step 6: Implementing intervention

Humans are complex occupational beings. The TRP guides therapists' understanding of the uniqueness of people's occupational experience. MOHO concepts form the basis for engaging a person in their meaningful occupations. This approach allows the therapist to consider interventions that work with a person's strengths and resources to

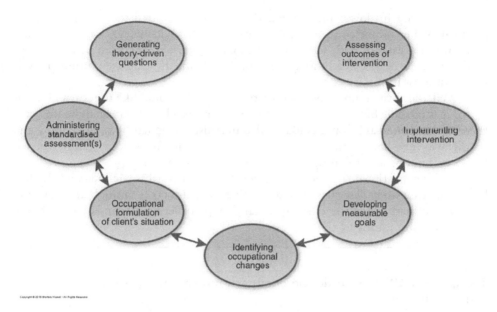

Figure 19.4 The MOHO Therapeutic Reasoning Process.

enable occupational performance. Health and well-being outcomes are achieved when a client can participate in their meaningful occupations.

Step 7: Assessing outcomes of intervention

This step can involve one or both of the following: reflecting on goal attainment (Step 5) and/or re-administering of standardised assessments (Step 2). This step may not be the final step in the therapeutic process. In many instances, this might be considered an opportunity to evaluate therapy and move through other steps in the therapeutic process, such as developing new measurable goals to reflect a client's change in circumstances or health status.

The next part of the chapter presents a case study and then applies the CPPF, the OTIPM and the MOHO. Table 19.1 summarises the main aspects of each process as it relates to the case study, highlighting the differences and similarities in each process.

Case study

Malcolm is a 66-year-old man who just retired from his job as a computer engineer. He was diagnosed with diabetic neuropathy ten years ago, which has meant the sensation in his lower limbs has progressively worsened. About two months ago an ulcer on his left foot became badly infected, resulting eventually in a left lower limb trans-tibial amputation. Malcolm also has a history of anxiety and depression which, at various parts of his life, has meant he needed treatment from a psychologist.

Following his lower limb amputation, he was admitted to the rehabilitation ward. When admitted to the rehabilitation ward, Malcolm was still in pain and required assistance with self-care and mobility. He also reported being anxious as having a new lower limb amputation and being in a new environment was stressful for him.

Malcolm lives at home with his partner Rod. He would like to return home as soon as possible but is worried about how he and Rod will manage if he isn't able to move around as he once could. Malcolm is also passionate about gardening and this was how he saw himself enjoying his retirement. As such, he is now worried he will not be able to engage in this important occupation.

The occupational therapist on the rehabilitation ward is Melinda and the following case study describes the journey that Malcolm takes through his admission to rehabilitation and three occupational therapy processes Melinda could choose to guide this journey.

Using the CCPF to guide the occupational therapy process with Malcolm

Table 19.1 describes how the CPPF can be used with Malcolm. An important aspect of the CPPF is remembering that it takes place within a societal context taking into consideration cultural, institutional, physical and social environmental factors. For example, Malcolm has a key social support in his partner Rod. He has been admitted to a rehabilitation ward where he is expected to engage in rehabilitation.

The CPPF also acknowledges that the practice context is important. In this case, the rehabilitation ward is the practice context that includes the physical environment (ward, gymnasium, common dining area) that is being staffed by a multidisciplinary team. Both Malcolm and Melinda have personal factors such as experience, beliefs, skills and knowledge that will shape the practice context and the therapeutic relationship.

Importantly, Melinda uses frames of reference (FOR) to guide her reasoning. For example, Melinda uses a compensatory FOR when thinking about what aids/equipment Malcom can use to compensate for his amputation. When Malcolm becomes anxious about his new situation, Melinda focuses on maximising his successes in rehabilitation using a psychological FOR. Throughout Melinda uses a biomechanical FOR to understand how a lower limb amputation alters how Malcolm can physically engage in occupation.

Using the OTIPM to guide the occupational therapy process with Malcolm

The transaction model of occupation guides Melinda to think about the geopolitical, sociocultural, and temporal elements that provide situational context to the interaction such as the expectations of a person admitted to the rehabilitation ward. Melinda thinks about Malcolm's physical and social environment including the rehabilitation environment described above and Rod as a key support person. Being aware of the client elements enables Melinda to incorporate Malcolm's habits, routines, rituals and roles into the goal setting and to offer support during periods of heightened anxiety.

Table 19.1 Application of the CPPF, OTIPM and the MOHO-TRP

	CPPF	OTIPM	MOHO
	Malcom is admitted to the slow stream rehabilitation ward. On the same day Melinda introduces herself, explains the role of an occupational therapist, helping Malcolm to understand her role and how that is different to other professionals in the multi-disciplinary team. Malcolm explains to Melinda his concerns about doing self-care occupations for himself in hospital and then being able to return home again, particularly to tend to his garden. Malcolm explains that he is anxious in hospital as it is a new environment and he is unsure of what to expect. Through this sharing of information, Melinda outlines what occupational therapy can offer to him and Malcolm accepts the offer to engage in occupational therapy. Melinda seeks to build rapport and a therapeutic relationship throughout this process.		
Assessment, goal setting and planning	**Set the stage** Melinda seeks to understand Malcolm as an occupational being, gathering an occupational history and seeking to understand how environmental and personal contexts influence performance. **Assess** Melinda uses The Functional Independence Measure (FIM)® Guide for the Uniform Data Set for Medical Rehabilitation (1997) to establish a baseline measure of performance in self-care occupations, as per ward procedures. She uses several frames of reference to guide her decisions in the assessment and intervention when working with Malcolm. Malcolm and Melinda use the Canadian Occupational Performance Measure (Law et al., 2014) to define several occupation-based issues and goals that are based around being independent with all self-care in the short term, managing anxiety while on the ward and a long-term goal of returning home and gardening.	**Gather initial information** Melinda uses the Transactional Model of Occupation to understand Malcolm as an occupational being and the complex interplay between Malcolm's occupations and situational contexts. This step concludes with Malcolm identifying occupations that he wishes to prioritise. **Implement Performance Analyses** Malcolm has prioritised self-care and gardening. An Assessment of Motor and Process Skills (AMPS) (Fisher & Bray Jones, 2011) establishes the client-centred performance context. Malcolm completes two tasks: 1) upper body grooming and total body dressing, and 2) watering plants and removing dead leaves. Melinda and Malcolm discuss the occupational performance from each of their perspectives and discrepancies are noted.	**Generating theory-driven questions** Melinda generates MOHO theory-driven questions about Malcolm as an occupational being to guide the occupational therapy process. For example: 'What is Malcolm's daily routine at home? What impact do the opportunities, resources, constraints and demands of Malcolm's home environment have on how he thinks, feels and approaches his activities? To what extent did Malcolm establish a pattern of participation as a retired person before his surgery that reflects his occupational identity?' **Administering standardised assessments** Using her MOHO theory-driven questions, Melinda considers what standardised assessments will support her to answer these questions. She administers the MOHOST (Parkinson et al., 2006) and the Functional Autonomy Measurement System SMAF (Rai et al., 1996). These assessments provide a structured method of collecting information on many MOHO elements, thereby providing an overview of his occupational functioning. She combines these assessments with the occupational therapy department's home visiting checklist to assist with identifying resources and demands in the environment.

(Continued)

	CPPF	OTIPM	MOHO
	Agree on objectives Goals are collaboratively developed using the COPM (Law et al., 2014) and the Goal Attainment Scale (Kiresuk et al., 1994) is used to break down the long-term goal of home gardening into smaller goals that are graded to allow for improvement in Malcolm's mobility. **Plan** Malcolm and Melinda plan to meet the short-term self-care goals by beginning a program of self-care retraining each day. They also plan a graded gardening program initially on the ward and then progressing to the ward courtyard.	**Finalise evaluation** The information gathered during the initial interview and the results of the performance analyses, including discrepancies, are discussed and Malcolm's occupation-focused goals are finalised in the areas of personal self-care and gardening. **Select model(s) or practice and plan** Malcolm and Melinda identify that compensatory and acquisitional approaches are required when planning the intervention. This includes the provision of an appropriate wheelchair and a graded training approach.	**Occupational formulation/identifying occupational changes** The assessment results provide the foundation for the occupational formulation. Assessment data indicates much of Malcolm's current anxiety is related to him being a burden to his partner to Rod (*personal causation*). He has also experienced a change in his performance capacity since his lower limb amputation. **Developing measurable goals** A short-term goal was made to prioritise a meeting with Rod within the week. Malcolm's goal was to be able to communicate openly with Rod the challenges of completing daily activities in their home. Malcolm also expressed a desire to increase his endurance for standing and mobilising to support with his return home. **Implement the plan** Melinda facilitates a meeting with Rod and Malcolm. Melinda used her therapeutic use of self to encourage both parties to discuss their hopes and concerns for Malcolm's return home.
Intervention	**Implement the plan/intervention** Melinda and Malcolm trial and choose an appropriate amputee frame wheelchair and accessories that support Malcolm to engage in occupations on the ward. With the physiotherapist, Melinda and Malcolm trial and choose techniques to safely transfer to the wheelchair, on/off a shower chair, and to bath, dress and toilet. These selfcare occupations are practised each day. Malcolm's partner brings in some gardening activities that involve cutting and pruning that he can do while sitting down. This achieves the aim of increasing the complexity and challenge of the daily occupations Malcolm engages in as his physical function improves.		
Case update	Malcolm receives a lower limb prosthesis and the physiotherapist teaches him how to walk with it. Malcolm is soon independent with transferring, walking with a prosthesis, and with self-care. This means that Malcolm can access more of his environment and his goals and plan are modified to address goals around being independent in meal preparation, community mobility, and more complicated gardening tasks.		

Monitor and modify

It is around this time that Malcolm is ready to return home, so a home assessment is completed using the Westmead Home Safety Assessment (Clemson, 1997). Following this assessment, Melinda suggests some modifications to Malcolm's home. She recommends equipment that would improve his safety and improve access into and around his home and, importantly, how to manage gardening tasks that are safe and meaningful.

Re-establish occupation-focused goals

The AMPS is repeated with more challenging tasks within Malcolm's home environment included: 1) weeding and raking grass cuttings or leaves; and 2) preparing a hot drink and toast. Rod is present during the home visit, and Malcolm, Rod and Melinda discuss plans for discharge and concerns or questions. They agree that some modifications and assistive equipment could enhance occupational performance within the home and the garden and possible options are identified. Melinda continues to apply a compensatory and acquisitional approach, including discussions with Malcolm and Rod about a graded training approach in the kitchen and garden.

Melinda utilises the OT kitchen with Malcolm to make simple meals, working on his volition to be more independent in meal preparation. Grading tasks enables him to increase his performance capacity by standing for longer periods each session. Melinda uses his interest in gardening to further increase his participation through a 'kitchen garden' group. He selects herbs and vegetables from the raised garden for the group to cook. His volition for gardening sees him standing for longer periods whilst being outdoors, and engaging with familiar gardening tasks which aims to reduce his anxiety. Melinda orders equipment to modify Malcolm's home environment in anticipation for discharge.

Assessing outcomes of intervention

A discharge date for Malcolm is set for next week. The MOHOST is readministered with Malcolm which provides evidence of his progress, aiding in the reduction of his anxiety. Melinda discusses his original SMART goals and they reflect on his achievements. He reports feeling relieved when Rod expressed his unconditional love and support during their family meeting. Melinda makes a referral to the outpatient team to work with Malcolm post discharge to continue his positive occupational adaptation in retirement and living with an amputation.

Evaluation

Re-evaluation

Malcolm was able to meet the goals he set in collaboration with Melinda both in the short term (self-care and transferring) and longer term (returning home to gardening). When he was discharged, he scored 7/7 for all self-care items on the Functional Independence Measure®. He was also able to meet the expected outcomes on the Goal Attainment Scale for gardening tasks. Potential falling hazards were removed or modified after administering the Westmead Home Safety Assessment (Clemson, 1997).

Re-evaluation and determine outcomes

Further evaluation with AMPS and discussion regarding occupational performance identify that all current goals have been met. It is agreed that inpatient rehabilitation is no longer required, and that Malcolm is ready for discharge to home.

Conclude/exit

Malcolm was discharged home after five weeks. Prior to his discharge Malcolm and Melinda met with the community occupational therapist. He was referred to the community occupational therapist to continue to work towards his goal of landscaping part of his garden.

Terminate services

It is identified that it is best for Malcolm to continue occupational therapy within his own home environment. Malcolm consents to a referral to a community occupational therapist.

Using the MOHO-TRP

For her Therapeutic Reasoning Melinda will process the incoming information on Malcolm under the MOHO constructs of volition, habituation and performance capacity. This will support her to form a good understanding of Malcolm as a complex occupational being. This means Melinda will strive to understand Malcolm from multiple and dynamic perspectives of his volition, habituation, performance capacity and environment. Initially she will see him in the context of the hospital ward environment; however, she will adapt her understanding to include the demands and resources of his home and social environment that he shares with Rod. Therapeutic reasoning supports Melinda to work collaboratively with Malcolm, taking his experiences and strengths as foundations for therapy planning and intervention whilst on the ward.

So far in this chapter, an overview and application of three therapeutic practice process models have been presented. These are commonly used to guide and inform Australian occupational therapists in their professional decision making and actions. Understanding these models occurs in a progression that first requires the learner to identify the stages of the model, be able to apply the model in a specific context (as with Malcolm above) and finally analyse and evaluate the effectiveness of a model to the applied situation. Using the case study of Malcolm, the table below demonstrates how each model can be used with the same person and context. The table aligns each model's stages to highlight their similar and contrasting features.

Conclusion

Practice processes support the occupational therapist to work collaboratively with the client through the core elements of assessment, intervention and evaluation. There are a range of practice processes available to the occupational therapist and in this chapter we have presented three examples, the CPPF, OTIPM and MOHO-TRP. A case study has demonstrated how the interactions between the occupational therapist and the client are guided with each of the processes. The purpose was to highlight that each practice process could be applied for the same client. The occupational therapist may adopt a preferred practice process based on their guiding conceptual practice models, or workplace requirements, or based on the characteristics and needs of the client and so forth. Although we have presented a case study example that relates to working with an individual, it is important to remember that the occupational practice process can be applied to working with groups and communities.

Summary

- The occupational therapy process is a way that occupational therapists can apply to support occupation-centred thinking and action when interacting with individuals, groups, communities or populations.
- The Occupational Therapy Intervention Process Model (OTIPM) (Fisher & Maraterella, 2019) outlines the steps required to implement occupation-centred reasoning throughout all phases of the occupational therapy process.
- The Canadian Practice Process Framework (Polatajko et al., 2007) is an occupation-focused, client-centred framework where the client can be an individual, group, community or population.

- The Therapeutic Reasoning Process (Forsyth, 2017) is an occupation-focused, client-centered practice model that embeds the four elements of the Model of Human Occupation at each step of occupational therapy.

Review questions

1. What are the eight practice process points of the CPPF?
2. What are the three practice phases in the OTIPM?
3. What are the seven steps of the MOHO-TRP?
4. Name three similarities and three difference between the CPPF, OTIPM and the MOHO-TRP.

References

Clemson, L. (1997). *The Westmead Home Safety Assessment*. Coordinates Publications.

Craik, J., Davis, J., & Polatajko, H. (2013). Introducing the Canadian Practice Framework (CPPF): Amplifying the context. In E. A. Townsend & H. J. Polatajko (Eds.), *Enabling occupation II: Advancing an occupational therapy vision for health, well-being, and justice through occupation* (pp. 229–246). CAOT Publications ACE.

Fisher, A. G., & Bray Jones, K. (2011). *Assessment of Motor and Process Skills: Vol 1; Development, standardisation and administration manual* (7th revised edn). Three Star Press.

Fisher, A. G., & Maraterella, A. (2019). *Powerful practice: A model for authentic occupational therapy*. Center for Innovative OT Solutions.

Forsyth, K. (2017). Therapeutic reasoning: Planning, implementing, and evaluating the outcomes of therapy. In R. R. Taylor & G. Kielhofner, G. (Eds.), *Kielhofner's Model of Human Occupation: Theory and application* (5th edn, pp. 159–172). Lippincott Williams & Wilkins.

Guide for the Uniform Data Set for Medical Rehabilitation, Version 5.1. (1997). State University of New York at Buffalo.

Helman, C. (2007). *Culture health and illness* (5th edn). Oxford University Press.

Kiresuk, T. J., Smith, A., & Cardillo, J. E. (1994). *Goal Attainment Scaling: Applications, theory, and measurement*. Lawrence Erlbaum Associates.

Law, M., Baptiste, S., Carswell, A., McColl, M. A., Polatajko, H., Pollock, N., & Toomey, M. (2014). *Canadian Occupational Performance Measure* (5th edn). CAOT Publications ACE.

Parkinson, S., Forsyth, K., & Kielhofner, G. (2006). *The Model of Human Occupation Screening Tool (MOHOST)* (Version 2nd edn). University of Illinois at Chicago.

Polatajko, H. J., Craik, J., Davis, J., & Townsend, E. (2007). Canadian Practice Process Framework. In E. A Townsend & H. J. Polatojko (Eds.), *Enabling occupation II: Advancing an occupational therapy vision for health, well-being and justice through occupation*. (p. 229–246). CAOT Publications ACE.

Rai, G. S., Gluck, T., Wientjes, H. J. F. M., & Rai, S. G. S. (1996). The Functional Autonomy Measurement System (SMAF): A measure of functional change with rehabilitation. *Archives of Gerontology and Geriatrics*, *22*(1), 81–85. https://doi.org/10.1016/0167-4943(95)00680-X

20 Core business

Task, activity and occupation analysis

Lynette Mackenzie, Gjyn O'Toole and Louise Gustafsson

Chapter objectives

Upon completion of this chapter, the reader will be able to:

*   Define and differentiate between task analysis, activity analysis and occupation analysis.
*   Identify how occupational therapists can use occupation analysis.
*   Identify factors to consider when conducting an occupation analysis.

Key terms

occupation; activity; task; analysis; meaning; environment

Introduction

When gathering information about a client or person, the occupational therapist seeks to understand the daily life of that person. The therapist explores the perspective of the client or person about their most important or meaningful occupations. This essential phase of the occupational therapy practice process involves analysis of these important occupations. This analysis is called occupation or occupational analysis. There are three different levels of analysis in daily practice: an occupation analysis, an activity analysis or a task analysis. This chapter provides an overview of these three forms of analysis, along with illustrative practical examples; and to conclude the chapter, there is a specific example of an occupation analysis of showering. Although some may learn about occupational analysis, the preferred term for this chapter is occupation analysis, to ensure a focus on the occupation, not the analysis.

Occupation, activity and task analysis

Occupation is the focus of occupational therapy (Chard & Mesa, 2017), making occupation analysis an important aspect of practice. A review of occupational therapy literature indicates occupation and activity analysis are used in multiple ways. In particular occupation analysis is either considered synonymous with activity analysis (American Occupational Therapy Association [AOTA], 2014; Wilson & Landry, 2014) or each distinctly different from each other (Boyt Schell et al., 2019; O'Toole, 2011). While these terms

Table 20.1 Definitions of occupation analysis, activity analysis and task analysis

Occupation analysis	'The process of exploring the transactional relationship between the characteristics of an occupation, the personal meanings attributed to the occupation by individuals, groups and communities, and the contribution of various factors to the performance of an occupation.' (Mackenzie & O'Toole, 2011, p. 383)
Activity analysis	'The examination of the demands of an activity that stipulates the required skills and component tasks for successful completion of the activity.' (Mackenzie & O'Toole, 2011, p. 378)
Task analysis	'The exploration of individual actions required by each of the components of an occupation.' (Mackenzie & O'Toole, 2011, p. 385)

may be used interchangeably in practice and in some literature, this chapter considers them as different. See the definitions in Table 20.1.

Occupation analysis examines engagement in a preferred occupation, while simultaneously considering the effect of and the dynamic relationship between personal factors and the particular contexts and environments of each unique individual/client (Boyt Schell et al., 2019; O'Toole, 2011). An occupation analysis is a comprehensive process designed to understand the values and meaning a person assigns to engagement in specific occupations within their particular environments (Thomas, 2015). The person is central in this analysis with consideration of their body functions and structures, life experiences, habits, routines, values and goals, along with the demands of the particular occupation within their unique environments and context for performance (Boyt Schell et al., 2019; O'Toole, 2011). It is essential to remember occupation analysis involves observing the person completing their preferred occupation, where possible in their particular environments.

Activity analysis identifies the overall demands of performing an activity within daily life, but unrelated to the individual. It isolates and sequences the required actions; the typically used equipment while performing the activity; and the required skills to perform the activity (Boyt Schell et al., 2019; Breines, 2012). These skills are typically more than physical skills, potentially including cognitive, emotional, perceptual, sensory and sometimes social skills (Perlman & Bergthorson, 2017). An activity analysis does not typically relate to the specific skills of the individual or their unique environment or contexts. It is conducted when seeking to understand the sequence of steps, the required equipment and skills to engage in the particular activity. It does not relate to the meaning attributed to a particular activity or occupation, nor to the unique personal factors and contexts of an individual. An activity analysis identifies potential areas of difficulty; ways of grading and adapting the activity; and the possible required supports to promote completion of the activity (Perlman & Bergthorson, 2017).

Task analysis is the examination of the set of actions required to achieve a specific outcome within an occupation. It may involve a more detailed observation and analysis of the exact actions of a specific individual within their particular contexts to complete the task. Alternatively, a task analysis may involve analysis of a specific set of actions to perform the task, unrelated to any individual. In either situation, the purpose of the analysis is to obtain a detailed understanding of the specific demands of the task and thus the required skills.

To empower readers in analysis of occupations, activities and tasks, two examples of analysing common activities of daily living follow: the first is making a cup of tea and the second is bathing.

The example of making a cup of tea

The occupation of making a cup of tea is commonly used to illustrate the three levels of analysis. Figure 20.1 illustrates these levels, with the following section providing a more detailed description of each level of analysis for making a cup of tea.

How an individual makes a cup of tea, the specific method and required objects depends upon the cultural context, the personal preferences and the environment of the specific person. Therefore, an occupation analysis empowers the occupational therapist to explore the meaning, habits, routines and preferences of a person, in addition to observing the person performing the occupation in their own environment. In contrast, an activity analysis of making a cup of tea, allows the occupational therapist to consider the typically required skills, equipment and component tasks of making a cup of tea within a particular culture. For example, making a cup of tea using a tea bag can be quite different to using a teapot to make tea. However, to assemble and prepare tea making items for these different procedures may involve any of the following tasks: boiling the water; putting tea into a pot; pouring hot water into the pot or cup; choosing the drinking vessel; and then pouring and drinking the tea. The task analysis of tea making allows the occupational therapist to consider and observe each component task and the required action of that task to make the tea. It is important to remember that these three levels of analysis require consideration of specific skills and attributes, such as vision, reach, grasp, strength, body awareness, sensation, cognition and so forth. These skills are components of a detailed occupation analysis. This is described further in the next example: bathing.

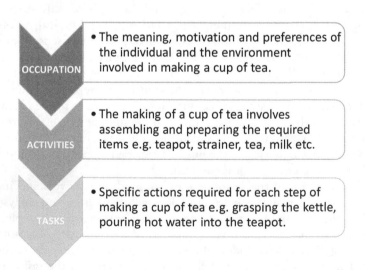

Figure 20.1 Levels of analysis involved in making a cup of tea.
Source: Creek (1996); Fair & Barnitt (1999); Hannam (1997)

The example of bathing

The occupation of bathing may vary substantially between individuals depending on their cultural backgrounds and personal values (McGraw & Drennan, 2009) and their individual environments. Bathing (or showering) is defined as 'obtaining and using supplies; soaping, rinsing, and drying body parts; maintaining bathing position; and transferring to and from bathing positions' (AOTA, 2008, p. 631). This example provides a more detailed description of the three levels of analysis, including examples of when they may be applicable.

Occupation analysis of bathing

Bathing will vary in its meaning for different individuals and for the same individual throughout their lifespan. For instance, a child may find bathing with toys the highlight of the day; while an adolescent may not value bathing as much as other activities or may want to stay in the shower for extended periods of time. Some individuals may value a hot shower or bath before going to bed in order to relax and sleep; some use a shower to rouse themselves in the morning; while others might complete bathing merely as part of their daily routine. For some people bathing must be done every day, while for others this is not considered necessary. Therefore, when conducting an occupation analysis, it is important to establish the personal preferences, routines, values and beliefs affecting the choices of each person, and therefore the meaning of particular occupations.

The particular environments will influence the occupation of bathing. This indicates the importance of considering environments in an occupation analysis. Typically, occupational therapists assess physical environments concerned with bathing, sometimes neglecting other equally relevant environments such as temporal, cultural, social, institutional and political. In some countries bathing occurs in a public bath house, including relaxing in a heated room to promote perspiration, then a massage; full body wash and finally relaxing in a cool quite room. Therefore, it is often the specific environments that significantly impact engagement and the manner of performing or participating in bathing. For example, a person who lives in a drought-affected location may value water highly, therefore choosing to use it sparingly, and only for specific occupations. In this instance, the environmental context may drive the use of a bucket for bathing.

When assessing a child bathing or recommending physical modifications to a bathing environment, it is important to consider other family members, the time of bathing, the duration of the activity, whether there is only one shared bathroom, and both the individual and family routine. Similarly, political and institutional contexts affect opportunities to bathe. For instance, limited length of showering at specific times due to lack of water or the cost of heating; or the availability of bathing assistance in the community may be limited to certain times of the day. The dynamic relationship between the occupation, the person and their environments must be central to occupational therapy practice to ensure recommendations or interventions are consistent with the unique preferences, values and needs of the individual (Polatajko et al., 2013; Whalley Hammell, 2013).

Activity analysis of bathing

An occupational therapist may conduct an activity analysis to generate the typical sequence of steps, tools and required skills for bathing. The analysis generates a predetermined set of expectations regarding how to complete the activity of bathing, thereby supporting the occupational therapist to readily understand the possible need for further assessments and/or apply the therapeutic skills of grading and adapting within intervention planning. Another example of activity analysis of bathing occurs when working with individuals who are not within their own environment, e.g., when a person is in hospital. A bathing assessment within a hospital environment is conducted to establish the level of independence of the individual in this occupation, or to identify the need for equipment or assistance (perhaps prior to discharge home from hospital). Throughout the activity analysis, the occupational therapist seeks to determine if the person performs the anticipated sequence and required skills independently within the hospital environment. This analysis identifies the personal (individual) or environmental factors limiting performance, thereby informing subsequent assessment and/or intervention, possibly including a graded therapeutic program, adaptation of a task, or introduction of assistive equipment.

Task analysis of bathing

There are particular tasks associated with bathing. Imagine an occupation analysis of a person bathing. During the activity of washing hair, a person identifies difficulties with the task of accessing shampoo and condition. The occupational therapist would then seek to determine the specific actions causing the difficulties with washing hair (e.g., squeezing shampoo into the hand, reaching to place shampoo in hair). They would then systematically identify required tools and skills to perform the actions. A task analysis therefore supports an observation and assessment regarding a specific, difficult aspect of bathing for the person. Not unlike an activity analysis, this information would inform subsequent assessment and intervention planning including a graded therapy program or adaptation of the task to enable hair washing.

Factors involved in conducting a comprehensive occupation analysis

When conducting a comprehensive occupation analyses it is essential to consider three fundamental components. These are the individual or personal factors, the contexts (environments), and the factors relating to the occupation. The complex dynamic relationship between these three components are recognised as key contributors to occupational performance by conceptual practice models such as the Canadian Model of Occupational Performance and Engagement (Polatajko et al., 2007); the Person–Environment–Occupational Model (Law et al., 1996); and the Person–Environment–Occupation–Performance Model (Baum & Christiansen, 2005). It is important to recognise that an occupational therapist may apply the components from within their chosen conceptual practice model when conducting an occupation analysis. For example, if applying the components from the Canadian Model of Occupational Performance and Engagement, the individual factors are spirituality, physical, cognitive and affective, while the contexts would be physical, social, cultural and institutional. This chapter applies the components of the model of occupation analysis developed by O'Toole (2011), as discussed below.

Individual components

Individual components are the intrinsic aspects of the individual typically interwoven with the contextual components. This dynamic personal system consists of the expected roles of the individual, their personal values and beliefs, their spirit and their personality. Attributes and traits such as gender, age, weight, height, skills (physical, cognitive, communication, social, etc.), motivation and emotional regulation are interwoven within the dynamic personal system. This system and the interwoven personal attributes determine choices, expectations, capacities and decisions when performing occupations (O'Toole, 2011).

Contexts

Contexts position the individual to perform occupations and may act as barriers or facilitators. The contexts of occupations (Table 20.2) include the cultural context, spiritual context, political and institutional context, social context, physical context (natural, build and temporal), technological contexts and socio-economic contexts (O'Toole, 2011). These interrelate and will have varying effects on the individual at a given time in their lifespan.

Table 20.2 Contexts considered in a comprehensive occupation analysis

Cultural	Provides the setting for and expectations of the occupation from within a cultural group, e.g., using your right hand to eat with your fingers or eating only leavened bread.
Spiritual	Provides the values and beliefs sustaining and motivating the individual, e.g., eating only after sunset during Ramadan *or* separation of thoser utensils for touching milk products from those used to touch meat products.
Political and institutional	Affects the availability and management of environments to allow performance of occupations within these environments, e.g., road rules and licensing facilitate driving occupations.
Social	Includes the influence of family, friends, colleagues, pets, neighbours and so on. They can be complex, sometimes producing unconscious expectations of occupational engagement and may significantly affect occupational performance, e.g., being obliged to continue family sporting traditions not necessarily reflecting personal skills or preferences.
Physical	The built, natural and temporal environments of the occupation. For some people there may be valued occupations, which are associated with particular locations; or times of the day/times of the year, e.g., swimming only at the beach, jogging early in the morning or eating Christmas pudding at Christmas time.
Technological	A significant force affecting modern-day occupations, e.g., demands of computer use for productive occupations require an individual to sit and focus on a computer screen for extended periods.
Socio-economic	Affect the availability of resources and access to occupations, e.g., not owning a car will necessitate accessing alternate forms of transport such as a public transport or walking.

Occupation

Occupation is the key to occupational performance. Understanding the occupation itself provides the basis for the beginning of an occupation analysis. This includes consideration of 'the doing' within the typical context in which the person performs the occupation and an understanding of their values, structures, circumstances and environments of the occupation. The occupational structure of an occupation consists of the expectations relating to the occupation, typically determined by governments, society or social groups (O'Toole, 2011). Such structures affect the availability of some occupations for specific individuals, e.g., an individual cannot legally drive a car, nor gain employment until a particular age in many countries. Other structures such as family routines inform occupational engagement and/or performance, e.g., in some families children must bathe before going to bed and must be in bed asleep by a particular time. Certain circumstances or environments also affect the time of performing individual occupations, e.g., undertaking household tasks or gardening early in the mornings or in the evenings during the height of summer.

How to conduct an occupation analysis

1. *Selecting the occupation to analyse:* Determining which occupation to analyse must be a collaborative process involving the person. As occupations fundamentally relate to individual meaning and motivation, it is essential that the decision to and process of analysing an occupation is collaborative and person-centred.
2. *Be careful not to assume anything about the occupation:* An occupational therapist must be aware of their personal opinion or idea of what is important or meaningful in an occupation. This awareness ensures that the personal values and expectations of the therapist do not affect the occupation analysis being conducted for and with another person.
3. *Occupation analysis needs to be consistent with person-centred goals:* It is essential that the occupation analysis undertaken is consistent with person-centred goals when developing occupational therapy interventions.
4. *Conduct an interview with the person (or significant others if appropriate) to determine priorities for occupation analysis:* This is an important step to identify the personal meaning for certain occupations held by the person and therefore the priority for analysis and any interventions as a result of the analysis. An interview will also enable the therapist to understand how and where an occupation is usually performed, and the typical use of equipment.
5. *Consult with any significant others:* It may be useful to consult any family members or other carers who may be able to provide an important perspective on the usual practices of the person and their capacity to undertake occupations.
6. *Observation of engagement in the occupation:* One way to gather information for an occupation analysis is to observe the person undertaking the occupation, and to record how the person is able to perform each of the observable components of the occupation. This process would ideally be conducted in the environment where the person typically performs the occupation, but on occasions may need to be in a simulated environment, for example in a hospital or community centre.
7. *Collect any assessment findings of relevance to the occupation:* Some assessment results will provide information about the capacity of the person to undertake some of the required actions of the occupation—for instance, range of movement of different joints, endurance capacity, memory, etc.

Case study: A completed occupation analysis with Harold

Harold is a 73-year-old man who was brought into the emergency department by ambulance, having fallen on the road while out walking his dog. Harold fractured his right humerus in his dominant arm, which required surgery and internal fixation with a pin and plate. Harold experiences extreme pain from the fracture and his right (dominant) arm is in a lightweight plaster cast. Harold also experiences short-ness of breath with any exertion. Harold is able to walk but is very unsteady. He lives alone in the two-storey terrace house where he lived with his wife for 30 years, until her death three years ago. He has no family support. Harold is a retired schoolteacher who requires glasses to read. He prides himself on his appearance. He is active in his local community and volunteers at the local library. Harold has identified that his priority is being able to shower himself independently. Harold has a shower over the bath with a curtain, with the toilet and shower in the same room, upstairs.

Table 20.3 Occupation analysis of showering

Component	Aspects of analysis
The occupation of showering	**Activities involved:** • Assembling items required for showering (towel, change of clothes, etc.) • Accessing the bathroom, the shower recess or the shower over the bath • Operating taps • Setting the water temperature • Undressing • Stepping into the shower area • Accessing toiletries • Lathering • Washing body • Washing hair • Rinsing • Turning taps off • Stepping out of shower area • Drying body • Dressing Note: If observing and analysing different individuals, these may vary, possibly including further steps (such as washing and drying the shower screen immediately after use) or may perform steps in a different order. **Required skills:** • Physical skills such as standing or sitting balance. Harold must step over the edge of the bath to shower, and has only one arm to assist with the transfer, especially if there are no rails to assist. Pain may limit his endurance. Observing Harold dressing will identify any difficulties he may have dressing or undressing. • Hand function and strength. Harold has only one hand to use and has to use a plastic bag to encase his cast when showering. Harold may have difficulty accessing and holding shampoo or body wash, as well as managing the towel to dry himself with two hands. • Cognitive skills, e.g., motor planning, memory and problem solving. Harold plans these activities to carry them out successfully. • Adequate vision and sensation, e.g., Harold may have difficulty reading labels with small print without glasses on in the shower.

(Continued)

Component	Aspects of analysis

Required values:
Harold prefers to shower first thing in the morning to invigorate himself for the day, and to prepare for going out.
Note: Other people choose to shower in the morning and the evening to feel clean.
Occupational structures:
Harold lives alone so can take his time showering although will have to be much more aware of safety precautions. Harold can also organise his own system for storing towels and clothing during showering. Note: Other people may need to consider the requirements of other members of the family or household.
Circumstances:
Time and age: Harold did not want homecare assistance for showering as his preference was having a shower early in the morning and such assistance could not be arranged at a particular time.
Place: The shower over the bath for Harold is situated in the bathroom on the same level as his bedroom.
Season: Harold wanted to be independent in showering so he could have additional showers if needed in hot weather. Note: Other people may choose to shower less frequently, e.g., when living in colder climates.
Equipment and safety: Harold had a shower hose and was willing to accept a bath board and purchase a non-slip bathmat to make his showering safer. Harold preferred not to use a sponge bath at a sink as an alternative.
Note: There are different cultural and environmental expectations for showering. Others may use a bowl of water to wash, rather than using plumbed-in shower facilities; or use communal showers, e.g., in public change rooms in sporting facilities. Each of these methods of showering requires different behaviours and abilities when showering.

Individual factors relevant to showering

Roles: The role of self-maintainer and volunteer were important to Harold.
Meaning and values: Harold values his appearance and has a history of formal relationships with others from his teaching role. He values showering for his appearance and presentation.
Spirituality: Harold prioritises showering as this occupation underpins his understanding of himself as a presentable, formal person, therefore providing confidence to interact successfully with others.
Note: Others may have different ideas about the importance of showering.
Age, gender and personal skills: Harold has always valued and been able to shower independently throughout his life.
Note: These factors may also affect how, why, when and where an individual will shower.
Motivation: Harold was motivated to engage in showering, as self-presentation was important to maintain his roles.
Cognition: Harold needed to be able to plan showering and needed to know and remember the sequence of steps and the required equipment when showering.
Note: Others may need to adapt to different showering 'set-ups', if showering is conducted in an environment including others, and communication (verbal and non-verbal) is needed to access bathrooms, e.g., when other members of the household share the same bathroom.
Physical status: Harold experiences pain; has the use of only one arm; experiences shortness of breath and is unsteady on his feet. Thus, he will take longer to shower, will have to be careful to maintain safety and will have to adapt his dressing techniques.
Emotional regulation: It is important to consider the emotional response Harold has to his difficulties when showering, especially if experiencing pain during this occupation.
Note: For others, there may be a variety of sensory feedback perceived as either enjoyable or uncomfortable when showering.

Component	Aspects of analysis
The contexts relevant to showering	**Cultural context:** Harold had cultural expectations about cleanliness, insisting on showering despite his physical status. He also valued his privacy, preferring not to have assistance with showering. Note: Others may have different expectations and norms about the occupation of showering. For instance, in circumstances where water is difficult to transport or is scarce, people may carry their water, which will limit how they shower, or if they shower. In addition, cultural norms about privacy vary in different cultures, e.g., where communal showering is typical. **Spiritual context:** Harold has no spiritual beliefs affecting his showering. Note: Spiritual values may determine where and when they wash, e.g., washing their feet immediately before going to bed or before entering a home. **Institutional context:** The following regulations require consideration when assisting Harold to shower, especially if he requires modifications to his showering environment. Regulations about temperature of hot water, water restrictions and usage, design of shower recesses and bathrooms (building codes and standards), costs of a water supply and so on may affect showering, or possible adaptations. **Social context:** Harold lives alone so there are limited effects from this context. Note: Family expectations, peer expectations and general societal expectations can influence the expectations of showering. **Physical context:** Harold has a shower over his bath and thus requires a bath board or bath seat and training in how to safely transfer using the bath seat to shower. **Technological context:** Currently Harold does not have any technical changes such as water-saving devices, methods of temperature control or automated devices such as tap sensors in his bathroom. **Socio-economic contexts:** This will affect the resources available for Harold to undertake showering or pay for assistive equipment.

For occupational therapists, safety is an essential priority for an occupation analysis of showering. Therefore, they will focus on the physical context, and how to modify the physical structure to promote safe showering. However, the other contextual aspects of showering may be equally important to enable an individual to engage fully in showering. Understanding this means the occupational therapist will collaborate intentionally with an individual to ensure any modifications or equipment recommendations are effective and acceptable to the individual.

Conclusion

Occupation, activity and/or task analysis is an essential competency for every occupational therapist, thereby enabling individuals to engage in chosen occupations. This analysis forms the basis of understanding the demands of all occupations in which a person engages; the pertinent aspects of the person; and the environmental challenges or facilitators inhibiting or supporting participation in occupations. This analysis enables grading and adapting of the occupations or development of focused and relevant interventions to assist individuals to better engage in meaningful occupations. Occupation analysis underpins all aspects of the occupational therapy process. This includes assessing the level of individual occupational engagement, by analysing relevant occupations, establishing meaningful and relevant occupation-focused goals, and providing interventions to enable a person to achieve desired occupational outcomes.

An occupation analysis is needed when an individual has an impairment that may prevent occupational performance, so that occupations can be adequately adapted or graded to enable participation.

Summary

- Occupation analysis considers the dynamic relationship between the occupation, the person and the contexts/environments.
- Individual values and skills, occupational structures and particular circumstances affect the occupation.
- Aspects of the person including their designated roles; their motivation; values; and cognitive, communicative, emotional, physical (including sensory) and social skills inform an occupation analysis.
- The particular contexts including cultural, spiritual, political and institutional, social, physical (natural, built, temporal), technological and socio-economic support occupation, which is an important component of an occupation analysis.

Review questions

1. State the relevance of an occupation analysis to occupational therapy practice.
2. What is the difference between an occupation analysis, an activity analysis and a task analysis?
3. Choose two contexts and suggest how they might support occupational performance.
4. List three aspects of the person to be incorporated into an occupation analysis. Suggest how they might be incorporate in practice.
5. Choose an occupational structure and explain how it affects occupational choices.

References

American Occupational Therapy Association. (2008). Occupational Therapy Practice Framework: Domain and Process, 2nd edition. *American Journal of Occupational Therapy, 62*, 625–683. https://doi.org/10.5014/ajot.62.6.625

American Occupational Therapy Association. (2014). Occupational Therapy Practice Framework: Domain and Process, 3rd edition. *American Journal of Occupational Therapy, 68*(Supp. 1), S1–S48. https://doi.org/10.5014/ajot.2014.682006

Baum, C. M., & Christiansen, C. H. (2005). Person–Environment–Occupation–Performance: An occupation-based framework for practice. In C. H. Christiansen, C. M. Baum, & J. Bass-Haugen (Eds.), *Occupation therapy: Performance, participation and well-being* (pp. 243–266). SLACK Inc.

Boyt Schell, B. A., Gillen, G., Blesedell Crepeau, E., & Scaffa, M. E. (2019). Analysing occupations and activity. In B. A. Boyt Schell & G. Gillen (Eds.), *Willard & Spackman's occupational therapy* (13th edn, pp. 320–334). Wolter Kluwer.

Breines, E. B. (2012). Therapeutic occupations and modalities. In H. Pendleton & W. Schultz-Krohn (Eds.), *Pedretti's occupational therapy: Practice skills for physical dysfunction* (7th edn, pp. 658–684). Elsevier Mosby.

Chard, G., & Mesa, S. (2017). Analysis of occupational performance: Motor, process and social interaction skills. In M. Curtin, M. Egan, & J. Adams (Eds.), *Occupational therapy and physical dysfunction: Promoting occupation and participation* (7th edn, pp. 217–243). Elsevier.

Creek, J. (1996). Making a cup of tea as an honours degree subject. *British Journal of Occupational Therapy, 59*(3), 128–130. https://doi.org/10.1177/030802269605900310

Fair, A., & Barnitt, R. (1999). Making a cup of tea as part of a culturally sensitive service. *British Journal of Occupational Therapy, 62*(5), 199–205. https://doi.org/10.1177/030802269906200504

Hannam, D. (1997). More than a cup of tea: Meaning construction in an everyday occupation. *Journal of Occupational Science: Australia, 4*(2), 69–73. https://doi.org/10.1080/14427591.1997.9686423

Law, M., Cooper, B., Strong, S., Stewart, D., Rigby, P., & Letts, L. (1996). The Person–Environment–Occupation model: A transactive approach to occupational performance. *Canadian Journal of Occupational Therapy, 63*(1), 9–23. https://doi.org/10.1177/000841749606300103

McGraw, C., & Drennan, V. (2009). Assisting older people with bathing. *Journal of Community Nursing, 12*, 15–16. Retrieved from http://search.proquest.com/docview/208560794/

Mackenzie, L., & O'Toole, G. (Eds.). (2011). *Occupation analysis in practice.* Wiley-Blackwell.

O'Toole, G. (2011). What is occupation analysis? In L. Mackenzie & G. O'Toole (Eds.), *Occupation analysis in practice* (pp. 1–24). Wiley-Blackwell.

Perlman, C., & Bergthorson, M. (2017). Task, activity and occupational analysis. In M. Curtin, M. Egan, & J. Adams (Eds.), *Occupational therapy for people experiencing illness, injury or impairment* (7th edn, pp. 192–206). Elsevier.

Polatajko, H. J., Craik, J., Davis, J., & Townsend, E. (2007). Canadian Practice Process Framework. In E. A. Townsend & H. J. Polatojko (Eds.), *Enabling occupation II: Advancing an occupational therapy vision for health, well-being and justice through occupation* (p. 229–246). CAOT Publications ACE.

Polatajko, H. J., Davis, J., Stewart, D., Cantin, N., Amoroso, B., Purdie, L., & Zimmerman, D. (2013). Specifying the domain of concern: Occupation as core. In E. A. Townsend & H. J. Polatajko (Eds.), *Enabling occupation II: Advancing an occupational therapy vision of health, well-being and justice through occupation* (2nd edn, p. 13–36). CAOT Publications ACE.

Thomas, H. (2015). *Occupation-based activity analysis* (2nd edn). SLACK Inc.

Whalley Hammell, K. R. (2013). Client-centred practice in occupational therapy: Critical reflections. *Scandinavian Journal of Occupational Therapy, 20*(3), 174–181. https://doi.org/10.3109/11038128.2012.752032

Wilson, S. A., & Landry, G. (2014). *Task analysis: An individual, group, and population approach* (3rd edn). American Occupational Therapy Association.

21 Understanding human occupations

Self-care, productivity, leisure, play, education, sleep and social participation

Ted Brown, Aislinn Lalor, Luke Robinson and Alana Hewitt

Chapter objectives

Upon completion of this chapter, the reader will be able to:

- Provide an overview of the types of daily occupations people typically engage in or perform.
- Define occupation, occupational performance and engagement.
- Define occupational adaptation, participation, competence and identity.
- Provide an overview of different ways of classifying human occupation.
- Describe self-care, productivity, work, play, leisure, recreation, education, sleep and social participation occupations.
- Outline how occupations may change across the lifespan.
- Identify and describe occupational performance issues and challenges.

Key terms

occupational performance; occupational engagement; occupational adaptation, competence and identity; self-care; productivity; play; leisure; recreation; education; sleep; social participation; micro, meso and macro levels of occupational development; occupational repertoires; occupational possibilities; occupational exposure; occupational expectations; occupational performance issues; occupational performance challenges

Introduction

All humans engage in and perform occupations on a daily basis, and this is often referred to as occupational performance. There are a variety of occupations that a person can engage in or perform including self-care, work, volunteering, play, leisure, education, sleep and social participation. The types and range of occupations engaged in or performed change from childhood through adulthood to older age. Occupational performance is also impacted by a variety of factors external and internal to each person. Occupational therapists aim to promote and maximise client, family and community health, well-being, life satisfaction, dignity, independence and social-connectedness through occupational performance and engagement. This chapter will provide an overview of occupational performance, the types of occupations people engage in or perform, the concepts of occupational adaptation, occupational competence and occupational identity, occupational performance issues and challenges, as well as how individual occupational performance and engagement may vary throughout the lifespan.

Defining human occupation and occupational performance

There are various definitions of human occupation and occupational performance. Regardless of the variation in these definitions, human occupation and occupational performance include the core components of everyday life for each individual. It is the unique components of an individual that an occupational therapist explores and focuses on in their professional practice. Larson et al. (2003) define human occupation as 'the activities that comprise our daily life experience and can be named in the culture' (p. 16), while another definition states that human occupation refers to 'the daily life activities in which people engage' (American Occupational Therapy Association [AOTA], 2014, p. S6). It has been reported that 'occupation gives meaning to life; occupation is an important determinant of health, well-being, and justice; occupation organizes behaviour; occupation develops and changes over a lifetime; occupation shapes and is shaped by environments; and occupation has therapeutic potential' (Canadian Association of Occupational Therapists, 2016, para 5).

Different practice models and frameworks suggest different components of occupational performance (Christiansen et al., 2015). In the Occupational Therapy Practice Framework—third edition (OTPF-III), occupational performance is defined as the 'act of doing and accomplishing a selected action (performance skill), activity, or occupation … that results from the dynamic transaction among the client, the context, and the activity' (AOTA, 2014, p. S43). In the Person–Environment–Occupation–Performance (PEOP) Model by Baum et al. (2015), occupational performance is described as 'the doing of meaningful activities, tasks, and roles through complex interactions between the person and the environment' (p. 52). Christiansen and Townsend viewed occupational performance as 'the task-oriented, completion, or doing aspect of occupations; often, but not exclusively, involving observable movement' (2010, p. 421).

The Model of Human Occupation (MOHO) views engaging in an occupation at three different levels, that is, occupational participation, occupational performance and occupational skills (Taylor & Kielhofner, 2017). Occupational participation refers to 'engaging in work, play, or activities of daily living (ADL) that are part of one's sociocultural context and that are desired and/or necessary to one's well-being' (Forsyth et al., 2019, p. 605). Occupational performance denotes performing tasks connected to participating in key areas of life while occupational skills are the actions that make up occupational performance. In the context of the MOHO, occupational performance stems from the components of the person (specifically, volition, habituation and performance capacity) and the environment (Taylor & Kielhofner, 2017). As such, occupational performance is constantly changing in a dynamic manner in response to environmental demands.

Occupational adaptation represents a person's 'doing, thinking, and feeling under certain environmental conditions in the midst of therapy or as a planned consequence of therapy' (Forsyth et al., 2019, p. 605). According to the MOHO, two key elements of occupational adaptation are occupational identity and occupational competence. Occupational identity is the 'cumulative sense of who people are and who they wish to be as occupational beings' (Forsyth et al., 2019, p. 605), while occupational competence is the extent to which people are able to maintain their blueprint of performing occupations that puts into action their occupational identity.

Types of occupations

There are also different definitions of occupations that share overt similarities and have subtle but distinct differences. In part, this is a result of the growth of the body of occupational therapy discipline knowledge; expansion of the research evidence base relative to occupational therapy practice; the increasing focus on occupational functioning of human beings and understanding of how people benefit from occupational therapy services; and different occupational therapy authors conceiving, publishing and investigating occupation-focused practice models, theories and frameworks (Baker & Tickle-Degnen, 2019; Cohen, 2019; Hooper & Wood, 2019).

In the OTPF-III, occupation refers to 'the daily life activities in which people engage' (AOTA, 2014, p. S6). In the Canadian Model of Occupational Performance and Engagement (CMOP-E), occupations refer to:

> groups of activities and tasks of everyday life, named, organized, and given value and meaning by individuals and a culture; occupation is everything people do to occupy themselves, including looking after themselves (self-care), enjoying life (leisure), and contributing to the social and economic fabric of their communities.
>
> (Polatajko & Townsend, 2013, p. 369)

Accordingly, the CMOP-E identifies self-care, productivity and leisure as the key components of occupational performance, whereas the OTPF-III categorises occupations as education, play, work, activities of living (ADLs), instrumental activities of daily living (IADLs), leisure, rest/sleep and social participation (AOTA, 2014) (see Figure 21.1). In the World Health Organization's (WHO, 2001) International Classification of Functioning, Health and Disability (ICF), daily occupations occur in the two categories of activities (defined as 'the execution of a task or action by an individual' [WHO, 2001, p. 123]) and participation (defined as 'involvement in a life situation' [WHO, 2001, p. 123]).

Within the occupational therapy and occupational science literature there are various means of delineating human occupation. Common classifications of human occupation consider categories such as self-care, leisure and productivity (Polatajko et al., 2013a; 2013b). Harvey and Pentland (2010) identified four types of occupations: necessary; contracted; committed; and free time. While these categories help us to understand the type of occupations performed, consideration also needs to be given to other important dimensions of occupation, such as individual meaning, purpose and value in one's life (Bar & Jarus, 2015; Johnson & Dickie, 2019).

The way in which our occupations structure our time is also worth consideration. For instance, occupations such as paid work, attending classes at school, sleeping, or engaging in voluntary activities, all provide a structure to our daily lives around which our social and leisure activities commonly occur. Time-use, however, varies between individuals influenced by factors such as individual health, roles, habits, family commitments and life stages (Pemberton & Cox, 2011). For instance, people living with a disability may spend an increased amount of time performing self-care occupations while people with care responsibilities are found to spend less time in paid work and leisure occupations (Backman, 2010; Eklund et al., 2009).

Self-care occupations

In the OTPF-III, self-care occupations are often referred to as activities of daily living (ADLs), basic activities of daily living (BADLs), or personal activities of daily living (PADLs). ADLs are 'activities oriented towards taking care of one's own body' (AOTA, 2014, p. S19), while instrumental activities of daily living (IADLs) are activities that 'support daily life within the home and community that often require more complex interactions than those used in ADLs' (AOTA, 2014, p. S19). Examples of ADLs include bathing, showering, toileting, dressing, eating, functional mobility, personal hygiene and grooming, and sexual activity; whereas IADLs include care of others or pets, child rearing, financial management, home management, meal preparation and shopping (Howe, 2014; James & Pitonyak, 2019; Meriano & Latella, 2016; Mlinac & Feng, 2016). Occupational therapists often assist clients who present with difficulties in completing their ADLs and IADLs, e.g., providing toilet training strategies to a parent of a child with autism spectrum disorder, or teaching adapted ways to prepare a meal to a person who has had a stroke with resultant upper extremity weakness.

Productivity occupations: working and volunteering

According to Christiansen and Townsend, work consists of 'labor or exertion; to make, construct, manufacture, form, fashion, or shape objects; to organize, plan, or evaluate services or processes of living or governing; committed occupations that are performed with or without financial reward' (2010, p. 342). Work involves any activity that a person engages in where they are paid, but can also include unpaid activities such as volunteering (Cook & Lukersmith, 2010). It can also include both part-time and full-time work. Referring to the OTPF-III, work involves employment interests and pursuits, employment seeking and acquisition, job performance, retirement preparation and adjustment, and volunteer exploration and participation (AOTA, 2014). It is an important factor in relation to the development of morale, self-esteem, self-worth, dignity, competence and sense of belonging (Blank et al., 2015; Dorsey et al., 2019).

Work may involve variation in skills levels or requirements (e.g., an air traffic controller has a complex number of skills required to manage simultaneously while a supermarket checkout operator may require a different set of technical skills). Work may occur in many different environments such as working in an office or from home, inside or outside (e.g., nurse working in a hospital versus a surf lifesaver working at a local beach), in an individual or group context, or in a structured/unstructured, formal/informal manner. Different types of work may require an extensive period of preparatory education in addition to an apprenticeship or internship, whereas other positions have fewer skill requirements (Snodgrass, 2014). Work hours also vary from a few hours per week to many hours seven days per week. Similarly, work may occur in specific shifts or time periods. For example, a paramedic might work during the day or have a night shift, and work weekdays and weekends. Occupational therapists often assist clients in returning to work after an injury or provide guidance about considering alternative work opportunities post-injury (e.g., vocational rehabilitation).

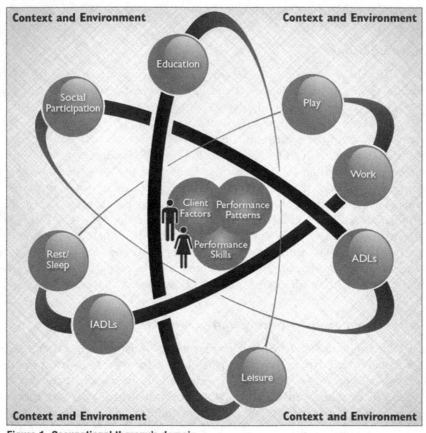

Figure 1. Occupational therapy's domain.
Note. ADLs = activities of daily living; IADLs = instrumental activities of daily living.

Figure 21.1 Categories of occupations in the Occupational Therapy Practice Framework—
third edition (OTPF-III).
Source: AOTA (2014, p. S5). Reproduced with permission from the author (Copy Clearance Centre
Licence Number 3799701405555)

   Volunteering usually involves participating in an unpaid activity, chosen specifically
by the person. Volunteering Australia (2015) defines volunteering as 'time willingly
given for the common good and without financial gain' (p. 1). People choose to engage
in volunteer activities for a variety of reasons including gaining practical experience;
personal satisfaction or gratification; meeting a personal need; a sense of obligation; or
'giving back' to the community (Black & Living, 2004). Volunteering can be short or
long term, formal or informal, or individual or group-based. Often people who have
retired from paid employment or who have had a major life role change (e.g., children
have grown up and left home or death of a spouse) may choose to assume a volunteer
position (Cole & Macdonald, 2011). Likewise, high school students who are investigating potential career options may opt to volunteer in different work sectors to see if
they enjoy aspects of the career they are selecting. It is interesting to note, however, that
according to the Australian Bureau of Statistics (2017), the following forms of unpaid

work are not considered voluntary: taking part in community work under mutual obligation, school-arranged/assigned work experience or an unpaid work trial, a community service order, a student placement or emergency work during an industrial dispute.
Occupational therapists may assist people to plan or prioritise volunteer activities in
order to assist with organising time; providing a routine and structure; or connecting
clients and families with volunteer organisations if they require additional assistance.

Play, leisure and recreation occupations

Play is defined as 'any spontaneous or organized activity that provides enjoyment, entertainment, amusement or diversion' (Parham & Fazio, 2008, p. 448) and includes play
exploration and play participation (AOTA, 2014). It is often considered the 'work' or
'productive role' of children since it provides a prime opportunity for them to learn
about many different aspects of daily life. Play assists children to develop key social,
emotional, cognitive, motor and psychological skills. There are several different types
of play including (among others) solitary play, spectator/onlooker play, parallel play,
associate play, cooperative play, pretend play and symbolic play. Children will often
engage in different types of play depending on their developmental level. For example, younger children (e.g., age 24 months to 36 months) might engage in spectator/
onlooker play or parallel play, whereas older children (e.g., age 48 months and older)
with more developed social awareness may engage in cooperative play with their peers
(Bundy & Du Toit, 2019).

Play can take many different forms including team play, indoor play, outdoor play,
imaginary play and sports play (Stagnitti, 2010). Similarly, play may be performed individually, in pairs, or in medium to large groups (e.g., playing video games on a computer tablet individually, playing chess with another person, playing on a football or
netball team). It can be resource intensive or undertaken with little or no equipment.
Play often occurs when someone 'loses themselves' in an activity, is experienced as relaxing or restorative, and based solely on freedom of choice.

Play is often influenced by culture, socio-economic status, outdoor landscape, accessible indoor facilities and gender (Bundy & Du Toit, 2019). Participating in a polo
match requires more financial resources than going swimming at a local beach. Occupational therapists often use play therapeutically to engage children in activities to promote skill development (Kuhaneck et al., 2013). For example, an occupational therapist
might encourage catching, throwing and bouncing a tennis ball, and walking forwards
and backwards on a balance beam in the context of a 'Simon Says' game for a child
presenting with poor eye–hand coordination and dynamic balance skills. Occupational
therapists often teach parents and caregivers about ways to play with their children to
promote skill development. Leisure is often synonymous with play; however, people
participate in leisure pursuits across the lifespan. Leisure includes 'non obligatory ac
tivity that is intrinsically motivated and engaged in during discretionary time, that
is, time not committed to obligatory occupations such as work, self-care, or sleep'
(Parham & Fazio, 2008, p. 447), including leisure exploration and participation (AOTA,
2014; Blacker et al., 2008). Leisure occupations, in a similar way to play, are often dependent on a variety of factors including culture, gender, socio-economic status, skill
level and living environments (Gross & Tascione, 2016; Olsen, 2014). For example,
comparing a young adult living on a farm in a rural region with another young adult
living in an urbanised area suggests different opportunities to engage in different types

of leisure activities. Culture can also influence leisure activities; for example, take the sport of cricket. Cricket is very popular in countries that have a British colonial heritage (Australia, New Zealand, South Africa, Pakistan, India and some Caribbean islands), whereas in other countries it is virtually non-existent (e.g., Germany, Japan, United States, Brazil, Egypt, China) (Stellar & Stanley, 2010).

Again, occupational therapists will utilise leisure occupations to promote skill development, life satisfaction, health and well-being in clients. For example, an occupational therapist could introduce wheelchair basketball to a construction worker who sustains a spinal cord injury to his thoracic region with resultant paraplegia, following a fall from scaffolding while at work who had played sports previously.

Education occupations

According to the OTPF-III, education is defined as 'activities needed for learning and participating in the educational environment' (AOTA, 2014, p. S20). Education can be formal or informal, as well as structured or unstructured. It usually involves learning a new set of skills or applying skills and knowledge that people have been exposed to previously. In addition, education can occur at any life stage (Swinth, 2019). For example, children attending primary and secondary school often study a variety of specific subjects such as mathematics, English, history, science and geography, whereas students studying at university level may enrol in a professional course (such as nursing or law) or choose to study a specific subject in more depth (e.g., English literature, art history, philosophy or physics). Adults may engage in educational activities to upgrade their skills or retrain for a new job. Occupational therapists will often collaborate with children, adolescents and adults about issues related to education, e.g., a therapist might provide guidelines for children with poor handwriting skills or assist an adult in structuring new work-related tasks that involved new learning (Swinth, 2019).

Sleep and rest occupations

Sleep can be defined as 'a natural, periodic state of immobility where the individual is relatively unaware of the environment and unresponsive to external sensory stimuli' (Paterson, 2012, p. 18). In the OTPF-III, rest and sleep are linked and defined as 'activities related to obtaining restorative rest and sleep to support healthy, active engagement in other occupations' (AOTA, 2014, p. S20). There are many variables that contribute to sleep and its function, with sleep being crucial for health, well-being and overall brain function. Day-time sleepiness and fatigue can significantly impact on an individual's cognition, work performance and absenteeism, and have increased risk of accidents, particularly whilst driving (Alford & Wilson, 2008). Likewise, day-time sleepiness has also been linked to increased risk of psychiatric disorders, substance use and health-related financial burden, as well as poorer prognosis and social functioning (Roth, 2015).

Typically, nocturnal sleep periods cycle between two types of sleep: 'non-rapid eye movement' (non-REM) and 'rapid eye movement' (REM) sleep (Kryger et al., 2017). Non-REM sleep is composed of three stages of slow-wave sleep, namely N1 and N2 (considered to be light sleep) and N3 (deep sleep) during which rapid eye movements and dreaming do not usually occur. Over the course of one night, a person alternates in cycles of approximately 90 minutes between non-REM and REM stages. Non-REM sleep accounts for approximately 75 per cent of the sleep period and is more prevalent during the first third of the night for a healthy adult, while REM sleep is more prevalent in the last third of sleep. As people age their total sleep time decreases and the quantity of N1 and N2 (light sleep) stages increases (Ohayon et al., 2004). Generally, the appropriate sleep duration for school-aged children is between nine to eleven hours, eight to ten hours for teenagers, and seven to nine hours for young adults and adults (Hirshkowitz et al., 2015).

Adequate rest and sleep are essential for individuals to be able to complete their daily occupational performance requirements (Solet, 2019). Studies have shown that poor sleep quality or sleep loss affects individual cognitive performance, particularly in relation to attention, memory and executive functions, which are most important for completion of activities of daily living (ADLs) by any individual (Duclos et al., 2015). In 2008, Green reported that sleep has been previously overlooked within occupational therapy practice, stating it is an important area for consideration, especially with a lack of sleep negatively impacting work performance, quality of life, social functioning, and essentially all aspects of activities of daily living. Occupational therapists need to recognise sleep as an occupation for exploration with children, adults and older adults, especially considering the impact of sleep issues upon day-to-day functioning. For example, a therapist may explore the sleep routine of an older adult, returning home after experiencing disrupted sleep in hospital, to enable them to regain their usual sleep pattern and re-engage in their usual leisure, self-care and productive occupations.

Social participation occupations

Social participation involves engagement in daily occupations, promoting connectedness with family, peers, friends, neighbours, co-workers and community members. It can occur 'in person or through remote technologies such as telephone calls, computer interaction, and video-conferencing' (AOTA, 2014, p. S21). Humans are instinctively social beings, making social participation essential in their daily life. Social participation includes social interactions with others and promotes social interdependence (Khetani & Coster, 2019). Studies have shown the connection between social isolation and increasing episodes of poor health (Hawton et al., 2011). Social participation influences the type of occupations performed by individuals. This might include attending a religious activity once a week; being a member of a monthly book group; being active in a political party; or being a member of a club with members who have a specific interest (e.g., collecting memorabilia, playing bridge or mah-jong, or being involved in a social club centred around playing a sport).

The common thread is that people gather to socialise with each other. Often with ageing, the opportunities for active social participation decrease due to ill health, disability, family and friends passing away, fewer social opportunities, or inability to access a social group to participate. Social participation can be influenced by culture, religious beliefs, region where one lives, and available financial resources and transportation options. Occupational therapists often work with clients and their families to promote social engagement opportunities (Leigers et al., 2016).

Occupational development: occupations across the lifespan

Occupational development is defined as 'the systematic process of change in occupational behaviours across time, resulting from the growth and maturation of the individual in interaction with the environment' (Townsend & Polatajko, 2013, p. 370). Occupations can change and evolve throughout the lifespan (Wiseman et al., 2005). The occupations a pre-schooler engages in or performs while playing in the local park are different to those of a young adult starting their first job.

Davis and Polatajko (2010) described three levels of occupational development: micro, meso and macro. The three levels of occupational development consider changes in individual occupational behaviours along a continuum of occupational competence from novice to mastery (Davis & Polatajko, 2010). At the micro level, occupational development is viewed at the level of occupation, with a beginning, middle and ending, moving from novice competence to mastery. 'The development of occupational competence is an iterative process, with the progression from novice to mastery repeated again and again, with the addition of each new occupation' (Davis & Polatajko, 2010, p. 140).

The next level is the meso viewpoint that considers occupational repertoires at the level of the individual. Occupational repertoires 'change continuously throughout the lifespan, sometimes expanding, and sometimes shrinking' (Davis & Polatajko, 2010, pp. 140–141). Macro is the final level of occupational development. It considers changes in occupational behaviours at the level of the species and 'humankind's occupational possibilities—that is, the set of occupations that exist in any given place and at any given time across the evolution of the occupational human that provide opportunities for engagement and participation' (Davis & Polatajko, 2010, pp. 140–141). Considering the micro, meso and macro perspectives, occupational development can be viewed as 'the systematic process of change in occupational behaviours across time resulting from the interaction of person, environment, and occupation at the level of the occupation, individual, and species' (Davis & Polatajko, 2010, pp. 140–141). Occupational therapists have a key role in promoting opportunities for optimal occupational development of clients and their families at the micro, meso and macro level.

With our sense of who we are, shaped by the occupations and our pattern of daily participation in these occupations, consideration to occupational identity and occupational competence of individuals is important (Altit et al., 2019). Over time our occupational identity and competence may change as one's capacity alters across the lifespan, during life transitions such as becoming a new parent, or influenced by the support or constraints of the context within which our occupations occur (Andrew et al., 2019). Maintaining one's sense of occupational identity and competence is underpinned by the notion of occupational adaptation (Grajo et al., 2018; Grajo & Boisselle, 2019). The outcome of these disruptions is influenced by an individual's capacity for occupational adaptation (Johansson et al., 2018). These concepts illuminate the ways in which our occupations reflect a sense of who we are as individuals, the importance of competence in being able to participate in occupations that reflect our identity, and the importance of being able to adapt to personal and/or contextual changes that may disrupt our occupational competence and occupational identity developed over time (Rudman & Dennhardt, 2008).

Factors affecting occupational performance

There are a variety of factors that can affect individual occupational performance. These may include age, gender, socio-economic status, religious beliefs, culture, ethnicity, living environment (e.g., urban, rural, low- and lower-middle-income countries), composition of family, political views, social connectedness, community participation, physical and mental health status, languages spoken, access to technology and intelligence, to name a few. When one or more of these factors impact, or have the ability to impact, an individual's ability to successfully 'choose, organize, and satisfactorily perform meaningful occupations', they have encountered an occupational performance issue (OPI) or challenge (Townsend & Polatajko, 2013, p. 181). Considerations and examples of occupational performance issues or challenges (OPICs) in the domains of productivity (education and work), self-care (ADLs and sleep and rest) and leisure (social participation and leisure/play activities) are illustrated in Figure 21.2.

Davis and Polatajko (2010) refer to three occupational determinants potentially affecting occupational performance: occupational possibilities, occupational exposure and occupational expectations. Occupations are constantly evolving, thereby increasing the occupational possibilities of humans. With occupations continually evolving, the occupational possibilities are constantly developing. This increases the opportunities for exposure of individuals to a range of occupations. This expanding occupational exposure may increase the motivation to enlarge occupational performance repertoires. Occupational expectations, underpinned by societal or cultural norms, influence the occupations one engages in at different ages and determines those considered culturally and socially acceptable.

Case study 1: Human occupation in action—Tim

Tim is a five-year-old boy who has just begun his first year of school. Tim enjoys spending time with his classmates during recess in the playground. However, he sometimes finds it challenging to settle and focus on table activities in his classroom. His teacher has reported that Tim is fidgety, not always appearing to pay attention to verbal instructions. He lives with his mother, father and older twin sisters in a detached single storey house. Tim plays soccer on a team that his father coaches. He also enjoys playing with his two best friends in the sandpit in his backyard and kicking a football around with them. Tim also enjoys being active, particularly enjoying swimming and riding his bicycle in the local park. Tim has difficulty settling to go to sleep at night and does not like getting up for school during the week. His mother describes Tim as 'not a morning person' and a 'child who constantly tests his behavioural limits'. His parents expect Tim to keep his room tidy, hang up his school uniform at the end of each day and feed the family pet dog after arriving home from school. He usually takes the family dog for a walk each evening with his father. Tim receives $5 per week as pocket money after successfully completing his assigned chores. Tim has no difficulty with his bowel and bladder routine; he occasionally requires a reminder to brush his teeth and comb his hair; he dresses independently and eats most things. Tim does have difficulty tying his shoelaces and differentiating his left from his right. He does not like activities that require the use of his hands to complete small, coordinated motor movements such as putting puzzles together, cutting and pasting, colouring, using a knife and fork in a synchronised manner to eat his food, and doing up buttons on a shirt.

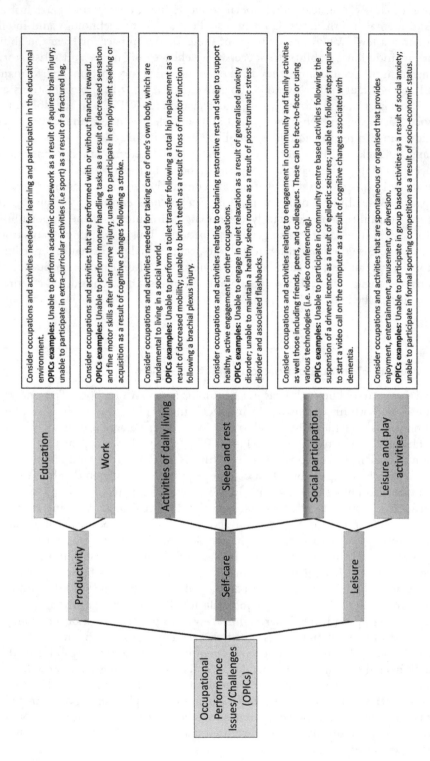

Figure 21.2 Examples of occupational performance issues or challenges (OPICs) in the domains of productivity, self–care and leisure.

Occupational participation analysis of case study 1—Tim

ADL: Tim is able to dress and feed himself but does find tying his shoelaces and using a knife and fork together challenging. Tim also finds doing up buttons challenging. He has a good bowel and bladder routine and can brush his teeth by himself.

IADL: Tim places his weekly pocket money in his moneybox and walks the family dog with his father after school each day.

Play: Tim enjoys playing with his friends and engaging in team sports. He enjoys physical activities including riding his bicycle, playing soccer and swimming. Tim also enjoys playing with his two friends in his sandpit and kicking a football back and forth. Tim appears not to enjoy engaging in play activities involving fine motor movements but appears skilled at participating in sports that primarily use large muscle abilities.

Sleep: Tim has difficulty falling asleep and often wakes up feeling tired.

Education: Tim is attending prep at his local primary school. Prep/kindergarten exposes students to a variety of necessary skills for success in the classroom setting (e.g., printing; paying attention in a classroom situation; following verbal instructions). Tim appears to have difficulty paying attention in a classroom setting and also completing certain types of table activities. He is learning the life role of being a student.

Work: Tim is attending prep/kindergarten where he is learning foundation skills for year one, his next year at school. In other words, his 'job' is being a student learning new skills at school. Tim also assists with several house chores at home including keeping his room tidy, taking out the rubbish bins and walking the family pet dog with his father. Tim is also paid an allowance by his parents for successfully completing these tasks each week.

Social participation: Tim engages in social activities with his friends, family and soccer team. He is actively involved in several social situations including his school classroom, local community, soccer team, family and his two friends with whom he plays in the sandpit and kicks a football.

Case study 2: Human occupation in action—Rose

Rose, an 82-year-old woman, lives alone in her own single-storey home with no community aged-care services in place. A typical week for Rose includes playing lawn bowls twice a week and bridge (a card game), attending her local Country Women's Association and volunteering at the local opportunity thrift shop. Rose completes her grocery shopping on her way home from volunteering on a Friday.

Rose drives herself to all activities and picks up a friend from the lawn bowls club who no longer drives to enable her continued involvement with the club. Rose is independent with all self-care occupations (e.g. showering, dressing, drying herself with a towel, grooming, toileting), meal preparation, house cleaning and laundry. Once a month Rose has a private gardener come to mow her lawn, complete larger gardening tasks such as pruning trees, and carry out minor repairs and house maintenance.

Each year Rose also pays someone privately to clean the gutters of her house. Rose has three children and eight grandchildren. Two of her children, and their families, live interstate. Rose collapsed early one morning while making her bed and woke up to find herself on her bedroom floor unable to move her right arm and with a cut to her forehead. Unable to get up off the floor, Rose used her personal alarm to call for assistance. Following review by attending paramedics, Rose was transported to hospital by ambulance for medical treatment. She was admitted to hospital to undergo surgery for her fractured right wrist. She received stitches to her forehead and had surgery to insert a pacemaker to help manage her bradycardia (slow heart rate), the cause of her fainting.

Following her surgery, Rose had restricted use of her right wrist for approximately six weeks to allow her fracture to heal and was unable to return to driving during this period. Rose was also not able to hold a pen or to write, since she was right-hand dominant, while her wrist healed. In hospital, it was identified that Rose required moderate assistance with her self-care occupations (such as showering, drying, dressing and grooming). Rose also needed to have her meals cut up and had to hold her fork or spoon with her left hand following the restrictions when using her right hand.

With the occupational performance issues identified, Rose living alone and with no aged-care support services currently in place, the acute care occupational therapist recommended Rose be transferred for inpatient rehabilitation to work on increasing her independence with self-care occupations and activities of daily living necessary to return home. Thus, once medically stable, Rose was transferred for two weeks of inpatient rehabilitation. During her admission the occupational therapists worked with Rose to set goals to form the focus of her occupational therapy sessions. These goals included:

- Increase independence in self-care occupations (e.g., showering, drying, dressing, grooming and toileting) through education of one-handed techniques and provision of equipment such as shower chair, grab rail and over-the-toilet frame;
- Increase independence with eating through education of one-handed techniques and provision of utensils to support one-handed eating and drinking;
- Increase independence with meal preparation through education of one-handed techniques and adjustment in cooking tasks (e.g., using individual steam vegetable packs, one-handed utensils, use of kitchen trolley to move items around kitchen and between kitchen and dining table);
- Referral to MyAgedCare (the starting point for older adults to access Australian Government-funded aged-care services to assist them to remain living in the community and transition to residential aged-care service) to have an assessment for community aged-care services to assist with housework, heavy laundry tasks (e.g., changing bed sheets) and shopping tasks to enable discharge home;
- Complete a home assessment to review and set up the necessary equipment and ensure appropriate accessibility (e.g., front access, amount of internal and external stops, removal of loose rugs or carpets) to minimise the risk of falls and enable safe and independent discharge home.

Following discharge from inpatient rehabilitation, Rose was referred for community-based rehabilitation to commence following approval from her managing medical team to begin using her right wrist in functional tasks. Community-based rehabilitation focused on supporting Rose to increase range of movement and strength in her wrist to enable her to return to, and increase independence with, meal preparation, shopping and light laundry tasks, driving, playing lawn bowls, attending Country Women's Association and volunteering in the opportunity thrift shop. Rose continued with home help to assist with housework following the healing of her right wrist.

Conclusion

Occupation and occupational performance are key concepts guiding occupational therapists as part of their profession. Occupational performance is the engagement with and completion of purposeful and meaningful activities. Occupations can be classified within several different categories (e.g., self-care, productivity, education, play/leisure, sleep and social participation). Occupational development refers to how individual occupations change and evolve throughout the lifespan and can occur at micro, meso and macro levels. Determinants of occupational development include occupational possibilities, occupational exposure, and occupational expectations that are in turn impacted by a person's occupational identity, competence and adaptation. It is essential for occupational therapists to be conversant with the types of occupation, to understand occupational development along with the factors that impact occupational performance.

Summary

- Occupational performance involves all the activities that human beings engage in or perform for health, well-being, social-connectedness, life satisfaction, economic necessity, and pleasure and enjoyment.
- Specific types of occupations include self-care, productivity, play, leisure, recreation, education, sleep and social participation.
- The types and repertoire of occupations for healthy people throughout their lifespan change and evolve, often starting with a limited range during young childhood, expanding upon reaching adulthood, and then shrinking again with ageing.
- Occupational development can occur at the micro, meso and macro levels.
- Occupational adaptation, competence and identity are key concepts related to occupational performance.
- Determinants of occupational development include occupational possibilities, occupational exposure and occupational expectations.
- A variety of factors can impact individual occupational performance including: socio-economic status; employment status; level of education; intelligence, skills and aptitudes; gender; religious beliefs; age; culture; ethnicity; living environment; composition of family; political views; social-connectedness; community participation; physical and mental health status; and so forth.

- Occupational performance issues or challenges (OPICs) can occur in the domains of productivity (education and work), self-care (ADLs and sleep and rest) and leisure (social participation and leisure/play activities).

Review questions

1. What is occupational performance and how is it relevant to the practice of an occupational therapist?
2. What are four types of occupations that a typically developing ten-year-old boy would perform?
3. What are four daily occupations that an 85-year-old woman with limited mobility might find challenging to complete?
4. What are four factors that may limit or inhibit the ability of a person to engage in their desired self-care and leisure occupations?
5. What are the three levels of occupational development proposed by Davis and Polatajko (2010), and include an example of each level?
6. Compare and contrast the types of occupations a typically developing three-year-old girl would engage in/perform with those of a typically developing 15-year-old girl.

References

Alford, C., & Wilson, S. (2008). Effects of hypnotics on sleep and quality of life in insomnia. In J. C. Verster, S. R. Pandi-Perumal, & D. L. Streiner (Eds.), *Sleep and quality of life in medical illnesses* (pp. 56–66). Humana Press.

Altit, T. P., Shor, R., & Maeir, A. (2019). Occupational identity, competence, and environments among adults with and without attention deficit hyperactivity disorder. *Occupational Therapy in Mental Health, 35*(2), 205–215. https://doi.org/10.1080/0164212X.2019.1588833

American Occupational Therapy Association. (2014). Occupational Therapy Practice Framework: Domain and Process, 3rd edition. *American Journal of Occupational Therapy, 68*(Supp. 1), S1–S48. https://doi.org/10.5014/ajot.2014.682006

Andrew, C., Phillipson, L., & Sheridan, L. (2019). What is the impact of dementia on occupational competence, occupational participation and occupational identity for people who experience onset of symptoms while in paid employment? A scoping review. *Australian Occupational Therapy Journal, 66*(2), 130–144. https://doi.org/10.1111/1440-1630.12535

Australian Bureau of Statistics. (2017). *Discussion paper: Information needs for volunteering data, April 2017.* Australian Bureau of Statistics. https://www.abs.gov.au/ausstats/abs@.nsf/mf/4159.0.55.004

Backman, C. (2010). Occupational balance and well-being. In C. H. Christiansen & E. A. Townsend (Eds.), *Introduction to occupation: The art and science of living* (2nd edn, pp. 231–249). Pearson.

Baker, N., & Tickle-Degnen, L. (2019). Evidence-based practice: Integrating evidence to inform practice. In B. A. Boyt Schell & G. Gillen (Eds.), *Willard & Spackman's occupational therapy* (13th edn, pp. 498–512). Wolters Kluwer.

Bar, M. A., & Jarus, T. (2015). The effect of engagement in everyday occupations, role overload and social support on health and life satisfaction. *International Journal of Environmental Research and Public Health, 12*(6), 6045–6065. https://doi.org/10.3390/ijerph120606045

Baum, C., Christiansen, C., & Bass, J. (2015). The Person–Environment–Occupation–Performance (PEOP) model. In C. H. Christiansen, C. M. Baum, & J. D. Bass (Eds.), *Occupational therapy: Performance, participation, and well-being* (4th edn, pp. 49–56). SLACK Inc.

Black, W., & Living, R. (2004). Volunteerism as an occupation and its relationship to health and well-being. *British Journal of Occupational Therapy, 67*(12), 526–532. https://doi.org/10.1177/030802260406701202

Blacker, D., Broadhurst, L., & Teixeira, L. (2008). The role of occupational therapy in leisure adaptation with complex neurological disability: A discussion using two case study examples. *NeuroRehabilitation, 23*(4), 313–319. https://doi.org/10.3233/NRE-2008-23404

Blank, A. A., Harries, P., & Reynolds, P. F. (2015). 'Without occupation you don't exist': Occupational engagement and mental illness. *Journal of Occupational Science, 22*(2), 197–209. https://doi.org/10.1080/14427591.2014.882250

Bundy, A. C., & Du Toit, S. H. J. (2019). Play and leisure. In B. A. Boyt Schell & G. Gillen (Eds.), *Willard & Spackman's occupational therapy* (13th edn, pp. 805–827). Wolters Kluwer.

Canadian Association of Occupational Therapists (CAOT). (2016). *Occupational therapy values and belief.* CAOT Publications. https://caot.ca/site/aboutot/whatisot_test

Christiansen, C. H., Baum, C. M., & Bass, J. D. (2015). Health, occupational performance, and occupational therapy. In C. H. Christiansen, C. M. Baum, & J. D. Bass (Eds.), *Occupational therapy: Performance, participation, and well-being* (4th edn, pp. 7–21). SLACK Inc.

Christiansen, C. H., & Townsend, E. A. (2010). *Introduction to occupation: The art and science of living* (2nd edn). Pearson.

Cohen, H. S. (2019). Scholarship in occupational therapy. In B. A. Boyt Schell & G. Gillen (Eds.), *Willard & Spackman's occupational therapy* (13th edn, pp. 84–97). Wolters Kluwer.

Cole, M. B., & Macdonald, K. C. (2011). Retired occupational therapists' experiences in volunteer occupations. *Occupational Therapy International, 18*(1), 18-31.

Cook, C., & Lukersmith, S. (2010). Work rehabilitation. In M. Curtin, M. Molineux, & J. Supk-Mellson (Eds.), *Occupational therapy and physical dysfunction: Enabling occupation* (6th edn, pp. 391–408). Elsevier.

Davis, J. A., & Polatajko, H. J. (2010). Occupational development. In C. H. Christiansen & E. A. Townsend (Eds.), *Introduction to occupation: The art and science of living* (2nd edn, pp. 135–170). Pearson.

Dorsey, J., Ehrenfried, H., Finch, D., & Jaegers, L. A. (2019). Work. In B. A. Boyt Schell & G. Gillen (Eds.), *Willard & Spackman's occupational therapy* (13th edn, pp. 779–804). Wolters Kluwer.

Duclos, C., Beauregard, M-P., Bottari, C., Ouellet, M-C., & Gosselin, N. (2015). The impact of poor sleep on cognition and activities of daily living after traumatic brain injury: A review. *Australian Occupational Therapy Journal, 62*, 2–12. https://doi.org/10.1111/1440-1630.12164

Eklund, M., Leufstadius, C., & Bejerholm, U. (2009). Time use among people with psychiatric disabilities: Implications for practice. *Psychiatric Rehabilitation Journal, 32*(3), 177–191. https://doi.org/10.2975/32.3.2009.177.191

Forsyth, K. et al. (2019). The Model of Human Occupation. In B. A. Boyt Schell & G. Gillen (Eds.), *Willard & Spackman's occupational therapy* (13th edn, pp. 601–621). Wolters Kluwer.

Grajo, L., & Boisselle, A. (2019). *Adaptation through occupation: Multidimensional perspectives.* SLACK Inc.

Grajo, L., Boisselle, A., & Dalomba, E. (2018). Occupational adaptation as a construct: A scoping review of literature. *The Open Journal of Occupational Therapy, 6*(1). https://doi.org/10.15453/2168-6408.1400

Green, A. (2008). Sleep, Occupation and the Passage of Time. *British Journal of Occupational Therapy, 71*(8), 339–347. https://doi.org/10.1177/030802260807100808

Gross, M. R., & Tascione, P. (2016). Leisure. In C. Meriano & D. Latella (Eds.), *Occupational therapy interventions: Function and occupations* (2nd edn, pp. 403–431). SLACK Inc.

Harvey, A., & Pentland, W. (2010). What do people do? In C. H. Christiansen & E. A. Townsend (Eds.), *Introduction to occupation: The art and science of living* (2nd edn). Pearson.

Hawton, A., Green, C., Dickens, A. P., Richards, S. H., Taylor, R. S., Edwards, R., Greaves, C. J., & Campbell, J. L. (2011). The impact of social isolation on the health status and health-related quality of life of older people. *Quality of Life Research, 20*(1), 57–67. https://doi. org/10.1007/s11136-010-9717-2

Hirshkowitz, M., Whiton, K., Albert, S. M., Alessi, C., Bruni, O., DonCarlos, L., Hazen, N., Herman, J., Katz, E. S., Kheirandish-Gozal, L., Neubauer, D. N., O'Donnell, A. E., Ohayon, M., Peever, J., Rawding, R., Sachdeva, R. C., Setters, B., Vitiello, M. V., Catesby Ware, J., Adams Hillard, P. J. (2015). National Sleep Foundation's sleep time duration recommendations: Methodology and results summary. *Sleep Health, 1*(1), 40–43. https://doi.org/10.106/j. sleh.2014.12.010

Hooper, B., & Wood, W. (2019). The philosophy of occupational therapy: A framework for practice. In B. A. Boyt Schell & G. Gillen (Eds.), *Willard & Spackman's occupational therapy* (13th edn, pp. 43–54). Wolters Kluwer.

Howe, T. H. (2014). Self-care occupations. In J. Hinojosa & M. L. Blount (Eds.), *The texture of life: Occupations and related activities* (pp. 337–352). American Occupational Therapy Association.

James, A. B., & Pitonyak, J. S. (2019). Activities of daily living and instrumental activities of daily living. In B. A. Boyt Schell & G. Gillen (Eds.), *Willard & Spackman's occupational therapy* (13th edn, pp. 714–754). Wolters Kluwer.

Johansson, A., Fristedt, S., Bostrom, M., & Bjorklund, A. (2018). The use of occupational adaptation in research: A scoping review. *Occupational Therapy in Health Care, 32*(40), 422–439. https://doi.org/10.1080/07380577.2018.1526433

Johnson, K. R., & Dickie, V. (2019). What is occupation? In B. A. Boyt Schell & G. Gillen (Eds.), *Willard & Spackman's occupational therapy* (13th edn, pp. 2–10). Wolters Kluwer.

Khetani, M. A., & Coster, W. J. (2019). Social participation. In B. A. Boyt Schell & G. Gillen (Eds.), *Willard & Spackman's occupational therapy* (13th edn, pp. 847–863). Wolters Kluwer.

Kryger, M. H., Roth, T., & Dement, W. C. (Eds.). (2017). *Principles and practice of sleep medicine* (6th edn). Elsevier Saunders.

Kuhaneck, H. M., Tanta, K. J., Coombs, A. K., & Pannone, H. (2013). A survey of pediatric occupational therapists' use of play. *Journal of Occupational Therapy, Schools, & Early Intervention, 6*(3), 213–227. https://doi.org/10.1080/19411243.2013.850940

Larson, E. A., Wood, W., & Clark, F. (2003). Occupational science: Building the science and practice of occupation through an academic discipline. In E. B. Crepeau, E. S. Cohn, & B. A. Boyt Schell (Eds.), *Willard & Spackman's occupational therapy* (10th edn, pp. 15–26). Lippincott Williams & Wilkins.

Leigers, K., Meyers, C., & Schneck, C. (2016). Social participation in schools: A survey of occupational therapy practitioners. *American Journal of Occupational Therapy, 70*(5). https://doi. org/10.5014/ajot.2016.020768

Meriano, C., & Latella, D. (2016). *Occupational therapy interventions: Function and occupations* (2nd edn). SLACK Inc.

Mlinac, M. E., & Feng, M. C. (2016). Assessment of activities of daily living, self-care, and independence. *Archives of Clinical Neuropsychology, 31*(6), 506–516. https://doi.org/10.1093/arclin/ acw049

Ohayon, M. M., Carskadon, M. A., Guilleminault, C., & Vitiello, M. V. (2004). Meta-analysis of quantitative sleep parameters from childhood to old age in healthy individuals: Developing normative sleep values across the human lifespan. *Sleep, 27*(7), 1255–1273. https://doi. org/10.1093/sleep/27.7.1255

Olsen, L. (2014). Leisure occupations. In J. Hinojosa & M. L. Blount (Eds.), *The texture of life: Occupations and related activities* (4th edn, pp. 285–316). American Occupational Therapy Association.

Parham, L.D., & Fazio, L. S. (2008). *Play in occupational therapy for children* (2nd edn). Mosby Elsevier.

Paterson, L. M. (2012). The science of sleep. In A. Green & A. Westcombe (Eds.), *Sleep: Multi-professional perspectives* (pp. 18–40). Jessica Kingsley Publishers.

Pemberton, S., & Cox, D. (2011). What happened to the time? The relationship of occupational therapy to time. *British Journal of Occupational Therapy*, 74(2), 78–85. https://doi.org/10.4276/030802211X12971689814043

Polatajko, H. J., Backman, C., Baptiste, S., Davis, J., Eftekhar, P., Harvey, A., Jarman, J., Krupa, T., Lin, N., Pentland, W., Laliberte Rudman, D., Shaw, L., Amoroso, B., & Connor-Schisler, A. (2013a). Human occupation in context. In E. A. Townsend & H. J. Polatajko (Eds.), *Enabling occupation II: Advancing an occupational therapy vision for health, well-being and justice through occupation* (pp. 37–61). CAOT Publications.

Polatajko, H. J., Davis, J., Steward, D., Cantin, N., Amoroso, B., Purdie, L., & Zimmerman, D. (2013b). Specifying the domain of concern: Occupation as core. In E. A. Townsend & H. J. Polatajko (Eds.), *Enabling occupation II: Advancing an occupational therapy vision for health, well-being and justice through occupation* (pp. 13–36). CAOT Publications.

Polatajko, H. J., & Townsend, E. A. (2013). Glossary. In E. A. Townsend & H. J. Polatajko (Eds.), *Enabling occupation II: Advancing an occupational therapy vision for health, well-being and justice through occupation* (pp. 364–376). CAOT Publications.

Roth, T. (2015). Effects of excessive daytime sleepiness and fatigue on overall health and cognitive function. *Journal of Clinical Psychiatry*, 76(9), e1145. https://doi.org/10.4088/JCP.14019tx1c

Rudman, D. L., & Dennhardt, S. (2008). Shaping knowledge regarding occupation: Examining the cultural underpinnings of the evolving concept of occupational identity. *Australian Occupational Therapy Journal*, 55(3), 153–162. https://doi.org/10.1111/j.1440-1630.2007.00715.x

Snodgrass, J. & Gupta, J. (2014). Work occupations. In J. Hinojosa & M. L. Blount (Eds.), *The texture of life: Occupations and related activities* (4th edn, pp. 318–336). American Occupational Therapy Association.

Solet, J. M. (2019). Sleep and rest. In B. A. Boyt Schell & G. Gillen (Eds.), *Willard & Spackman's occupational therapy* (13th edn, pp. 828–846). Wolters Kluwer.

Stagnitti, K. (2010). Play. In M. Curtin, M. Molineux, & J. Supk-Mellson (Eds.), *Occupational therapy and physical dysfunction: Enabling occupation* (6th edn, pp. 371–390). Elsevier.

Stellar, B., & Stanley, M. (2010). Leisure. In M. Curtin, M. Molineux, & J. Supk-Mellson (Eds.), *Occupational therapy and physical dysfunction: Enabling occupation* (6th edn, pp. 358–369). Elsevier.

Swinth, Y. L. (2019). Education. In B. A. Boyt Schell & G. Gillen (Eds.), *Willard & Spackman's occupational therapy* (13th edn, pp. 753–778). Wolters Kluwer.

Taylor, R. R., & Kielhofner, G. (2017). *Kielhofner's model of human occupation: Theory and application* (5th edn). Lippincott Williams & Wilkins.

Townsend, E., & Polatajko, H. (2013). *Enabling occupation II: Advancing occupational therapy vision for health, well-being and justice through occupation* (2nd edn). CAOT Publications ACE.

Volunteering Australia. (2015). *New definition of volunteering in Australia*. https://www.volunteeringaustralia.org/wp-content/uploads/300715-Media-Release-New-Definition-of-Volunteering-FINAL.pdf

Wiseman, J. O., Davis, J. A., & Polatajko, H. J. (2005). Occupational development: Towards an understanding of children's doing. *Journal of Occupational Science*, 12(1), 26–35. https://doi.org/10.1080/14427591.2005.9686545

World Health Organization. (2001). *International Classification of Functioning, Disability, and Health*. WHO. https://www.who.int/classifications/icf/en/

22 The development of occupations across the lifespan

Reinie Cordier, Annette Joosten, Kylie Wales and Lindy Clemson

Chapter objectives

Upon completion of this chapter, the reader will be able to:

- Provide an overview of self-care, play, leisure and productivity including education, paid work and volunteerism across the lifespan.
- Discuss the importance of occupation to the development of routines and rituals, values, health and well-being, engagement, personal identity and roles.
- Outline key points of transitioning occupations across the lifespan.

Key terms

occupation; lifespan; roles; identity; engagement

Introduction

Engagement in occupations commences in early infancy and occupational roles and identities develop and change across the lifespan as a result of maturation, experiences, and the interaction between person, environment and occupation (Rodger & Kennedy-Behr, 2017). Play is one of the first occupations to develop and remains the primary occupation of childhood, whereas self-care and student roles develop in the child's early years and continue alongside other roles such as being a worker, volunteer and carer. Occupations change throughout our lives. While establishing occupations is influenced by parents' views, values, resources, motivations and purposefully generating opportunities during early life, it is the child's active participation in their own development that is essential to controlling their life course from birth (Smet & Lucas, 2020). The trajectory of occupational development is not linear with people starting engagement in occupations at different stages, for different reasons, and as part of being a community member (Humphry & Womak, 2019). Occupational development can be interrupted following significant events, such as family breakup, loss of financial security, injury, illness or disability, and experiencing trauma. Such interruptions not only alter the way we engage in activities, but also the time and the priority we dedicate to those occupations. Ageing can significantly influence the maintenance of many occupations, but later life also provides opportunities to engage in occupations based on both individual strengths and capacity (Källdalen et al., 2013).

This chapter provides the reader with a snapshot of how occupations, occupational roles and occupational identities evolve across the lifespan. In particular this chapter focuses on providing an overview of the occupations of play, leisure and social participation, self-care occupations, such as dressing and sleep, and the productivity occupations of being a student and worker, paid or unpaid, and how these occupations develop and diversify across the lifespan. Given the multitude of occupations, in this chapter we have only provided a snapshot of common everyday occupations. We will illustrate these with the case study of James as we follow him at critical time points across his lifespan. In this chapter we have adopted a broad occupation-focused approach to lifespan development to illustrate how patterns change across the lifespan. However, there may be differences in cultural influences and expectations around occupational roles and independence in occupations as individuals use their own primary culture and communities to shape their values and beliefs (Cronin & Mandich, 2016). Occupations are always contextual and develop and change in response to physical and social environmental demands and resources across the lifespan (Smet & Lucas, 2020).

Play and leisure

Play is the main occupation of early childhood and remains an important occupation throughout our lives. Play is difficult to define but a widely accepted definition of play is that it is a transaction between the individual and the environment, and is intrinsically motivated, internally controlled, free of some unnecessary constraints of reality, and requires the ability to frame the transaction as being play (Bundy & Du Toit, 2019; Cordier & Bundy, 2009). Sometimes the words play and playfulness are used interchangeably. For the purpose of this text playfulness refers to the tendency or disposition to play, and play is the transaction or the occupation (Bundy & Du Toit, 2019). Play is usually chosen freely and results in fun and enjoyment. Children bring many things to the play transaction, such as particular interests, relative playfulness and developmental abilities. The play environment is influenced by cultural expectations and resources and can either inhibit or facilitate play opportunities and occupational therapists often adapt the play environment to facilitate play, so as not to disrupt the play transaction. For example, placing recyclable materials not designed as play objects, such as milk crates and car tyres, increased physical activity and opportunities for play in school playgrounds (Bundy et al., 2017).

When a very young baby watches his mother's face, follows her voice with his eyes and responds to her with a smile—he is engaging in his first play transaction. These early interactions lead to the child's first games such as 'peek-a-boo'. These transactions between mother and child are important for the establishment of joint attention, which is the ability to focus and share attention on an object or event with at least one other person, and are critical to the development of attachment to the child's mother and significant others. These small but important play transactions are foundational to the development of current and future relationships.

In the first 12 months of life, from accidently bumping a toy suspended on a frame above a baby lying on a mat, to purposefully focusing on the toy, reaching out to hit it with one hand and eventually being able to grasp it with two hands, the child's play develops as his nervous system matures. Play skills emerge with the opportunity to lie, sit and then stand, while playing with a wide range of brightly coloured, often noisy, toys, which provide a variety of taste, touch, movement and other sensory experiences and opportunities for interaction with others.

In their second year, play becomes more physical as children learn to climb and run; they enjoy rough and tumble play, swings, slides and any movement through space. Children experience mastery of their environment as cognition, motor coordination and social skills develop. These skills are further enhanced through play as the child's nascent understanding of the world expands while exploring their environment. At this stage play is often alongside, or in parallel to, other children, but with limited interaction. Language and communication skills, together with the emergence of pretend and symbolic play, provide the means for the child to suspend reality. Children eagerly engage in constructing creative and imaginative games with pretend friends, imaginary characters and dress ups, and use everyday items in unconventional ways to replicate daily activity. Over time play becomes more associative, involving some sharing of items and ideas until the transaction evolves into cooperative play, where children interact with each other, share and build on each other's narrative, and play with a common focus and goal in mind.

Cooperative play emerges more fully by four to five years of age when children problem-solve, create scripts, begin to share ideas and take turns to understand rules and deal with winning and losing. Regulating emotions, dealing with frustrations and knowing how to initiate, respond and negotiate, become important elements of successful play in all the child's environments—home, child care, playgroups, kindergarten and in the community. Children begin to take risks and understand their physical limitations by learning to ride a bike or climb a tree, they can problem-solve when building a fortress out of blankets and pillows, and they learn empathy and negotiation when playing with friends and taking on others' ideas. Children often take pride in their role as player and being a teammate, but also have times where they might prefer to play alone.

Case study: James, five years of age

James is an active and sociable boy who likes to have friends over to play at his house. They play for hours in the backyard, building castles in the sandpit and climbing the apple tree where his dad has built him a cubbyhouse. The cubbyhouse stocks an array of treasures gathered during Viking raids of foreign lands. James and his best mate Johnno sail their langskip to conquer new territories and sail back on their knörr to hide their treasure. But perhaps James's favourite time of the day is early evenings when he gets to play Star Wars with his dad. He insists in taking on the character of Luke Skywalker. His dad takes on the character of Darth Vader and says in his deep baritone voice: 'Together we can rule the galaxy as father and son—hhhhhhhoooch whhhhhhhooo!' Sometimes the swordplay gets a bit out of hand, but James squeals with delight when he finally slays Darth Vader—and begs his dad to start the same pretend play sequence all over again.

James has also started participating in leisure activities and he is a team member of the local mini-soccer team. His coach recognises that James is cooperative in a team and that he is good at negotiating his needs. As a soccer player, he has learned how to be good at winning and losing—although he'd much rather win. At school he is often picked to join footy games at lunch break and he often gets invited to birthday parties.

By the time children start school, in Australia that is usually by six years of age, they have developed the fine motor skills, in-hand manipulation, eye–hand coordination and bilateral hand skills for construction, threading and tool use including cutting with scissors and drawing with pencils. Board games, team sports and more complex electronic games are all activities enjoyed by the older child and adolescent (Smet & Lucas, 2020).

More structured play activities share common attributes with competition and sport and in the early school years many children begin to engage in school sport teams or other team-based leisure activities, such as chess club, drama club or playing a musical instrument. These interests often form the foundation for lifelong leisure activities. Children's physical, cognitive and social skills continue to develop through mastery of the tasks required to play and engage with these activities. Of children under the age of 15 years in Australia, 63 per cent participated weekly in at least one out-of-school sporting or physical activity (Australian Sports Commission, 2019). The most popular sports for males are swimming, football (soccer) and Australian football, and for girls, swimming, dancing (recreational), netball and gymnastics. For Australian adolescents, leisure activities account for approximately 24 per cent of their time (Australian Bureau of Statistics, 2008), although their time spent engaging in sport and leisure activities is decreasing slowly over time and being traded for time spent working or screen time. Even though sport remains an important leisure occupation within the Australian context, it only accounts for about 12 hours a week on average for Australian adolescents. Engaging in passive leisure activities, such as watching TV and sedentary screen-based activities,only 1 in 5 (20 per cent) of adolescents aged 13–17 years were meeting the physical activity guidelines (Australian Institute of Health and Welfare, 2019). It is through informal leisure activities that adolescents participate in a social context where they form friendships and their first intimate relationships as they 'hang out', sit around, talk or listen to music. Online activities provide a social culture which also enables the development of friendships, but there is an increasing awareness of the influences of cyberbullying that requires parents to find a balance between monitoring online activity and allowing the child to manage their safety age appropriately (Child Family Community Australia, 2012).

Playing and engaging in leisure activities remain lifelong occupations, though they take on a different shape during adulthood. Adults become their children's first playmates and they continue to engage in both formal and informal leisure activities such as becoming a sports coach, playing for the masters hockey team, or joining the bowls club. Leisure for adults can still have elements of play, by engaging in activities in which one feels intrinsic motivation, internal control and freedom from constraints of reality. Being absorbed in these activities likely contributes to a sense of self-actualisation, which is the subjective nature of engagement in terms of productivity, pleasure and restoration (Bundy et al., 2018). Understanding the meaning of activity and the quality of engagement can give a clue to whether an activity is leisure.

Jonsson (2008) notes how in the absence of meaningful and highly engaging social occupations, described in terms of intensity and flow, activities such as reading or shopping can be interpreted as 'time-killing' to just pass the time and are seen as being of low significance for well-being. What is leisure for one person may be simply self-care or work for another. Engagement in valued leisure activities provides a sense of purpose, gives meaning and satisfaction to everyday life, and promotes a sense of belonging (Bundy et al., 2018). People develop an understanding of preferences and likes, of patterns of interacting, and build a connection through shared activity. The choice of leisure activities reflects one's personality and contributes to the formation of identity (Bundy et al., 2018). Leisure activities, 'doing together', can also be a way of developing and maintaining a relationship (Low, 2015). Leisure activities provide an outlet for the continued engagement in meaningful life activities which is especially important as older adults transition into retirement.

The health benefits of regular participation in leisure activities cannot be understated. Enhanced social contact, reduced risk of cognitive decline, enhanced quality of life and lower levels of depression are just some of the benefits for older adults. A group of Italian retirees in rural Australia (Pereira & Stagnitti, 2008) explained how their leisure, often revolving around a Bocce game, was intrinsically motivating and meaningful and was also reported to have health benefits. There is evidence that leisure activities can improve participation and increase psychological well-being of older people (Eakman et al., 2010). Leisure activities for older adults are limitless and may vary from active (e.g., gardening) to passive activities (e.g., reading books). Although older adults may spend significant proportions of their time on their own, a recent study highlighted that time alone can be a positive experience when the older adult has choice and control over how time is spent (Stanley et al., 2017).

Older people who experience frailty can encounter restriction in the amount and/or type of leisure activities that they can engage in. For example, driving cessation in later life can lead to restrictions in activities reliant on transportation (Liddle et al., 2012). Maximising opportunities for older adults to engage in meaningful leisure activities is seen as essential to their health and well-being. A number of government-based initiatives have been developed to promote continued engagement in leisure activities in later life, including Men's Sheds, which provide an environment for men to work on meaningful projects such as metal work or small joinery projects (Wilson & Cordier, 2013). This program provides older men with a choice of activities and allows for continued skill development, which are important motivators for participation.

Kubina et al. (2013) explored the experience of re-engaging in personally valued activities following a stroke. They found that key concepts that led to engagement were social connection and being in control (i.e., having a sense of internal control). Being in control may be deciding who and how much assistance is given, or being in control of what aspects the person would do or what would be an acceptable altered standard of performance. Important facilitators of participation were opportunities to problem-solve in context, getting buy-in from others, and support to take risks from significant others.

Intergenerational programs offer another mechanism for engaging older adults in leisure programs. A recent systematic review identified three models of intergenerational programs that bring together older adults and children (Radford et al., 2018). The first incorporates centre-based visits by child care services to aged care services, or vice versa; the second brings together child care and aged care services on a single site, allowing for shared service provision; and the third provides services to children and older adults in a residential home (Radford et al., 2018).

We all have a right to be active, and for some people with dementia they have much idle time and idle hands. Matching activity to preserved capacity and interest can transform even simple activities, such as small-number jigsaws or folding and sorting towels, into an engaging and absorbing task. A conversation with people with dementia and their families is the first step in identifying leisure pursuits (O'Connor et al., in press). Providing items that the person can see, touch and manipulate can elicit memories and an opportunity to reminisce. In addition to tapping into preferences, habits and roles, modifications to enhance engagement can encompass space demands such as lighting or ambient noise, social and communication modifications, such as specific praise, or perhaps limiting instructions or modifications related to issues of sequence and timing (Trahan et al., 2014).

Occupational therapists build on the strengths of an older person with dementia through matching activities and skills and harnessing habits to encourage participation. Incorporating families into activities, breaking down the task into achieveable componets and providing verbal cues and simple instructions are additional ways to enhance engagement in leisure activities for people with dementia (O'Connor et al., in press). For example, the Tailored Activity Program is a unique occupational therapy program, wherein the therapist identifies the preserved capabilities, deficit areas, and previous roles, habits and interests of the person with dementia and develops activity goals tailored to individual profiles. Family caregivers are then trained to set up and use activities and strategies to reduce task demands along with strategies in how to manage situational stresses (Gitlin et al., 2018). The program reduces behavioural symptoms, slows functional dependence and alleviates caregiver distress. A systematic review and meta-analyis provides clear evidence that occupational therapy services for people with dementia in the community should incorporate multiple components and be provided over multiple sessions (Bennett et al., 2019).

The role of occupational therapists when the occupations of play and leisure are disrupted

During early childhood, the role of the occupational therapist would be to work with parents to promote positive parent–child interactions. As the child matures and mobility increases, the occupational therapist increasingly focuses on developing the child's motor, social and cognitive skills required for play, and modifying the play environment to facilitate interaction and exploration. The occupational therapist also assists parents in understanding the importance of play and social interaction and on how they can develop the child's play skills. In early childhood and primary school age, the role of the occupational therapist shifts towards developing social play skills and facilitating the development of early friendships. In adolescence and adulthood and beyond, the occupational therapist focuses on facilitating participation in leisure activities as a means of enabling and maintaining social inclusion and participating in meaningful activities. This becomes particularly important as leisure time replaces salaried work activities in retirement, or when the older person is no longer able to participate in their previous leisure activities.

Personal self–care

Self-care and instrumental daily activities include occupations focused on caring for one's own body and on occupations required to manage one's home and community. Dressing is described in this chapter as one example of a daily self-care occupation that develops early in life, contributes to identity and remains important across the lifespan. Personal self-care occupations include toileting, dressing, hygiene, grooming, sleeping and feeding oneself (American Occupational Therapy Association, 2017). The ability to complete the required tasks and sequences is influenced by the child's personal attributes (e.g., perception, cognition, motor skills, motor planning and motivation) and by factors external to the child (Smet & Lucas, 2020). These external factors include the physical environment, cultural and family expectations, family routines, resources, opportunity and social expectations. From learning to lie still while a nappy is being changed to being able to assist at 12 to 18 months of age by putting out an arm or leg, the very young child becomes increasingly independent in dressing (Smet & Lucas, 2020). The pride evident in the two- to three-year-old who has dressed him or herself, even if the shirt is back-to-front or inside out and fastenings not completed, is evidence of the importance of these tasks—not just in developing independence, but in also contributing to a sense of achievement and self-efficacy.

Increasingly demanding tasks, such as lining up buttons and button holes and doing up and undoing buttons, joining the sides of a zipper on a jacket, reaching behind one's own back to tuck in clothing, and tying shoelaces, are all mastered by about seven years of age, resulting in the child being nearly independent in all aspects of dressing. In-hand manipulation, the ability to move or re-orientate small objects within the hand, develops considerably by about four years of age. It is the improved ability to isolate finger movement, oppose thumb to flexed fingers to hold and move objects, determine the correct force required to hold and move objects in the fingers and the ability to have a mobile radial side of the hand (thumb and index and middle finger) and a stable ulnar side of the hand that contributes to success in these tasks (Smet & Lucas, 2020). By the same age the development of a preferred and more skilled hand, and the ability to use both hands together with smooth coordinated movements in conjunction with visual and perceptual skills, also ensures success. These skills combine with the ability to motor plan (understand the requirements of the task and then plan, sequence and execute the steps of the task) and to problem-solve, to ensure children develop and maintain independence as their fashion choices begin to influence their clothing choices.

By the age of five to six years, children are able to remove and orient most clothing, put items in the correct order, e.g., underwear before pants, and do up and undo most fastenings (such as buttons, zippers and snaps). By this age children have the balance and fluidity of movements to dress independently, shift weight from one foot to the other without support or falling over as they dress the lower body. They also have the perceptual skills to identify items and orient them in relation to their own body and their fine motor skills become more refined (Shepherd & Ivey, 2020).

Dressing is no longer about how to get dressed and undressed for children in middle childhood, seven to 12 years of age and as they move into adolescence. At this stage the influence of family is superseded by the influence of peers who have more impact on the development of opinions and beliefs, and a sense of belonging and identity (Shepherd & Ivey, 2020). The young person's appearance and clothing choice become expressions of identity and belonging and are demonstrated by what they are wearing. In middle childhood and adolescence, young people spend most of their time in school or online with peers; dressing becomes more about what to wear, which in turn is strongly influenced by peers and what is deemed popular in media. Celebrities, their choice of fashion and their capacity to determine what is desirable in terms of body shape and appearance are major influences on adolescents and young adults. Such influence is not always positive and can create unrealistic beliefs about what one needs to be *normal* as fashion and appearance become the means of judging who you are and the worth of others.

This is often a time when new occupational roles develop, including becoming a secondary school student, being a team player in sporting activities, and art, music or drama activities that also influence their sense of identity and appearance. With adolescence and the development of secondary sexual characteristics and associated change of body shape, adolescence is a time of experimentation. Where mastery of and independence in tasks contributed to a young child's identity and self-esteem, identity at this age is often expressed as a statement through one's appearance. This can be about strict adherence to peer norms, or a statement to stand out and be individual, or an expression of sexual identity. Choice of clothing is complemented by the overall time spent on appearance with grooming, hair style, shaving, make-up and jewellery all adding to the time spent and the rituals of dressing in the teenage years. These choices are often strongly influenced by peers, and in recent years through the medium of social media.

Uniforms (in the forms of school uniforms and sports team uniforms) have often been the dress code imposed on school-aged children, with many finding ways to wear it to still express identity. Teenagers often have a great need for conformity, expressed in the latest fashions, but there are always some who adopt an alternate expression of dress that does not conform to fashion that is widely popular. Trends have included grunge, emo or hipster styles which all move away from mainstream fashion and are also associated with other lifestyle choices such as music, art and attitudes to consumerism and other mainstream views.

Case study: James, 20 years of age

His large plastic-rim glasses add the finishing touch to James's carefully *put-together look*. He has just spent the last 30 minutes dressing as if he didn't care—tight-fitting Levi jeans hugging his hips, check shirt and skinny, knitted cardigan, and worn classic Reeboks on his feet. With a last glance in the mirror, a tug at his forward fringe and running his hands through his short hair and beard on his face, James heads out the door to join his friends for dinner at their local wine bar that serves raw, organically sourced, vegan food.

With his favourite Indie rock band playing through the buds of his mobile phone in the pocket of his jeans, James's image is complete. At 20 years of age and in the second year of his arts degree, James's clothing and appearance identify him as the young, intellectual, politically progressive hipster who has rejected the popular fashions of the day. Without a label in sight it is not James who identifies himself a hipster—it's the tag given, sometimes derisively to reflect the subculture of independent thinkers quietly proud of being adopters of fashion that others will soon make their own.

For adults, fashion is often reflective of workplace, work role, income, culture and status. This expression of our identity continues through later life. Dressing is a valued occupation during adulthood and there are whole fashion and dressing accessory industries that are built on this valued occupation which often becomes intrinsically intertwined with identity and role. Adults are usually very adept in adjusting dress code from one occupational environment to the next. For some, the importance of individualism as expressed through dressing remains important, but perhaps now with greater sophistication.

Age-related physical and cognitive changes may affect older adults' ability to perform functional activities of self-care, such as dressing. Physical changes, such as arthritis, may limit one's fine motor skills, making it difficult to manipulate fastenings. Reduced flexibility, balance and strength may mean that older adults may need to sit to dress and take more time to dress (McIntyre, 2013). Cognitive changes, such as perceptual difficulties post-stroke, can lead to difficulties in planning and sequencing (Walker et al., 2012). For individuals residing at home, they may use compensatory strategies such as task modification and the use of equipment (e.g., shoe horn, sock gutter, dressing stick) or receive assistance from paid or informal services to complete activities of daily living such as dressing. For older adults admitted to hospital or residing in residential aged care facilities, the choice of clothing may be restricted. Enhancing choice in an activity such as dressing provides one with the ability to express oneself and promote independence from others. For most people, dressing remains an important occupation, reflective of independence and an expression of identity.

An aspect of self-care often neglected in occupational therapy practice is sexuality. For example, adults and older adults post-stroke, and their partners, often experience disruption to their sexuality due to physical and cognitive changes. Indeed, the development and expression of sexuality is key to all adults, their relationships and quality of life, and should be addressed in occupational therapy assessment and intervention (McRae, 2013). Therapists need to be aware of and reflect on their own views on ageing and sexuality, and on ageism more broadly. Davys (2008) explored perspectives of occupational therapists and students on attitudes toward ageing. She reported on the impact it can have on an occupational therapist's ability to involve older persons in program planning, evaluation and decision-making in a truly meaningful manner. Various approaches to reflexivity are proposed as a way to assist health care professionals and students, to better work with older adults and to make sense of their own learning processes within today's ageist society (Flores-Sandoval & Kinsella, 2020).

Occupational therapists also introduce or promote activities that focus on engagement in meaningful activities and facilitate those activities that maintain or improve functional outcomes. Through engagement, older adults enhance independence and maintain connections with community. The innovative LiFE program is an example of how to enhance functional outcomes and engagement through embedding balance and lower limb strength into habitual daily routines and activities (Clemson et al., 2014). This particular program takes on a unique occupational therapy perspective on improving strength and balance through occupations. Emerging trials are exploring the enhanced benefit of occupational therapists delivering a combined LiFE program with home safety or home modifications (e.g. Szanton et al., 2020).

The role of occupational therapists when self-care occupations are disrupted

The role of occupational therapists in developing the skills involved in dressing emerges when children are about two to three years of age. At this stage, the occupational therapist works closely with the carer to guide them in problem-solving and developing strategies to enable greater independence and participation in dressing. As the child matures physically and cognitively, the emphasis shifts towards modification of the task and the environment to facilitate independence in dressing. For those children with disabilities the emphasis shifts towards using compensatory techniques for dressing (e.g., teaching the child one-handed dressing techniques or using clothing that has Velcro fasteners). Another strategy is to modify the environment, so the individual is able to complete a task successfully. This role continues into late adulthood and may involve working with carers and support staff to maximise an individual's ability to participate in the task while also providing the assistance required.

Case study: James, 40 years of age

James and his wife Angela have two young children, Isabella (six) and Oliver (four). James is a doting dad, coaching his daughter's soccer team and taking Oliver to swimming lessons. James is also a carer for his elderly parents who live in the next suburb. James's Dad is a retired mechanic who has osteoarthritis and congestive heart failure and James's mum has type II diabetes mellitus. James supports his parents, tending to their lawn and garden maintenance once a fortnight and taking his mother and father to medical appointments as well as the local shops. James juggles these caring responsibilities with his full-time accountant role, a Dad of two children, and a husband.

Study and work

In Australia, child care centres and kindergartens are the first formal education settings with all children funded to attend kindergarten for between ten and 15 hours each week in the year prior to starting school, and some states are extending this program to children from the age of three years. The Early Years Learning Framework (Council of Australian Governments, 2009) is a government-funded initiative ensuring a play-based curriculum. It was designed to support the development of language and communication skills, early literacy and numeracy skills, and social and emotional development for children nought to five years in care and education settings. Children participate in activities to develop their play, communication and social skills, independence in self-care and looking after one's self and belongings (Council of Australian Governments, 2009).

The pre-school settings provide opportunities for learning across the day, including: counting, recognising colours and shapes, categorising items, picking up a book and understanding the words are connected to the pictures, starting to recognise and form numbers and letters, and writing their name on a drawing. Additionally, children are provided with the opportunity to learn school-related occupations such as the skills and behaviours of belonging to a group, sitting still, learning routines and rules such as being quiet when the teacher or others are speaking, putting their hand up to answer or ask questions, caring for and respecting others, and transitioning between activities. Experiences of shared meaning sustain occupations in new situations that challenge skills and require subtle adjustments in performance strategies (Humphry & Womak, 2019).

Children enter pre-primary the following year, and in Australia they must commence school by six years of age. Being a student involves participation in the roles of being a player, friend and learner. Children at school participate in activities as a school and class group, in small groups in the classroom setting and as friends in the playground and as an individual. Young children often participate in activities at *mat* or *circle* time and in table-top and out-of-class opportunities. Children need to learn to be listeners and doers and to work independently and cooperatively. From an early focus on learning to read and write, count and use numbers, children also learn about the world and their role as good citizens (Smet & Lucas, 2020).

Formal learning is structured based on key learning areas in the curriculum which increase in content and difficulty over time. Transitions create the need for new occupations as life circumstances change (Humphry & Womak, 2019). While the curriculum remains broad, as the child moves through secondary school, Years 7–12, they start to become selective in areas of study with a focus on what is needed and what 'they might do' once they leave school. During the school years, a child's engagement with learning occupations matures through various skill development and task mastery. In fact, experiencing a sense of mastery is one of the main drivers of development (Miller et al., 2015). Basic mathematical understanding develops into algebra, which contributes to later chemistry lessons. Spelling and grammar form the foundation for later essay structure, debate and creative thinking. School work and learning also happens after school hours, with increasing homework demands as children progress through their schooling years (Smet & Lucas, 2020).

School years are not just about school and study—these need to compete with the demands of leisure activities including sport, spending time with friends and even sleeping. Early rest and sleep routines are initially established and maintained by a caregiver. Rest and sleep become more independent and self-regulated as children mature. There is a bi-directional relationship between rest and sleep patterns and ADL performance. For example, rest and sleep occupational patterns often affect ADL performance, and ADL routines and patterns can impact rest and sleep, such as bath time influencing sleep onset and vice versa (Shepherd & Ivey, 2020).

Paid and unpaid work, as well as study, contribute to healthy development and assist with transitions from childhood to adolescence to adulthood. In school and work settings there are opportunities to interact with peers and other generations, to learn social behaviours, develop responsibility and shape individual values that guide later decision-making.

Many students begin their first paid casual employment during their senior years at school. In Australia, many get their first job at Maccas, Subway, Bunnings or Woolies, where they develop vocational skills such as taking orders, customer service and punctuality; but also softer vocational skills such as engaging with fellow workers and being collegial. Paid employment develops life skills, outside of those required for the specific job task. These include, but are not limited to, financial management, administrative management of accounts and paper work, establishing routines by organising time and commitments, using public transport and negotiating expectations and relationships with other people (Cleary & Persch, 2020).

After completing secondary school, many young adults choose to continue in their role as a student by enrolling in a university, polytechnic or a TAFE (Technical and Further Education) institute, or by completing an apprenticeship at a local college. Others enter the formal job market directly from high school. Economic independence is a cornerstone for moving away from dependence on parents and family for young adults, regardless of circumstances, and is an important milestone in assuming adult responsibilities. Choosing a particular career or job contributes to a sense of identity and promotes self-esteem. Many young adults also have their first experience of being a volunteer at a local charity or sports club.

Work is arguably the main occupation during adulthood, particularly during midlife (Australian Bureau of Statistics, 2017). Many adults are career-focused and spend most of their waking hours in formal employment and/or informal work such as engaging in child-rearing activities. For many adults, their work gives meaning to their lives and often their sense of identity is intertwined with their work. Adults start to plan for their futures post-retirement with particular emphasis on financial management, such as paying off the mortgage on their home and making payments into their superannuation.

Some adults adopt not only a caring role for their children, but also for elderly parents. Referred to as the sandwich generation, adults juggle the demands and role of parenthood with caregiving for older adults (Evans et al., 2016; Spann et al., 2020). Occupational therapists can support adults to utilise strategies such as nurturing social connections to help stabilise and manage role balance. Retirement is characterised with changing time structure. For some, a move from full-time to part-time hours helps lengthen their working career and prepares older workers for the move to retirement. As the transition moves forward, the structure of paid work is replaced with a slower pace and the ability for an older adult to have more choice over what activities they engage in (Pepin & Deutscher, 2011). Weekdays become filled with domestic duties, social engagement and participating in personally motivated activities, with weekends focused on relaxation and rest or looking after grandchildren while their parents work.

In the early stages of retirement, a honeymoon phase is often experienced. Early stages of retirement may be experienced as a 'holiday' (Jonsson et al., 2001). As this period ends there may be a sense of loss regarding the worker role (e.g., loss of social status and financial independence) and adjustment to newly established routines, life roles and activities (Pettican & Prior, 2011).

Case study: James, 65 years of age

James has been an accountant for 40 years and has made the decision with his wife Angela to retire in the coming year. James is looking to sell his share of an accountancy business to his business partner, Michael. James built the business after four years at university and interning in high-profile agencies in the city for another four years. James fondly remembers the highs and lows of running his business. He is looking forward to a long holiday in Europe with Angela once he retires. They have planned a 15-week adventure through Italy, France and Portugal that will allow them to leisurely explore the beautiful surrounds.

James has also organised to become involved in the local volunteer marine rescue team when he returns from his trip. James has recently been acting as the finance manager for the marine rescue board and hopes to become part of the rescue team. James has also offered to stay involved in his accountancy company through contract work at peak times, although James feels 'funny' about going back to the business he created as an employee and not a leader. The change of life roles is challenging but also less stressful. James also promised Angela that he would be more involved in family activities, especially with looking after the grandchildren.

Literature has identified that choice and freedom over how and when activities are completed is valued by older adults; however, the structure and commitments that are often associated with paid work are frequently missed. Volunteering activities may offer further structure and commitment for older adults and provide opportunities to actively engage in, and give back to, the community (Milbourn et al., 2018).

Helping and giving to others is highly valued as a meaningful activity for older people. Volunteering provides an opportunity for older adults to contribute, give back to their society and feel valued, and has shown to contribute to one's overall health and well-being. Older adults will often assume the role of a carer for a partner or a family member. The role of caring and how to care should form part of the occupational therapy assessment. The Care of People with Dementia in their Environments (COPE) is an example of how carers are integrated into occupational therapy interventions. Eight to ten occupational therapy consultations along with two nursing interventions are provided; all of which focus on the capabilities of the persons with dementia and include the care partner fully in the process (Clemson et al., 2018).

Even in residential care where residents are limited in what they can do for themselves, they can find a sense of well-being and accomplishment helping others and staying socially connected with their community (O'Rourke & Sidani, 2017). The principle of reciprocity describes how people report a greater sense of well-being if they also feel rewarded for their participation (Stephens et al., 2015).

Case study: James, 85 years of age

James cared for his wife Angela in the last decade of her life as she became blind and her dementia became severe. James is now in residential care since Angela passed away. His children all have busy lives so he 'cares' for the residential care staff, listening to all their concerns and their family ups and downs. In an ever-diminishing world he still walks with his walking frame to the dining room early to set up the table—Harold has two sugars ready in his cup, Mavis needs her cutlery in a certain order as her sight is failing, and Beryl needs her chair positioned so she can get in easily. James also goes to the front desk of the residential care facility each day to pick up the daily newspaper and delivers it to his two neighbours who have rooms next to him.

James spends most of his afternoons pottering in the recreation room, often reading and enjoying the sunshine streaming through the bay windows. Each Thursday James will set up the draughts board for a game with fellow resident, Merv. Their games are often forgotten as they both share stories about their time with the marine rescue team. James enjoys reliving his time with the team and often reminisces about jobs he did in the past, thinking of different ways things could have been done or his ability to get the clunky radio system to work when nobody else could. James is still in contact with the team, albeit once a year through their annual gala dinner. James also enjoys weekly visits from the local pre-school as part of an intergenerational program where James plays and reads to children. These meaningful activities, along with his caring role, provide a link to his past and are important to sustain him and maintain his self-identity.

Older volunteers are more likely to be from higher socio-economic status, those in good health, and those with easily accessible transport. In promoting volunteering opportunities, consideration must be given as to how to engage older volunteers. Failure to engage in volunteer activities may reinforce the inability to live up to social norms of reciprocity and may further exclude the older adult from their communities (Stephens et al., 2015). People with poor health, those who have a disability, poor access to transport or have reduced financial means are less likely to engage in volunteering activities, despite their potential for volunteering when matched to skill and capacity, as a meaningful and rewarding activity.

A balance of hours is needed to provide older adults with opportunities to engage without causing too much stress and demand (Jonsson et al., 2001). Through volunteering older adults are able to remain physically active and maintain skills (e.g., continuing wood lathing through participation in the Men's Shed) and give back to the community (e.g., fundraising). Volunteering can also provide a means for social interaction and further leisure opportunities.

The role of occupational therapists when productive occupations such as study and work are disrupted

Occupational therapists often work with children to help develop school readiness skills, including learning to participate in a group, looking after their belongings, managing their emotions and following directions. The occupational therapist also assists in developing pre-academic and school-related occupations, such as handwriting, task completion and more complex group skills (e.g., negotiating and dealing with competition); these supports may continue into early adolescence. Occupational therapists also work with children in school settings to ensure they have the necessary skills and supports to access all school activities and are able to participate in the curriculum. This may involve the use of technology and modification to the school or classroom environment. During adolescence, the emphasis shifts towards facilitating social participation, developing pre-vocational skills and transitioning from school to a work or educational setting. In post-school years, the occupational therapist's role involves providing support to young people in the work or educational setting and advocating for the young person's social inclusion. In adulthood, the occupational therapist may be involved in aspects such as rehabilitation to facilitate clients' return to work following injury and/or illness. In late adult life, the occupational therapist focuses on retaining independence, and enabling clients to participate in meaningful activities post-retirement through socialisation, leisure activities and community engagement.

Conclusion

This chapter focused on how occupations and associated occupational roles and identities evolve across the lifespan. The case studies of James illuminated how the occupations of play and leisure, dressing, and school and work change across the lifespan. James's occupational roles changed from being a player to being a student, an accountant, a volunteer and a retiree. Some of these roles gained greater prominence during different developmental stages and changed in relative importance and value. Similarly, associated occupational identities evolved, all intimately associated with a person's sense of belonging, health and well-being. Even though we used the occupations of play/leisure, personal self-care, study and work to exemplify how occupations evolve across the lifespan, the same principles can be applied to most occupations.

Summary

- Occupations contribute to our development, roles and identity at all ages.
- The type and meaning of occupations of play and leisure, rest and sleep, personal self-care, social participation, and study and work develop and evolve across our lifespan.
- Transitions to new occupational roles enable the development of new skills.
- Engaging in occupations of personal value and choice contributes to health and well-being.

Review questions

1. How does the concept of play and leisure change throughout the lifespan?
2. How do a person's unique characteristics influence the development of occupations?
3. What is the significance of clothing choice and the ability to dress oneself for a child, adolescent and older adult?
4. Describe how transitions to new occupational roles contribute towards the development of new skills.
5. Identify and explain barriers and enablers of transitioning to retirement from an occupation-focused perspective.

References

American Occupational Therapy Association. (2017). Occupational Therapy Practice Framework: Domain and Process, 3rd edition. *American Journal of Occupational Therapy, 68*(Supp. 1), S1–S48. https://doi.org/10.5014/ajot.2014.682006

Australian Bureau of Statistics. (2008). *How Australians use their time, 2006* (Catalogue number 4153.0). https://www.abs.gov.au/ausstats/abs@.nsf/mf/4153.0

Australian Bureau of Statistics. (2017). *Census of population and housing: Reflecting Australia—stories from the Census, 2016*. Cat. no. 2071.0. https://www.abs.gov.au/ausstats/abs@.nsf/mf/2071.0

Australian Institute of Health and Welfare. (2019). *Insufficient physical activity*. https://www.aihw.gov.au/reports/risk-factors/insufficient-physical-activity/contents/physical-inactivity

Australian Sports Commission. (2019). *Annual report 2018–2019*. https://www.sportaus.gov.au/__data/assets/pdf_file/0007/716119/ASC-Annual-Report-20182019.pdf

Bennett, S., Laver, K., Voigt-Radloff, S., Letts, L., Clemson, L., Graff, M., Wiseman, J., & Gitlin, L. (2019). Occupational therapy for people with dementia and their family carers provided at home: A systematic review and meta-analysis. *BMJ Open, 9*(11), e026308. https://doi.org/10.1136/bmjopen-2018-026308

Bundy, A. C., & Du Toit, S. H. J. (2019). Play and leisure. In B. A. Boyt Schell & G. Gillen (Eds.), *Willard & Spackman's occupational therapy* (13th edn, pp. 805–827). Wolter Kluwer.

Bundy, A., Du Toit, S., & Clemson, L. (2018). Leisure. In B. R. Bonder (Ed.), *Functional performance in older adults* (4th edn, pp. 805–827). F. A. Davis Co.

Bundy, A., Engelen, L., Wyver, S., Tranter, P., Ragen, J., Bauman, A., Baur, L., Schiller, W., Simpson, J. M., Niehues, A. N., Perry, G., Jessup, G., & Naughton, G. (2017). Sydney playground project: A cluster-randomized trial to increase physical activity, play, and social skills. *Journal of School Health, 87*(10), 751–759. https://doi.org/10.1111/josh.12550

Child Family Community Australia. (2012). *Parental involvement in preventing and responding to cyberbullying*. Paper No. 4. Australian Institute of Family Studies. https://aifs.gov.au/cfca/publications/parental-involvement-preventing-and-responding-cyberbullying

Cleary, D., & Persch, A. (2020). Transition services. In J. O'Brien & H. Kuhaneck (Eds.), *Case-Smith's occupational therapy for children and adolescents* (8th edn, pp. 659–679). Elsevier.

Clemson, L., Laver, K., Jeon, Y. H., Comans, T. A., Scanlan, J., Rahja, M., Culph, J., Low, L-F., Day, S., Cations, M., Crotty, M., Kurrle, S., Piersol, C., & Gitlin, L. N. (2018). Implementation of an evidence-based intervention to improve the wellbeing of people with dementia and their carers: Study protocol for 'Care of People with dementia in their Environments (COPE)' in the Australian context. *BMC Geriatrics, 18*(1), 108. https://doi.org/10.1186/s12877-018-0790-7

Clemson, L., Munro, J., & Singh, M. A. F. (2014). *Lifestyle-integrated Functional Exercise (LiFE) program to prevent falls: Trainer's manual*. Sydney University Press.

Cordier, R., & Bundy, A. (2009). Children and playfulness. In K. Stagnitti & R. Cooper (Eds.), *Play as therapy: Assessment and therapeutic interventions* (pp. 45–58). Jessica Kingsley Publishers.

Council of Australian Governments. (2009). *The early years learning framework for Australia*. Commonwealth of Australia.

Cronin, A. C., & Mandich, M. B. (2016). *Human development and performance throughout the lifespan* (2nd edn). Cengage Learning.

Davys, D. (2008). Ageism within occupational therapy? *British Journal of Occupational Therapy*, *71*(2), 72–74. https://doi.org/10.1177/030802260807100207

Eakman, A. M., Carlson, M. E., & Clark, F. A. (2010). The Meaningful Activity Participation Assessment: A measure of engagement in personally valued activities. *International Journal of Aging and Human Development*, *70*(4), 299–317. https://doi.org/10.2190/AG.70.4.b

Evans, K. L., Millsteed, J., Richmond, J. E., Falkmer, M., Falkmer, T., & Girdler, S. J. (2016). Working sandwich generation women utilize strategies within and between roles to achieve role balance. *PloS one*, *11*(6), e0157469–e0157469. https://doi.org/10.1371/journal.pone.0157469

Flores-Sandoval, C., & Kinsella, E. A. (2020). Overcoming ageism: Critical reflexivity for gerontology practice. *Educational Gerontology*, *46*(4), 223–234. https://doi.org/10.1080/03601277.2020.1726643

Gitlin, L. N., Arthur, P., Piersol, C., Hessels, V., Wu, S. S., Dai, Y., & Mann, W. C. (2018). Targeting behavioral symptoms and functional decline in dementia: A randomized clinical trial. *Journal of the American Geriatrics Society*, *66*(2), 339–345. https://doi.org/10.1111/jgs.15194

Humphry, R., & Womak, J. (2019). Transformation of occupation: A life course perspective. In B. A. Boyt Schell & G. Gillen (Eds.), *Willard & Spackman's occupational therapy* (13th edn, pp. 100–112). Wolter Kluwer.

Jonsson, H. (2008). A new direction in the conceptualization and categorization of occupation. *Journal of Occupational Science*, *1*(1), 3–8. https://doi.org/10.1080/14427591.2008.9686601

Jonsson, H., Josephsson, S., & Kielhofner, G. (2001). Narratives and experience in an occupational transition: A longitudinal study of the retirement process. *American Journal of Occupational Therapy*, *55*(4), 424–432. https://doi.org/10.5014/ajot.55.4.424

Källdalen, A., Marcusson, J., & Wressle, E. (2013). Interests among older people in relation to gender, function and health-related quality of life. *British Journal of Occupational Therapy*, *76*(2), 87–93. https://doi.org/10.4276/030802213X13603244419239

Kubina, L. A., Dubouloz, C. J., Davis, C. G., Kessler, D., & Egan, M. Y. (2013). The process of re-engagement in personally valued activities during the two years following stroke. *Disability and Rehabilitation*, *35*(3), 236–243. https://doi.org/10.3109/09638288.2012.691936

Liddle, J., Gustafsson, L, Bartlett, H., & McKenna, K. (2012). Time use, role participation and life satisfaction of older people: Impact of driving status. *Australian Occupational Therapy Journal*, *59*(5), 384–392. https://doi.org/10.1111/j.1440-1630.2011.00956.x

Low, L. F. (2015). *Live and laugh with dementia: The essential guide to maximizing quality of life*. Exisle Publishing.

McIntyre, A. (2013). Occupation and successful ageing—activity and participation. In A. Atwal & A. McIntyre (Eds.), *Occupational therapy and older people* (2nd edn, pp. 185—223). John Wiley and Sons.

McRae, N. (2013). *Sexuality and the role of occupational therapy*. https://www.aota.org/About-Occupational-Therapy/Professionals/RDP/Sexuality.aspx

Milbourn, B., Saraswati, J., & Buchanan, A. (2018). The relationship between time spent in volunteering activities and quality of life in adults over the age of 50 years: A systematic review. *British Journal of Occupational Therapy*, *81*(11), 613–623. https://doi.org/10.1177/0308022618777219

Miller, L., Ziviani, J., Ware, R., & Boyd, R. (2015). Mastery motivation: A way of understanding therapy outcomes for children with unilateral cerebral palsy. *Disability and Rehabilitation*, *37*(16), 1439–1445. https://doi.org/10.3109/09638288.2014.964375

O'Connor, C. M., Clemson, L., & Wesson, J. G. (in press). Active and engaged: Maintaining leisure activities in dementia. In L.-F. Low & K. Laver (Eds.), *Rehabilitation for dementia: A resource for health professionals, service planners and researchers*. Elsevier.

O'Rourke, H., & Sidani, S. (2017). Definition, determinants, and outcomes of social connectedness for older adults: A scoping review. *Journal of Gerontological Nursing, 43*(7), 43–52. https://doi.org/10.3928/00989134-20170223-03

Pepin, G., & Deutscher, B. (2011). The lived experience of Australian retirees: 'I'm retired, what do I do now?' *British Journal of Occupational Therapy, 74*(9), 419–426. https://doi.org/10.4276/030802211x13153015305556

Pereira, R. B., & Stagnitti, K. (2008). The meaning of leisure for well-elderly Italians in an Australian community: Implications for occupational therapy. *Australian Occupational Therapy Journal, 55*(1), 39–46. https://doi.org/10.1111/j.1440-1630.2006.00653.x

Pettican, A., & Prior, S. (2011). It's a new way of life: An exploration of the occupational transition of retirement. *British Journal of Occupational Therapy, 74*(1), 12–19. https://doi.org/10.4276/030802211X12947686093521

Radford, K., Gould, R., Vecchio, N., & Fitzgerald, A. (2018). Unpacking intergenerational (IG) programs for policy implications: A systematic review of the literature. *Journal of Intergenerational Relationships, 16*(3), 302–329. https://doi.org/10.1080/15350770.2018.1477650

Rodger, S., & Kennedy-Behr, A. (2017). *Occupation-centred practice with children: A practical guide for occupational therapists* (2nd edn). Wiley-Blackwell.

Shepherd, J., & Ivey, C. (2020). Assessment and treatment of activities of daily living, sleep, rest, and sexuality. In J. O'Brien & H. Kuhaneck (Eds.), *Case-Smith's occupational therapy for children and adolescents* (8th edn, pp. 267–314). Elsevier.

Smet, N., & Lucas, C. B. (2020). Occupational therapy view of child development. In J. O'Brien & H. Kuhaneck (Eds.), *Case-Smith's occupational therapy for children and adolescents* (8th edn, pp. 76–121). Elsevier.

Spann, A., Vicente, J., Allard, C., Hawley, M., Spreeuwenberg, M., & de Witte, L. (2020). Challenges of combining work and unpaid care, and solutions: A scoping review. *Health & Social Care in the Community, 28*(3), 699–715. https://doi.org/10.1111/hsc.12912

Stanley, M., Richard, A., & Williams, S. (2017). Older peoples' perspectives on time spent alone. *Australian Occupational Therapy Journal, 64*(3), 235–242. https://doi.org/10.1111/1440-1630.12353

Stephens, C., Breheny, M., & Mansvelt, J. (2015). Volunteering as reciprocity: Beneficial and harmful effects of social participation to encourage contribution in older age. *Journal of Aging Studies, 33*, 22–27. https://doi.org/10.1016/j.jaging.2015.02.003

Szanton, S. L., Clemson, L., Liu, M., Gitlin, L. N., Hladek, M. D., LaFave, S. E., Roth, D. L., Marx, K. A., Felix, C., Okoye, S. M., Zhang, X., Bautista, S., & Granbom, M. (2020). Pilot outcomes of a multicomponent fall risk program integrated into daily lives of community-dwelling older adults. *Journal of Applied Gerontology,* 733464820912664. https://doi.org/10.1177/0733464820912664

Trahan, M. A., Kuo, J., Carlson, M. C., & Gitlin, L. N. (2014). A systematic review of strategies to foster activity engagement in persons with dementia. *Health Education & Behavior, 41*(1 Suppl.), 70S–83S. https://doi.org/10.1177/1090198114531782

Walker, M. F., Sunderland, A., Fletcher-Smith, J., Drummond, A., Logan, P., Edmans, J. A., Garvey, K., Dineen, R. A., Ince, P., Horne, J., Fisher, R. J., & Taylor, J. L. (2012). The DRESS trial: A feasibility randomized controlled trial of a neuropsychological approach to dressing therapy for stroke inpatients. *Clinical Rehabilitation, 26*(8), 675–685. https://doi.org/10.1177/0269215511431089

Wilson, N., & Cordier, R. (2013). A narrative review of Men's Sheds literature: Reducing social isolation and promoting men's health and wellbeing. *Health & Social Care in the Community, 21*(5), 451–463. https://doi.org/10.1111/hsc.12019

23 Occupational therapy practice contexts

Annette Joosten, Susan Darzins, Geneviève Pépin, Natalie Roche, Liana Cahill and Rosamund Harrington

Chapter objectives

Upon completion of this chapter, the reader will be able to:

- Describe the client groups occupational therapists work with and the role of the occupational therapist in six practice contexts.
- Recognise that legislation and regulations affect access to, and provision of, occupational therapy services.
- Discuss a person-centred approach to working with clients on their prioritised occupational goals and potential outcomes across a range of practice contexts.

Key terms

practice contexts; care continuum; community-based services/primary care; hospitals; workplaces; schools; residential aged care facilities; vocational rehabilitation; neurological rehabilitation, occupational therapy services

Introduction

Occupational therapists work with people and communities to enable people's performance and participation in the occupations they want, need or have to do in their life (World Federation of Occupational Therapists [WFOT], 2012). Occupational therapists develop an understanding of people's life situations, experiences and priorities, and analyse the interaction between people and their environments. Consequently, occupational performance and participation may be enabled by acting on and facilitating change at the level of the person, the environment or the occupation (Turpin & Iwama, 2011). The context within which occupational therapy services are provided has a substantial impact on the extent, emphasis and even availability of occupational therapy.

Legislation and policy influences practice

Occupational therapists must have a strong working knowledge of laws and regulations relevant to their practice area, as national and state legislation and regulations influence service provision. For example, occupational therapists working in schools should be familiar with the Salamanca Statement and Framework for Action on Special Needs Education (United Nations Educational, Scientific and Cultural Organization [UNESCO],

1994) and the Disability Standards for Education (Commonwealth Government of Australia, 2006). Occupational therapists working in disability services should be familiar with the National Disability Insurance Scheme (NDIS) (National Disability Insurance Agency [NDIA], 2014) and the *Disability Discrimination Act 1992* (Commonwealth Government of Australia, 1992). The NDIS was rolled out in July 2016 and has changed service delivery in the disability sector. Based on insurance principles, NDIS takes a lifetime approach and aims to provide eligible participants with the necessary and reasonable supports to participate in mainstream services in their local environments (NDIA, 2014). NDIS is a system that offers participants choice and control over the services they receive.

Occupational therapists working in vocational rehabilitation need to be familiar with their own state or territory laws as they do differ between jurisdictions. Information about the relevant laws in each jurisdiction is available on the Australian Government's Safe Work Australia website (Safe Work Australia, 2019). These laws influence the type of services available to clients and how they are provided by occupational therapists. Occupational therapists working with elderly people should be aware of the Australian Government's Living Longer Living Better aged care reform and the subsequent amendments to the *Aged Care Act 1997* (Commonwealth Government of Australia, 2014; 2015a). The Australian Government's Aged Care Quality and Safety Commission website (Commonwealth of Australia, 2020a) and the My Aged Care website (Commonwealth of Australia, 2020b) provide online access to information about aged care services in Australia and outline obligations and responsibilities of aged care providers for services with older adults.

Occupational therapists working in mental health should be familiar with the Fifth National Mental Health and Suicide Prevention Plan (Council of Australian Governments [COAG], 2017) and be aware of the National Review of Mental Health Programmes and Services conducted by the National Mental Health Commission (NMHC, 2014). Other state legislation exists, such as the *Victoria Mental Health Act* 2014 (Victoria Government, 2014) which aims to put people with mental illness at the centre of the decision-making processes, to determine safeguards, and to protect the rights, dignity and autonomy of people with a mental illness.

Working solo or in teams

Across the range of practice settings, occupational therapists may work as the only therapist or allied health professional or as part of a larger team. They may also receive referrals from, or refer to, other health professionals. Different models of teamwork exist across different work settings. Bell et al. (2009) described the identifying features of different teams, which are discussed below.

Multidisciplinary teams involve a separate but complementary professional relationship between team members that results in discipline-specific assessment and intervention, although team members collaborate and communicate to share client information on common aims. For example, in hospital settings occupational therapists often work in a multidisciplinary team led by a paediatrician, geriatrician, psychiatrist or rehabilitation consultant. Team members may include other medical practitioners and specialists, nurses, physiotherapists, social workers, speech pathologists and others.

Interdisciplinary teams involve the client and all team members in decision-making processes. Together, team members work collaboratively to set common goals and each team member continues to provide discipline-specific care for the client to achieve their overall goal(s). Team members will communicate frequently and may also work alongside each other with the client.

Transdisciplinary teams, sometimes called inter-professional teams, involve members sharing their expertise to the extent that professionals do not work within their discipline-specific roles. In these teams, professionals have ongoing communication and each needs to be aware of the specific skills of other team members. They need to be able to carry out interventions that cross discipline boundaries. Assessment is often carried out by one professional, commonly known as a client's case manager or key worker. This person may be the only, or main, professional with direct contact with the client.

Influences on occupational therapy services

Policy and government-led priorities influence workplaces and services within which occupational therapists provide occupational therapy services. Occupational therapy service delivery is different across nearly every context: between organisations, and within and between each state and territory in Australia. Three examples are provided here.

The first example is occupational therapists working with older adults. The central focus of the occupational therapy role working in hospitals is in supporting older people to remain, or return to, living in the community, particularly following an injury or illness. Geriatric Medicine Units and Transition Care Programs (TCP) are two types of specialised sub-acute care service teams (which include occupational therapists) that focus on assessment, intervention, discharge planning and case management of older people's health and care needs. Government funding and policies determine the frequency, duration and types of services that can be delivered in each jurisdiction. For example, occupational therapists may work in Aged Care Assessment Teams (ACAT), or Aged Care Assessment Services (ACAS), conducting assessments to determine a person's eligibility for government aged care services such as a home care packages, respite care, entry into a TCP or residential aged care facility (Commonwealth of Australia, 2020a).

In another example, occupational therapists who work with children may work in the child's home, childcare settings, kindergarten, in schools or in early intervention services and may work on their own in private practice. Services may be delivered through not-for-profit, non-government agencies or through state or federal government services. Early intervention for children is typically provided by multidisciplinary or transdisciplinary or inter-professional teams including the occupational therapist, physiotherapist, speech pathologist, psychologist and early educators. Funding policies, available resources and context determine the model of service delivery. For example, NDIS guidelines and the funding received from NDIS will determine how and where the child's individual care plan will be implemented and the supports and services that the occupational therapist can provide (NDIA, 2014).

The third practice context example is mental health settings, where occupational therapists often work in transdisciplinary teams. Whether they practise alone or within a team, occupational therapists also work closely with other people important to the client's context. In this role they aim to create opportunities in the person's environment/community that promote well-being and occupational engagement while limiting barriers to engagement and participation. In mental health settings occupational therapists frequently work alongside consumer consultants and carers in line with recommendations from the Fifth National Mental Health and Suicide Prevention Plan (COAG, 2017).

Family, person-centred and consumer-directed care

The context in which occupational therapists practise also determines the overall approach to service delivery. When working with children occupational therapists use a family-centred framework to meet the child and the family's needs. Family-centeredness refers to a combination of beliefs and practices that define the ways of working with families that are consumer driven and competency enhancing (Rosenbaum et al., 1998). This framework recognises that parents/caregivers are the constant in the child's life and have valuable insights into their child's abilities, likes and needs. This approach is both enabling and empowering for families and health care workers (Rosenbaum et al., 1998).

Occupational therapists working with adults provide person-centred intervention plans, programs and services developed with the client and their family, with consideration also given to their environment and community. Person-centred care is based on understanding and respecting what is important to the person, their families and communities and is achieved by working together to share decisions and decide the care plan (Australian Commission on Safety and Quality in Health Care, 2018). Occupational therapists working in mental health and aged care need to understand how the environment affects occupational performance. They also need an understanding of specific strategies and reforms in this area that support using a client-centred approach such as the National Review of Mental Health Programmes and Services (by the NMHC) (Commonwealth Government of Australia, 2015b) and the Australian Government's Living Longer Living Better aged care reform, which was founded on the principle of consumer-directed care (Australian Institute of Health and Welfare [AIHW], 2013). Consumer-directed care extends person-centred care and refers to the person receiving care being the chief decision-maker and director of their plan and is currently available for all Home Care Packages (Australian Government, 2019).

Practice contexts

An overview of the occupational therapy role across six practice contexts is provided in this section, with each one illustrated by a case study.

Children in early intervention

Participation in occupations can be restricted when external risk factors such as poverty, neglect, parental mental health or cognitive status, abuse, war and other world events interfere with typical development. Internal risk factors related to the child's physical and mental health and development and genetic factors, or chronic illness can also reduce the child's participation. Children might have a developmental delay in one area: cognition, social, communication, fine or gross motor skills, or a more global delay across all, or several, areas of development. These delays or disabilities can restrict participation in self-care, playing and communicating with peers, and learning.

In contrast, some children have a developmental disability/disorder which is distinguishable from delay in that the child, before the age of 18 years, meets a set of criteria for a lifelong diagnosis, for example, cerebral palsy, autism spectrum disorder, Down syndrome or intellectual disability. Additionally, many occupational therapists work with children who do not have a disability and assess as typically developing but who do not learn as quickly or easily as other children, resulting in participation restrictions. Some common difficulties experienced by these children include being clumsy or having poor coordination, difficulty with maintaining attention or in following instructions.

The NDIS provides for opportunities for early intervention for eligible children (aged 0–6 years) with developmental delays or disability to develop the skills they need to participate in daily activities. Families engage with Early Childhood Partner organisations who link the family to individuals or organisations who deliver support or services using the Early Childhood Early Intervention (ECEI) approach (NDIA, 2020). Occupational therapists, either individually or as part of a transdisciplinary team, work with the child and their family to achieve their goals in their home, day care, preschool, kindergarten or other environments.

NDIS funding support can enable the occupational therapist to work with the child to achieve their goals in areas such as play, social interaction, self-care and participation in all daily occupations, and will also focus on building parent and other care givers capacity. Educational funding may be available in early education settings to enable the occupational therapist to collaborate with the educator and other team members to adapt the curriculum or the environment to meet the child's educational needs. Occupational therapists use a range of family-centred and evidence-based interventions including coaching to develop the parents' problem-solving skills so they can build their child's capacity to participate in meaningful activities and environments (Graham et al., 2009).

Case study: Tara

Tara is a four-year-old girl with autism spectrum disorder (ASD) and mild intellectual disability who lives with her mother, Fiona, and father, Andrew, and her two-year-old sister, Sophie. Tara has recently commenced preschool two days per week and she also attends long day care two days a week. Tara enjoys playing outside, although her motor skills are not well developed, and she is not yet able to pedal her bike with training wheels. Tara loves to play with her figurines, and she enjoys looking at books. Her paternal grandparents live close by and she enjoys spending time at the park with her grandpa, although she is hesitant to go on the swings or slides. Tara was recently assessed as eligible for an individualised funding plan with the NDIS and referred to a local multidisciplinary service provider to implement her plan. The occupational therapist was appointed as her key worker and commenced monthly home visits. Tara's childcare agreed to the occupational therapist attending the childcare for six sessions. Tara's plan has goals related to her self-care, particularly dressing, mealtimes and toileting. The plan also has goals related to her play and social interactions with peers, her communication with adults and children, and her tantrums when things do not go her way.

Using coaching strategies, the first two home sessions have focused on Tara becoming more independent with dressing/undressing herself, and on using a spoon or fork to feed herself. Together with her mother they have worked out that picture cards, rather than too many verbal prompts, help her understand the next step and help her stay focused on the task. Using 'first you do' and 'then you can …' strategies have helped Tara complete non-preferred activities, such as getting dressed, before she can play with her figurines, without having a tantrum. At home and with her grandpa the occupational therapist will provide activities and strategies to develop Tara's gross motor skills and to introduce her to movement activities to build her confidence and skills using the playground equipment. In day care the occupational therapist will collaborate with the educators to help Tara initiate interaction with other children, share and take turns without tantrums, participate at meal times, and manage her clothing and hand washing at toilet time, implementing the strategies used at home. The preschool has agreed to the occupational therapist attending their program support meeting to share strategies with the therapists and educators who will work with Tara in that setting.

Children in school

Occupational therapists working with school-aged children must work collaboratively with teachers and others to assess and support the child to have access to, and to participate in, the classroom and all school environments (Rens & Joosten, 2014). It is important for occupational therapists to see the child in the school environment to assess the interaction of the student (person), environment and occupational demands to maximise participation. For the child with physical disabilities this might focus on access to, and modification of, the physical environment and assistive technology, positioning of the child throughout the day and modification of the tasks. For other children the focus might be on their classroom behaviours, attention to task, organisational skills, ability to follow instructions, ability to work in a group and their social skills in and out of the classroom. For some students the focus may be on the impact of delayed motor skills on their ability to play, write or complete the self-care skills that are an important part of the school day. As a student progresses through school the focus shifts to supporting successful transitions from primary to secondary school and then preparing for life after school. Active engagement in the educational setting enables the occupational therapists to make realistic recommendations, work collaboratively with the teacher, student and family, and to set shared goals that will optimise classroom and school participation. NDIS funding for School Leaver Employment Supports can enable occupational therapists to work collaboratively with the student and their family, school transition support personnel, employment service and employers to support a successful transition from school to work.

Case study: Mark

Mark was in his final year of school and wanted to get a paid part-time job, but was unsure how to find a job, or what type of work he would like to do. Mark enjoyed school and was well liked by his classmates. Although he sometimes had difficulties understanding instructions, he learnt best through practical demonstration of new tasks, clear step-by-step visual prompts, and by completing tasks repeatedly. Mark lacked confidence in new social situations and became anxious in unfamiliar environments. However, he knew his way around his local neighbourhood and walked to school by himself each day.

Mark had worked with an occupational therapist many times since he was diagnosed with an intellectual disability at age three. Since Mark entered school, school-based occupational therapists have worked collaboratively with him, his parents and teachers to set goals and develop strategies to support his participation in school and extra-curricular activities. Each time, the occupational therapist had collected information from a variety of sources, including interviews, observations in the classroom, samples of Mark's work, behavioural checklists and formal assessments, including the *Pediatric Evaluation of Disability Inventory* (PEDI) (Haley et al., 1998)—now the PEDI-CAT (Haley et al., 2012)—completed by Mark's parents when he entered school, and the *School Function Assessment* (SFA) (Coster et al., 1998) completed with Mark's teacher in year three to support her understanding of Mark's performance and participation in school. The *Child Occupation Self-Assessment* (COSA) (Keller et al., 2005) was completed with Mark when supporting his transition to secondary school. Mark's therapist used this information to make recommendations regarding: specific skills to teach Mark (e.g., using a colour-coded school timetable to aid organisation); changes to the physical and social environment to optimise learning; changes to tasks and the way instructions were delivered; and curriculum adjustments required to support Mark's participation at school.

Mark had been progressing well at school with an Individual Education Plan (IEP). However, he experienced difficulties meeting expectations while completing school-organised work experience placements because of the inadequate level of on-the-job support. Subsequently, School Leaver Employment Supports (SLES) were included in Mark's most recent NDIS participant plan to help him achieve his goal of getting a paid part-time job. Mark's SLES provider arranged some worksite visits and work experience placements. When Mark decided that he would like to work at a local coffee shop, his SLES provider arranged a work trial and engaged an occupational therapist to conduct a workplace assessment and develop a plan for supporting Mark in the workplace. The occupational therapist interviewed Mark and contacted Mark's parents, teacher and school-based occupational therapist to gather information about the environmental supports and modifications which had been most successful in enabling his participation in the past. He visited the coffee shop with Mark to conduct a workplace assessment, speak to the manager about workplace expectations, and complete task analyses while observing the tasks Mark would be required to do. The occupational therapist used this information to develop a plan to support Mark before, during and after work.

Mark started working a few hours, three days a week, clearing customer tables and helping to stack the coffee shop dishwasher. His parents helped him plan what he would wear to work each day, get ready on time, and purchase a travel card. Mark's SLES provider caught the bus to work with him each day and provided on-the-job support to help Mark get to know his co-workers, demonstrate new tasks, and provide verbal and visual prompts using the visual task schedules developed by Mark's therapist. Mark worked hard to learn new tasks and after an initial period of shyness made friends with other workers. The occupational therapist followed up with Mark's parents, SLES provider and employer to ensure the plan was working and to adjust as required. After several weeks Mark was offered an ongoing position, achieving his goal of getting a paid job. His next goal is to learn to use public transport to get around town independently.

People with mental illness

Over the past 28 years, the Australian federal government has changed focus from institutionalised care of people with mental illness to the development of mental health service initiatives and programs that focus on care in the community. Gradually, access to the right services within a reasonable time frame, and increased foci on the ability of people with mental illness to participate in employment, education and training, and community activities was added to mental health plans and strategies. More recently, coordination and continuity of care, quality improvement and innovation as well as accountability and measuring and reporting progress have been introduced (NMHC, 2014). In 2017, the Council of Australian Governments (COAG) released *The Fifth National Mental Health and Suicide Prevention Plan.* This plan further supports the vision of a mental health system that 'enables recovery, prevents and detects mental illness early, and ensures that all Australians with a mental illness can access effective and appropriate treatment and community support to enable them to participate fully in the community' (COAG, 2017, p. 2). More specifically, the fifth plan identified areas of priorities, strategies and performance indicators that will achieve integrated planning and service delivery of mental health- and suicide prevention-related services (NMHC, 2020).

This vision for mental health systems is congruent with core principles of occupational therapy where clinicians support and promote clients' participation in meaningful occupations such as employment and education. Furthermore, recovery, which underpins mental health service delivery, also shares similarities with occupational therapy core concepts. Whether we consider the vision for mental health services or the core principles of our profession, providing individualised and person-centred interventions and empowering the client in taking responsibility for their recovery is encouraged (COAG, 2017; NMHC, 2020; Townsend & Polatajko, 2013).

If occupational therapists work in mental health or other settings, their overall goal is similar: to promote health and well-being through engagement in the occupations people want, need or are expected to do (WFOT, 2012). More specifically, in a mental health setting, occupational therapists will assess the impact of mental illness on a person's daily life. This includes the ability to engage in meaningful and important occupations such as self-care, school, work, leisure activities and social interactions. Engagement in these occupations can enhance or re-establish important life skills and roles supporting the development of a strong and supportive social network. In addition, strong therapeutic use of self and knowledge of functional implications of mental illness are specific aspects of mental health practice (Scanlan et al., 2015).

Assessment and intervention choices are influenced by different factors such as the setting in which the occupational therapist works, the impacts of mental illness on the client's life, and their needs. For example, in an acute mental health setting, where the length of stay is short, the occupational therapist will identify the impact of the mental illness on the person's occupational performance and participation in meaningful occupations (Mahaffey & Holmquist, 2011). This can be achieved by using assessments that will describe the occupational profile of the client, measure their performance, document their participation in activities of daily living, and their sensory processing. This information, with the input of the other members of the team such as psychiatrist, psychologist, nurses and social worker, will determine the best intervention and discharge plans. Some particularities to mental health practice include being familiar with the different government plans, the Mental Health Act 2014, as well as national strategies and guidelines for mental health services. With the implementation of the NDIS, there are opportunities for occupational therapists to contribute meaningfully to the recovery of people with mental illness. However, this requires that occupational therapists become aware of the approaches and priorities of the NDIS, keeping in mind that they might be slightly different to those in the mental health system.

Case study: Emily

Emily is 16 years old. She lives at home with her father Josh, her mother Carrie and her older sister Elizabeth. Just over 20 months ago, Emily's mother noticed changes in her behaviours around food and her social interactions. Emily became more withdrawn and anxious around mealtime, started exploring diets online, and often said to her sister that her thighs were too big and that all she wanted was to have a really flat stomach. After rapid weight loss and increased anxiety, irritability and social isolation, Emily's mother took her to their general practitioner (GP). The GP suspected there was something more complex than typical teenage behaviour. After weeks of tests and waiting for a referral to see a child psychiatrist, Emily was diagnosed with anorexia nervosa.

Emily is hospitalised in an inpatient eating disorders service. The eating disorders team includes a psychiatrist, a psychologist, a nurse, a dietitian and Abby, an occupational therapist. The eating disorder team implements Family Based Treatment (FBT). FBT is supported by robust evidence and its effectiveness in successfully treating most people with anorexia nervosa has been demonstrated (Hurst & Zimmer-Gembeck, 2019). However, for some of these young people, their eating disorder symptoms and psychological distress remains during and post FBT (Wufong et al., 2019). While Abby completed her training in FBT and delivers FBT, she noted that Emily experienced distress and anxiety before and after mealtime. Abby met with Emily and shared her observations while they were working together to identify meaningful goals for Emily. One of Emily's goals was to feel less stressed and scared of eating food she felt was 'bad'.

Abby considered using sensory approaches with Emily to help her regulate her emotional responses, arousal and distress level. Abby knows there is evidence supporting the use of sensory approaches in mental health settings in regulating emotional responses and levels of arousal and distress (Bailliard & Whigham, 2017; Scanlan & Novak, 2015; West et al., 2017). Abby completed the *Adolescent/ Adult Sensory Profile* (Brown & Dunn, 2002) with Emily and results suggested that Emily is sensory avoiding. It became apparent that the fast-paced environment of the ward accentuated Emily's anxiety especially around mealtime. Together, Emily and Abby identified sensory supportive spaces and strategies such as dimming the lights, aromatherapy and soft music with a repetitive rhythm. Emily integrated the strategies and felt increasingly comfortable using them when she felt her emotional and anxiety levels were increasing. In the next occupational therapy sessions, Abby will work with Emily towards occupation-based goals like re-engaging in meaningful social activities and her role as a student. For Abby, combining evidence-based eating disorders interventions with client-centred practice and occupational therapy-specific strategies helped her consolidate and maintain her professional identity.

People in the workplace

Being productive and contributing to the world in which we live is central to human values and our existence. The term *work* refers to paid employment, volunteer activities, care-giving activities, or any other productive occupation, which involves people contributing to their community and to society (AOTA, 2014). Participation in productive occupations is important to people not only because of financial security and independence that arises from paid work, but also because productive occupations offer people a sense of role identity, fulfilment, satisfaction, self-worth and social status. Work is considered beneficial to health and well-being (Waddell & Burton, 2006).

Occupational therapists are well positioned to use a biopsychosocial approach based on The International Classification of Functioning, Disability and Health (ICF) (World Health Organization [WHO], 2001) which is commonly used in vocational rehabilitation contexts to improve the health and participation of working-age adults in productivity-related occupations. Occupational therapists providing vocational rehabilitation and/or injury prevention services typically work in private practices or as part of specialised rehabilitation services within larger health care organisations. Occupational therapists who provide vocational rehabilitation services assist clients who have physical, cognitive and/or mental health impairments impacting on their work performance. Services occur predominantly in people's work environments but may also occur in clinical settings and in people's living environments, as it is important to address people's occupational performance issues in self-care and domestic life activities of daily living prior to addressing return-to-work, work readiness and job seeking activities. In vocational rehabilitation contexts, occupational therapists form part of a broad team of service providers assisting people to return to work. Team members may include medical practitioners, physiotherapists, psychologists, employers and workers' compensation insurers.

Vocational rehabilitation involves establishing short- and long-term work goals in consultation with the person, their current or future employer, and other treating health professionals. Frequently, return-to-work programs are developed to assist an injured worker returning to their pre-injury role. This involves commencing with suitable or modified duties within their demonstrated capabilities; and monitoring, reviewing and evaluation of the outcomes of the return-to-work program. Occupational therapists may also conduct home assessments to identify the need for support in self-care and domestic-life activities of daily living, which may enable participation in work-related activities. Occupational therapists may also assist job seekers with physical, cognitive and/or mental health to gain suitable employment. This often involves integrating a range of strategies such as environmental modification, job redesign, employer education and graded work programs.

In order to develop person-centred work goals, occupational therapy assessment usually focuses on the person, their occupations and their home and work environments. An initial assessment provides baseline information about the person that is relevant to setting their work-related goals. Assessment of the person's current or future work environment and work activities are also required to evaluate the physical, social and cognitive job demands. Assessment of the person's physical, cognitive and/or affective status, frequently called a functional capacity evaluation, provides information about the person's current abilities. The occupational therapist uses reasoning to determine the areas where a person's abilities match job roles or work demands. Where there is disparity the therapist identifies if any modifications to the work tasks, equipment or environment are needed to enable the person to return to work or gain employment.

Case study: Malcolm

Malcolm is a 38-year-old electrician who has a partner and two small children aged four and six. Malcolm was electrocuted during an accident when he was exposed to live wires when repairing the antenna on the roof of a client's home. Malcolm sustained burns to both hands and arms and fell, fracturing his spinal vertebrae at levels L5 and S1. There was no damage to his spinal cord. Malcolm required several operations on both hands and forearms for skin grafting He required amputation of the fourth and fifth fingers on his right hand because of necrosis. Malcolm works with an occupational therapy hand therapist who is helping him to improve range of motion and strength in his fingers, hands and forearms; to minimise adhesions and oedema; and work towards independence in his activities of daily living. Malcolm wears a pressure garment on both hands to minimise scar tissue at the skin graft sites and to maintain the web spaces between the fingers of both hands. He must be careful of the fragile skin on his hands and forearms because healing is slow.

Malcolm experiences ongoing back pain. He can sit for approximately 30 minutes and needs to alternate between sitting, standing and walking through the day. The hand therapist has assessed Malcolm's level of independence with self-care and domestic activities of daily living several times over the six months since the accident. The hand therapist arranged for home supports to be provided, and funded, by Malcolm's employer's workers' compensation insurer.

Six months after the accident Malcolm had not been able to return to his electrician job, or resume normal domestic duties, placing a strain on family life. Because of Malcolm's back injury, hand and forearm injuries, he has been unable to pick up or play vigorous games with his children. Malcolm has not been able to play sport or to carry out several domestic and home maintenance tasks because such activities would pose a risk to the integrity of the skin on his hands and forearms. Malcolm has been depressed and pessimistic about his employment options. He sought psychological counselling to help him deal with the trauma of the accident as well as difficulties adjusting to his altered physical state, family situation and sense of competence as a partner, father, friend and worker. Malcolm feels hesitant to return to work due to the challenges/barriers he still experiences due to his injury; however, financial stress is motivating him to do so.

An occupational therapist recently commenced working with Malcolm to assist his return to employment. The occupational therapist assessed Malcolm's physical capacities through a functional capacity evaluation. The occupational therapist then assessed Malcolm's work duties through an onsite work assessment with Malcolm and his employer. Together, they established that he could not return to his former electrician duties; however, there was a need for a job estimator within the business and Malcolm could learn to perform this role. This job's demands primarily required Malcolm to drive a vehicle, walk, interact with potential customers, use a computer and write out information.

The role of the occupational therapist in this scenario was to devise a graduated return-to-work program that enabled Malcolm and his employer to work collaboratively to facilitate his learning of the new work tasks through on-the-job training. The occupational therapist assisted Malcolm and his employer to problem-solve how Malcolm would record necessary information with the aid of computer technology. Malcolm was referred for an occupational therapy driver assessment and was assessed for necessary vehicle modifications. The occupational therapist helped Malcolm and his employer to problem-solve how Malcolm would manage interactions with clients when faced with questions about his injury. A graduated return-to-work plan was devised to provide Malcolm the opportunity to continue his hand therapy and counselling, to gradually improve his endurance and strength for work, and to manage his home activities. Over the next six months Malcolm managed to return to full-time employment in his new role and find new ways to be involved in his family life again as he felt more positive and competent in his roles as worker, partner and father.

Adults with a neurological condition

Individuals with a neurological condition have experienced injury or disease to their central or peripheral nervous system. These conditions may have a sudden onset (such as stroke or traumatic brain injury) or may have an evolving presentation and be progressive in nature (such as multiple sclerosis, Parkinson's disease or motor neurone disease). Neurological conditions are prevalent in Australia. For example, by 2050 it is projected nearly one million Australians will be living with stroke (Deloitte Access Economics, 2017). As a result of the high prevalence, those living with a neurological condition comprise a large and significant occupational therapy client group.

The occupations of people living with a neurological condition can be severely affected by a change in physical, sensory, cognitive, communication or psychological function. Each person experiences a different constellation of symptoms with varying levels of severity from mild to severe. Common neurological impairments that can alter participation in life tasks and roles are hemiparesis, somatosensory loss, aphasia, visual impairment and executive dysfunction. Occupational therapists work in partnership with individuals with a neurological condition as part of a multi- or interdisciplinary team to provide neurological rehabilitation. Neurological rehabilitation is an active process that enables clients to reach their optimum level of function by providing skills and tools needed to attain independence and self-determination (WHO, 2001). Occupational therapy for individuals with 'sudden onset' conditions may focus on recovery and restoration of function while for those with progressive neurological conditions occupational therapy may aim to maintain function or compensate for lost function (British Society of Rehabilitation Medicine, 2019). Restorative therapy is based on concepts of neuroplasticity and occupational therapists' use the brain's capacity to change and adapt, to facilitate recovery after brain injury. Principles of neurological rehabilitation include client-centred goal setting, multidisciplinary team care and task-specific training (Langhorne et al., 2011). Occupational therapists in neurological rehabilitation work closely with colleagues such as physiotherapists, speech pathologists and social workers, and the team may involve professionals outside of health care, such as social services or the employment sector (Barnes, 2003).

Occupational therapists in this field may work in an acute hospital setting, an inpatient rehabilitation centre, outpatient department or clients' homes. Occupational therapy changes depending on the setting. For example, in an acute hospital an occupational therapist may focus on assessing a client's impairments that will impact on occupational performance, while in the community setting the focus may be on a client's community integration and participation of the client in their chosen activities. The evidence base for neurological practice has grown dramatically in recent years and clinical practice guidelines exist to guide the work occupational therapists do (Bayley et al., 2014; National Stroke Foundation, 2017; National Clinical Guideline Centre [NCGC], 2013). Neurological rehabilitation may involve upper limb retraining, cognitive rehabilitation, psychosocial support and intervention, prescription of assistive technology, home modifications, promotion of community re-integration and driver rehabilitation.

Case study: Teuila

Teuila is a 63-year-old woman originally from Samoa, who experienced a left hemisphere stroke. Her husband Peter called an ambulance after he returned from work and found Teuila with slurred speech and weakness on her right side. Peter reported that a week prior to her admission, Teuila mentioned an episode of transient right-hand weakness with difficulty putting on her earrings. After magnetic resonance imaging (MRI), it was determined that Teuila had an infarct in the region of the right middle cerebral artery. Teuila and Peter's four children live locally, and Teuila enjoys spending time with her seven grandchildren, aged between two and 12 years. Teuila works part-time as a practice manager at a local GP clinic and outside of work she enjoys organising Pasifika festivals with her daughter Sefina. She recently set up the WhatsApp on her phone to contact family in Samoa and enjoys keeping up to date with news online.

Teuila was transferred from the acute stroke unit to an inpatient rehabilitation facility where she met an occupational therapist who introduced their role to Teuila, Peter and Sefina. The occupational therapist read the handover notes from the acute stroke unit which detailed Teuila's medical and social background, home set-up and previous level of occupational performance (she was previously independent in all tasks). The handover noted Teuila's occupational performance and indicated she was having difficulty with self-care tasks due to right hemiparesis, impaired somatosensation of her right hand, mild expressive aphasia and short-term memory impairment.

On initial assessment, Teuila was found to be mobile around the ward with a single point stick with close supervision. The occupational therapist noted she had some mild subluxation at her right shoulder. At the end of the occupational therapist's assessment, it was noticed Teuila had difficulty feeding herself from a lunch tray with a fork in her right hand (her dominant hand). The occupational therapist discussed the potential for brain recovery with Teuila and her family and used a drawing to illustrate the potential for new brain pathways being strengthened through rehabilitation. The idea of setting goals was discussed and Teuila indicated her goal priority area was feeding herself independently, making a cup of coffee and sending text messages to her family. The occupational therapist completed components of the *Functional Independence Measure* (FIM) (Uniform Data System for Medical Rehabilitation, 2009) to discuss at the multidisciplinary team meeting that afternoon and initiated a discussion with Teuila about the possibility of participating in Constraint-Induced Movement Therapy (CIMT). Teuila consented to visiting the occupational therapy department the next day with Peter for a session focussed on retraining Teuila's left upper limb for independent eating and using her phone. The occupational therapist discussed plans for this session with the speech pathologist and physiotherapist on the team. At a case conference meeting the multidisciplinary team discussed Teuila's discharge home with home-based therapy after three weeks of inpatient rehabilitation.

Older adults

Older people are living longer and are entering later life in better health than past generations (AIHW, 2013). Ageing, however, is a complex process commonly associated with physical, psychological and social changes (Stav et al., 2012). Long-term (chronic) health conditions, such as arthritis, vision and hearing loss, osteoporosis, coronary heart disease, cerebrovascular disease, chronic obstructive pulmonary disease, high blood pressure, and Type II diabetes, are more common among older people and can cause disability (AIHW, 2014). Older people may also experience typical age-related changes, acute illness or injuries, most commonly from falls, that may result in hospitalisation impacting on their participation in meaningful occupations. Following recovery from an acute illness an older adult may become deconditioned, particularly during hospitalisation, and require rehabilitation. A common focus of occupational therapy intervention with an older person who is an inpatient is to work as a member of the health care team to support the person's transition from hospital to community living. This may involve modifying aspects of the person's living environment or adjusting aspects of their occupations to re-enable participation in daily life at home and in the community. For some older adults, returning home may not be possible, and thus the focus may shift to facilitating the transition to a residential aged care facility.

Most older people continue to make valuable contributions to their community, for instance, through volunteering, paid work, and through caregiving responsibilities (e.g., parents, spouse, children or grandchildren). Many older people engage in social and educational activities (e.g., University of the Third Age (U3A), Probus, sporting clubs and various interest groups). However, changes often associated with ageing may impact on an older person's participation in occupations they value and find meaningful. Common occupational changes include retirement from paid employment or driving cessation. Person-level changes may include reduced mobility or visual or hearing impairment. Situational changes could include loss of a partner or spouse, moving houses or moving into residential aged care. Occupational therapy intervention commonly focuses on addressing relevant person, occupation and situational factors that are important to the older person to support them to return to participation in self-care, productive and leisure occupations that they want or need to do.

When an older person enters an occupational therapy service an initial assessment is undertaken, providing an important opportunity to develop rapport with the person and identify their occupational participation issues and goals for therapy. Commonly, an understanding of the older person's current level of participation in self-care, productivity and leisure occupations is discussed, as well as supports available and home set-up. Supporting the person's participation in occupations such as meal preparation, self-care, community access, shopping, housework and gardening may be used as a means of restoring an older person's confidence, mobility, strength and independence. Interventions used to enable older people to achieve their goals may frequently include education, falls prevention strategies, carer support and education (e.g., equipment use, manual handling), home assessment and modifications, or provision of assistive technology.

Case study: Frank

Mr FH (Frank) is a 91-year-old retired factory worker who immigrated to Australia from Italy in 1954 and has been widowed for nine years. He lives alone in his own home and stopped driving about a year ago. One morning he felt weak and dizzy and was found by his son still sitting on his bed around lunchtime, when his son came to take him shopping. He was hospitalised for investigation of weight loss and generalised weakness. It was noted that Frank had lost about 8 kg over about a year, that his conversation was long-winded and that he was vague when discussing his situation. He had unkempt hair, long fingernails and was wearing a food-stained shirt, his spectacles were dirty, and his hearing aids were not working. Although he has several medical conditions, including hypertension, Type II diabetes, gout, osteoarthritis, hearing impairment and varicose veins, all his conditions appeared stable and there had been no changes to his medications. Extensive investigations did not reveal any clear cause for the weakness and weight loss. It was noted that in hospital Frank ate all meals and dietary supplements completely. There was a concern about his ability to return home; hence he was transferred from the acute hospital General Medicine Service to a Geriatric Medicine Unit.

When the occupational therapist first met Frank, he reported that some days he just could not be bothered with cooking for himself or even having much to eat and agreed with suggestions that lately he had not really been taking care of himself. The possibility of depression was considered by the medical team, as was that of dementia, but both were thought unlikely. He was thought to have mild cognitive impairment, but testing was difficult due to his old glasses and non-functioning hearing aids.

To gain further insights into his cognition the occupational therapist assessed Frank's functioning in the unit. The occupational therapist received a report from the nursing staff about Frank's continence and toileting (no clear problems identified), and his ability to wash himself. The occupational therapist observed Frank shave and clean his dentures and observed his ability to get dressed (after the occupational therapist had arranged for his son to bring in clothes and shoes for Frank). Frank's ability to make breakfast was assessed. These assessments showed that Frank was able to achieve all his personal care tasks, requiring just minimal prompting. After attending to his personal care, having his glasses cleaned and hearing aid batteries replaced, it was noted that Frank expressed his desire to return home. He had gained weight in hospital and was eager to talk to anyone who came near him.

The occupational therapist was the designated key contact person between the Geriatric Medicine Unit and Frank's family, both receiving information and providing it. The physiotherapist reported that Frank's gait now appeared safe and the medical team reported no further episodes of low blood pressure and noted no active medical problems. The occupational therapist conducted a home assessment, and even after it had been cleaned by his son, found it be moderately cluttered, with trip hazards in the worn carpet and some non-functioning interior lights; and the home was still relatively unclean.

Overall, it was thought that Frank's deterioration was due to mild cognitive impairment, with consequent self-neglect. The occupational therapist explained this to Frank and his son. Neither wanted community supports, but did accept Meals on Wheels, and agreed to liaise with Frank's General Practitioner about a My Aged Care assessment to get other possible services at home. The occupational therapist provided a detailed written summary of Frank's situation and called his GP to provide a verbal handover to facilitate Frank's discharge home.

Conclusion

Occupational therapists work with people, their family and communities, across the lifespan in a range of practice settings in urban, regional, rural and remote areas of Australia. Practice settings extend across the care continuum and include hospitals, homes, schools, non-government and private organisations, workplaces, residential aged care facilities, and community and rehabilitation centres. These health-related, education-based and community services may be funded by government, non-government and by private sectors. Some services address specific age groups. For example, tertiary paediatric hospitals provide health care services to children and young people from birth to 18 years. Other services focus on the needs of people with specific disorders or illness such as mental health disorders. Models of service delivery and practice within these settings vary greatly. This chapter provided an overview of the role of occupational therapists with a case example in six common practice areas: early intervention, school-based occupational therapy, mental health, vocational rehabilitation, adult neurological rehabilitation and practice with older adults.

Summary

Occupational therapists working with people across the lifespan in a range of contexts conduct a variety of standardised and observational assessments and interventions. Through the more detailed explanation of six practice areas and the use of case studies, this chapter provided evidence that:

- Occupational therapists work in a variety of settings.
- Enabling occupation and improving participation are the foci of occupational therapy.
- Despite frequently complex contextual differences, at the core of occupational therapists' practice is delivering client-centred, occupation-focused care.

Review questions

1. Describe three different practice contexts in which occupational therapists work.
2. What are the core similarities in the occupational therapy role across these environments?
3. Describe the key differences between multidisciplinary, interdisciplinary and transdisciplinary teams.

References

American Occupational Therapy Association. (2014). Occupational Therapy Practice Framework: Domain and Process, 3rd edition. *American Journal of Occupational Therapy, 68*(suppl. 1), S1–S48. https://doi.org/10.5014/ajot.2014.682006.

Australian Commission on Safety and Quality in Health Care. (2018). *Review of key attributes of high-performing person-centred healthcare organisations.* https://www.safetyandquality.gov.au/sites/default/files/migrated/FINAL-REPORT-Attributes-of-person-centred-healthcare-organisations-2018.pdf

Australian Government. (2019). *Ageing and aged care. Home care packages—reform.* https://agedcare.health.gov.au/aged-care-reform/home-care/home-care-packages-reform

Australian Institute of Health and Welfare. (2013). *Australia's welfare 2013.* AIHW. https://doi.org/10.25816/5eba34da74756

Australian Institute of Health and Welfare. (2014). *Australia's health 2014.* AIHW. https://doi.org/10.25816/5ec1e4122547e

Bailliard, A. L., & Whigham, S. C. (2017). Linking neuroscience, function, and intervention: A scoping review of sensory processing and mental illness. *American Journal of Occupational Therapy, 71*(5), 1–7. https://doi.org/10.5014/ajot.2017.024497

Barnes, M. P. (2003). Principles of neurological rehabilitation. *Journal of Neurology, Neurosurgery & Psychiatry, 74*(suppl. 4), iv3–iv7.

Bayley, M. T., Tate, R., Douglas, J. M., Turkstra, L. S., Ponsford, J., Stergiou-Kita, M., Kua, A., & Bragge, P. (2014). INCOG guidelines for cognitive rehabilitation following traumatic brain injury: Methods and overview. *The Journal of Head Trauma Rehabilitation, 29*(4), 290–306. https://doi.org/10.1097/HTR.0000000000000070

Bell, A., Corfield, M., Davis, J., & Richardson N. (2009). Collaborative transdisciplinary intervention in early years—putting theory into practice. *Child: Care, health and development, 36,* 142–148. https://doi.org/10.1111/j.1365-2214.2009.01027.x

British Society of Rehabilitation Medicine (2019). *Specialist neuro-rehabilitation services: Providing for patients with complex rehabilitation needs.* https://www.bsrm.org.uk/downloads/specialised-neurorehabilitation-service-standards--7-30-4-2015-pcatv2-forweb-11-5-16-annexe2updatedmay2019.pdf

Brown, C., & Dunn, W. (2002). *Adolescent/Adult Sensory Profile.* Pearson.

Commonwealth of Australia. (2020a). *Aged Care Quality and Safety Commission.* https://www.agedcarequality.gov.au

Commonwealth of Australia. (2020b). *My Aged Care.* https://www.myagedcare.gov.au/

Commonwealth Government of Australia. (1992). *Disability Discrimination Act 1992.* https://www.legislation.gov.au/Details/C2016C00763

Commonwealth Government of Australia. (2006). *Disability Standards for Education, 2005.* https://docs.education.gov.au/system/files/doc/other/disability_standards_for_education_2005_plus_guidance_notes.pdf

Commonwealth Government of Australia. (2014). *Aged Care and Other Legislation Amendment Act (1997) 2014.* https://www.legislation.gov.au/Details/C2020C00054

Commonwealth Government of Australia. (2015a). *Aged Care Reform*. https://www.dss.gov.au/our-responsibilities/ageing-and-aged-care/aged-care-reform.

Commonwealth Government of Australia. (2015b). *National Mental Health Commission: Leading, collaborating, advising, reporting*. http://www.mentalhealthcommission.gov.au/

Coster, W., Deeney, T., Haltiwanger, J., & Haley, S. (1998). *School Function Assessment*. Psychological Corporation.

Council of Australian Governments (COAG). (2017). *The Fifth National Mental Health and Suicide Prevention Plan*. https://www.coaghealthcouncil.gov.au/Portals/0/Fifth%20National%20Mental%20Health%20and%20Suicide%20Prevention%20Plan.pdf

Deloitte Access Economics. (2017). *No postcode untouched: Stroke in Australia*. https://strokefoundation.org.au/About-Stroke/Facts-and-figures-about-stroke#fn

Graham, F., Rodger, S., & Ziviani, J. (2009). Coaching parents to enable children's participation: An approach for working with parents and their children. *Australian Occupational Therapy Journal, 56*, 16–23. https://doi.org/10.1111/j.1440-1630.2008.00736.x

Haley, S. M., Coster, W. J., Dumas, H., Fragala-Pinkham, M. A., & Moed, R. (2012). *Pediatric Evaluation of Disability Inventory Computer Adapted Test (PEDICAT)*. Psychological Corporation.

Haley, S. M., Coster, W., Ludlow, L., Haltiwanger, J., & Andrellos, P. (1998). *Administration manual for the Pediatric Evaluation of Disability Inventory*. Psychological Corporation.

Hurst, K., & Zimmer-Gembeck, M. (2019). Family-based treatment with cognitive behavioural therapy for anorexia. *Clinical Psychologist, 23*(1), 61–70. https://doi.org/10.1111/cp.12152

Keller, J., Kafkes, A., Basu, S., Federico, J., & Kielhofner, G. (2005). *The Child Occupational Self-Assessment (COSA)* (version 2.1). University of Illinois at Chicago.

Langhorne, P., Bernhardt, J., & Kwakkel, G. (2011). Stroke rehabilitation. *Lancet, 377* (9778), 1693–1702. https://doi.org/10.1016/S0140-6736(11)60325-5

Mahaffey, L., & Holmquist, B. (2011). Hospital-based mental health care. In C. Brown, V. C. Stoffel, & J. P. Munoz (Eds.), *Occupational therapy in mental health: A vision for participation* (pp. 581–594). F. A. Davis Co.

National Clinical Guideline Centre (NCGC). (2013). *Stroke rehabilitation: Long-term rehabilitation after stroke*. Clinical guideline no. 162. NICE.

National Disability Insurance Agency. (2014). *What is the National Disability Insurance Scheme?* https://www.ndis.gov.au/understanding/what-ndis

National Disability Insurance Agency. (2020). *National Disability Insurance Scheme*. https://www.ndis.gov.au

National Mental Health Commission. (2014). *The National Review of Mental Health Programmes and Services*. https://www.mentalhealthcommission.gov.au/Monitoring-and-Reporting/national-reports/2014-Contributing-Lives-Review

National Mental Health Commission. (2020). *Monitoring mental health and suicide prevention reform: National Report 2019*. https://www.mentalhealthcommission.gov.au/

National Stroke Foundation. (2017). *Clinical guidelines for stroke management*. https://informme.org.au/Guidelines/Clinical-Guidelines-for-Stroke-Management-2017.

Rens, L., & Joosten, A. (2014). Investigating the experiences in a school-based occupational therapy program to inform community-based paediatric occupational therapy practice. *Australian Occupational Therapy Journal, 61*(3), 148–158. https://doi.org/10.1111/1440-1630.12093

Rosenbaum, P., King, S., Law, M., King, G., & Evans, J. (1998). Family-centred service: A conceptual framework and research review. *Physical and Occupational Therapy in Paediatrics, 18*(1), 1–20. https://doi.org/10.1080/J006v18n01_01

Safe Work Australia. (2019). *Safe Work Australia*. http://www.safeworkaustralia.gov.au/sites/swa/pages/default

Scanlan, J. N., & Novak, T. (2015). Sensory approaches in mental health: A scoping review. *Australian Occupational Therapy Journal, 62*, 277–285. https://doi.org/10.1111/1440-1630.12224

Scanlan, J. N., Pepin, G., Haracz, K., Ennals, P., Webster, J. S., Meredith, P. J., Batten, R., Bowman, S., Bonassi, M., & Bruce, R. (2015). Identifying educational priorities for occupational therapy students to prepare for mental health practice in Australia and New Zealand: Opinions of practising occupational therapists. *Australian Occupational Therapy Journal, 62*, 286–298. https://doi.org/10.1111/1440-1630.12194

Stav, W. B., Hallenen, T., Lane, J., & Arbesman, M. (2012). Systematic review of occupational engagement and health outcomes among community-dwelling older adults. *American Journal of Occupational Therapy, 66*, 301–310. https://doi.org/10.5014/ajot.2012.003707

Townsend, E., & Polatajko, H. (2013). *Enabling occupation II: Advancing occupational therapy vision for health, well-being and justice through occupation* (2nd edn). CAOT Publications ACE.

Turpin, M., & Iwama, M. K. (2011). *Using occupational therapy models in practice: A field guide.* Churchill Livingstone.

Uniform Data System for Medical Rehabilitation. (2009). *The FIM System® Clinical Guide, version 5.2.* UDSMR.

United Nations Educational, Scientific and Cultural Organization. (1994). *The UNESCO Salamanca Statement and Framework for Action of Special Needs Education.* https://unesdoc.unesco.org/ark:/48223/pf0000098427

Victoria Government. (2014). *Victoria Mental Health Act 2014.* https://www2.health.vic.gov.au/mental-health/practice-and-service-quality/mental-health-act-2014

Waddell, G., & Burton, K. (Eds). (2006). *Is work good for your health and well-being?* TSO (The Stationary Office).

West, M., Melvin, G., McNamara, F., & Gordon, M. (2017). An evaluation of the use and efficacy of a sensory room within an adolescent psychiatric inpatient unit. *Australian Occupational Therapy Journal, 64*(3), 253–263. https://doi.org/10.1111/1440-1630.12358

World Federation of Occupational Therapists. (2012). *Statement on occupational therapy.* https://www.wfot.org/about-occupational-therapy

World Health Organization. (2001). *International Classification of Functioning, Disability and Health* https://www.who.int/classifications/icf/en/

Wufong, E., Rhodes, P., & Conti, J. (2019). 'We don't really know what else we can do': Parent experiences when adolescent distress persists after the Maudsley and family-based therapies for anorexia nervosa. *Journal of Eating Disorders, 7*(5). https://doi.org/10.1186/s40337-019-0235-5

24 Emerging professional practice areas

Focus on technology

Marina Ciccarelli, Helen Bourke-Taylor, Claire Morrisby, Ian Cheok, Libby Callaway, Lisa O'Brien and Amy Barrett-Lennard

Chapter objectives

Upon completion of this chapter, the reader will be able to:

- Describe some contemporary examples of occupational therapy practice areas that have emerged to meet a community need and fill a service gap.
- Explain some innovative approaches to use of emergent technologies in service provision from the perspective of occupational therapists in Australia.
- Discuss the importance of remaining innovative and responsive through emerging occupational therapy practice areas in Australia.
- Demonstrate the role of research and evidence in the development and evaluation of emerging technologies in occupational therapy practice areas.

Key words

emerging practice areas; digital technologies; occupational therapy; service provision; remote service delivery; evidence-based practice

Introduction

Twenty-first century society in Australia is technologically advanced with access to excellent education, digital technology and health services. However, some Australians experience acute and chronic health conditions and social disadvantages that may be detrimental to participation in meaningful occupations. A theoretical underpinning of occupational therapy practice is that humans are occupational beings and that engagement in occupations is important to promote health and well-being (Wilcock, 2006). There have been significant national and international events, such as the 2020 Australian bushfires and the coronavirus disease (COVID-19) pandemic that have influenced the occupational engagement, and health and well-being of Australians, in recent times (Department of Health, 2020). Occupational therapy practice must evolve to remain relevant and responsive to community needs.

Occupational therapy is an evolving profession that is grounded in meeting people's occupational needs. Reflection on the history of occupational therapy (see Chapter 3) substantiates the profession's capacity to respond to the needs of individuals, families, groups, organisations and communities. As Australian society evolves, existing occupational therapy practice areas adapt, and new or emerging practice areas arise in response to changing needs. Some of the current societal trends influencing the development of the profession and emerging practice areas include:

- An ageing Australian population with high rates of disability and chronic medical conditions and key reforms like My Aged Care;
- Lifelong care and opportunities for people living with disability funded through the National Disability Insurance Scheme;
- Improved rates of survival for people living with catastrophic injury;
- An increasing emphasis on health promotion and prevention of disease and disability;
- Substantial increases in rates of mental health conditions across all ages and genders;
- Changes in the way people work, work-related health issues, and retirement;
- Emphasis on the relationships between culture, social disadvantage and health;
- Increasing use of technologies and remote access in the education and health sectors; and
- Increasing health and digital literacy among people of all ages.

These societal, population and professional trends have resulted in new funding approaches from Federal and State governments, and necessitated changes to service delivery models for occupational therapists working in these systems. For example, limits to funding for travel have caused some organisations to reconsider the cost-effectiveness of delivering therapy services in home or community settings, versus centre-based services.

In Chapter 18, the relationships among people, occupation and the environment are examined in detail. Another area of the environment that affect people and occupations is natural disasters such as fire, flood and environmental health emergencies. Natural disaster in the form of the extensive and prolonged bushfires across Australia in the summer of 2019-2020 resulted in the loss of lives, homes, possessions, businesses and livelihoods for thousands of people. There were major and immediate mental health needs of those affected by the bushfires, including emergency services personnel. Entire communities became displaced or had restricted access to health services. The coronavirus disease 2019 (COVID-19) pandemic in 2019–2020 (World Health Organization, 2019a) changed human physical interactions on a global and unprecedented scale. Limits on the number of people gathering in public spaces, social distancing rules, self-isolation requirements and restricted access to the elderly and immune-compromised people in health and residential care facilities (World Health Organization, 2019b) have caused significant occupational disruption (Mynard, 2020). These requirements have also expanded the need and opportunity for service redesign, including occupational therapy telehealth and digital delivery of individual and group programs, to ensure service continuity.

Now, more than ever, there is a growing need to re-imagine occupational therapy service provision to engage individuals in meaningful occupations and take advantage of the digital transformation created by emergent technologies. Digital transformation refers to new actors, structures, practices, values and beliefs that change, threaten, replace or complement the existing ways of working within organisations, fields or industries and that are the result of combined digital innovations (Hinings et al., 2018). Professional practice applications of these digital transformations may include telehealth; customisation and individualisation of technology-enabled products and interventions; and digital empowerment of individuals, families, organisations and communities through co-design. These new approaches are characterised in the re-imagined and rapidly emerging occupational therapy practice areas described in this chapter.

The eight applications of technologies emerging in contemporary occupational therapy practice are featured in this chapter under three main sections: (i) complementing face-to-face service delivery with digital technologies; (ii) using immersive extended realities to promote occupational engagement and performance; and (iii) designing with technology to improve participation in occupations.

These technologies have evolved in relation to diverse and often rapidly changing client, clinical and community needs in Australia. Some of the technology-enabled practice areas include innovations driven by ideas developed, delivered and evaluated by occupational therapists. In other areas of practice, occupational therapists contribute to the application and uptake of the technology by consumers and other stakeholders.

Complementing face-to-face service delivery with digital technologies

The roll-out of the National Disability Insurance Scheme (NDIS) (Department of Social Services, 2011) and My Aged Care (Commonwealth of Australia, 2013) funding systems have increased the need for service delivery models that are innovative, effective, sustainable, evidence-based and cost-efficient. A survey of Australians living in rural and remote areas identified 'poor access to health services' as the most significant issue impacting their communities (Bishop et al., 2017, p. 36). The challenges of low population density, geographical spread, limited infrastructure, difficulty retaining health care professionals and inflated costs of service delivery in rural and remote areas all significantly affect access to health care (Australian Institute of Health and Welfare, 2018).

Telehealth offers a means of providing assessment and intervention when face-to-face therapy supports are not possible due to distance or inaccessibility due to other factors, as experienced during the 2019–2020 bushfires and the 201—-2020 COVID-19 pandemic. For some marginalised or at-risk groups, the use of telehealth means the difference between receiving therapy services and not. Virtual connections with clients may be through free or low-cost smart device applications (e.g., for video calls), or more advanced subscription-based videoconferencing. Consideration of how a person receives telehealth supports becomes integral to the success of telehealth in occupational therapy practice. These include the type of device on which telehealth is delivered, device mounting and accessibility features, user interface and training required, software used, internet access and data allowances. Personal factors also impact delivery of telehealth services and include technology skills of the health professional delivering the online service and the consumer receiving the service, and ongoing support by another person such as a family member or formal carer.

The ROAM project: Remote Orientation and Mobility

Orientation and Mobility (O&M) is a field of practice focused on the movement and travel of people who are blind or vision impaired. O&M specialists work with people of all ages, with the aim of developing an individual's skills to enable them to move through an environment with confidence, safety and efficiency. As part of comprehensive assessment and interventions, O&M specialists offer highly skilled advice regarding mobility aids, orientation techniques, route planning, environmental accessibility, assistive technology and sensory awareness.

VisAbility is a community-based disability service organisation located in Western Australia and Tasmania specialising in blindness and vision impairment. VisAbility is funded primarily by State and Federal government grants, and the NDIS. The organisation is reliant on fundraising and philanthropy of guide dogs for people who are not eligible for the NDIS. Providing regular and consistent services to a client population spread over regional and remote areas presents challenges; especially when O&M staff are located mostly in metropolitan areas. In 2015, VisAbility commenced the ROAM (Remote Orientation & Mobility) Project to explore the viability of using dynamic video conferencing techniques to provide remotely O&M assessment and intervention. Task analysis, occupational performance, community participation and capacity building are fundamental to O&M training, and so occupational therapists are ideally positioned to collaborate with O&M specialists. The occupational therapists are often known to the clients and can help to overcome some of the challenges of remotely building rapport.

Occupational therapists located in VisAbility's regional offices in Western Australia (Broome, Karratha, Geraldton, Albany) were integral to the development of the ROAM program and its long-term success. By participating in the multidisciplinary ROAM service delivery model, the occupational therapists immerse themselves in O&M practices and further develop their own knowledge and skills for working with clients who are vision impaired. A three-month pilot with six visually impaired clients aimed to determine the feasibility of ROAM. Encouraging pilot results led to funding from the Western Australian Department of Communities Disability Services for a comprehensive two-year project. The project included 45 clients aged four months to 92 years living in regional and remote areas, and aimed to determine how ROAM was used effectively in a variety of O&M programs.

The basic ROAM method involves the O&M Specialist based at the office while the support person (occupational therapist) visits the client's home environment with a ROAM equipment kit. The occupational therapist sets up the equipment that includes a chest-mounted camera (see Figure 24.1).

After establishing a video-link, the O&M specialist commences the session as they normally would during a face-to-face assessment or intervention (see Figure 24.2); and the occupational therapist monitors the client's performance and safety, and provides information to the O&M Specialist as required. ROAM is intended to supplement and not replace face-to-face service delivery; and wherever possible, the client's O&M program includes a combination of remote and in-person assessment and intervention.

Evaluation of ROAM found a 24 per cent increase in the number of clients in regional areas receiving O&M services; a 67 per cent increase in the number of O&M service events; and a 101 per cent increase in hours of O&M services delivered. Clients in regional areas can now access O&M services that are thorough, better able to meet their O&M needs, and comparable with services delivered in the metropolitan areas. The duration of O&M programs is now determined by the clients' individual goals and not by how long the O&M specialist is in the rural or regional centre. ROAM project participants provided feedback about ROAM via telephone surveys. Eighty-six per cent of respondents reported increases in their mobility and travel skills, ability to access their local community, and confidence. All respondents reported they would recommend ROAM to others. As with any service incorporating digital technology, the ROAM

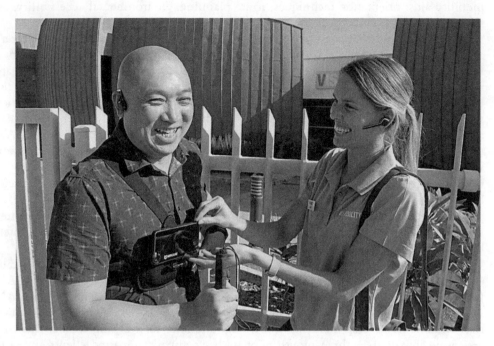

Figure 24.1 The client with the occupational therapist at a remote location, setting up
equipment for a ROAM session.
Image credit: VisAbility Engagement Marketing Team

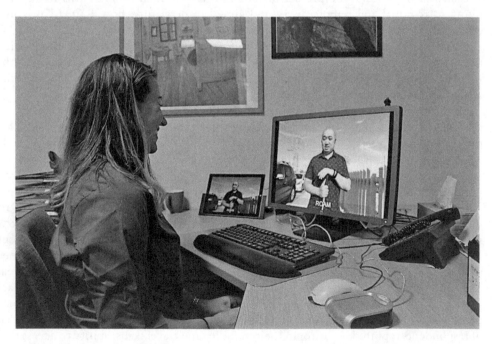

Figure 24.2 The O&M specialist providing remote instruction during a ROAM session.
Image credit: VisAbility Engagement Marketing Team

method will remain flexible and dynamic, integrating new developments in video conferencing equipment and technologies as required. There is compelling potential to apply ROAM best practices to a broad range of occupational therapy areas, and to expand access to therapies for other client groups using similar remote service delivery models.

Healthy Mothers Healthy Families

The Healthy Mothers Healthy Families (HMHF) program was developed in response to the health and well-being needs of Australian mothers of children with disability (Bourke-Taylor & Jane, 2018; Bourke-Taylor et al., 2019). The research is irrefutable that long-term caring can have negative repercussions on the mother and other family members with regards to finances, health and family relationships (Bourke-Taylor et al., 2012). Depression, anxiety and prolonged extreme stress are more common among mothers who are carers of children with disability (Commonwealth of Australia, 2011; Bourke-Taylor et al., 2012). A recent retrospective study investigated the cause of death in a large group of Australian mothers of children with disability compared to other mothers, who had died between 1983 and 2011. Findings identified a 40 per cent higher risk of death from cancer, a 150 per cent risk of death through cardiovascular disease, and a 200 per cent risk of death through misadventure—the mean age of the mothers at death was 42 years (Fairthorne et al., 2014).

Occupational therapists are experts in the needs and required supports of children and youth with a disability and are well positioned to team with other professionals to provide health and support services to families and carers. Occupational therapists can take a lead role in developing programs and accommodating the needs of carers in existing disability organisations by applying clinical knowledge and broader population-based approaches to health and well-being. One example is the HMHF program designed by occupational therapist, Dr Helen Bourke-Taylor, which is now available online. Other medical and health practitioners have contributed to the site, providing users of the online ten-module package with up-to-date professional information from general medical practice, dietetics, counselling, physiotherapy and occupational therapy.

Healthy Mothers Healthy Families is an evidence-informed program based on research that identified factors strongly associated with compromised well-being and caregiving capacity among mothers. These factors include lack of support and time for participation in healthy activities; lack of empowerment; child's behaviour; problems finding and accessing services; sleep; and paid work issues (Bourke-Taylor et al., 2012). Over eight years, HMHF workshops were delivered to groups of about 20 mothers by an inter-professional team and co-delivered with mothers of children with disability. In 2019–2020, seven mothers of children with disability were trained to facilitate the HMHF workshop, and 26 workshops were subsequently delivered to mothers across Victoria and Tasmania. Workshops occurred in local communities, thereby facilitating a local circle of support and connections with others. Aims of the HMHF program are for women to: be validated in their important and ongoing role as carers; be educated about women's health issues; learn strategies that will lead to empowerment and resiliency; learn about health services that may support their future health and well-being; and develop communication skills. Whilst interest in the program was high, about half the mothers cancelled their attendance at the workshop due to their caring requirements at home or their child's school.

Sustaining the HMHF program was also challenged by geographical disparity where many rural mothers did not have access to the program, and the number of mothers in need of the HMHF exceeded the number of trained facilitators available to deliver the program. Application of digital technology in the form of an online package proved to be the most feasible solution for program sustainability and upscale. The HMHF program now has a website (http://www.healthymothers-healthyfamilies.com) with the main sections of the workshop available online for mothers. Experts that were previously only available in the in-person workshops (i.e., health professionals and mothers with inspiring stories to tell) now share their information in the website via videos, worksheets and content within the ten modules. The online HMHF workshop content is accessible through any internet-enabled device, making the program accessible to an unlimited number of mothers and at their convenience.

The Australian Government targeted the health needs and service access of Australia's 2.7 million carers in 2020 through development of the Carer Gateway (https://www.carergateway.gov.au). The site provides carers with access to e-learning material specifically for carers and also various counselling (phone or online), coaching and skills courses. Carers who are often socially isolated and have limited time to access resources due to their carer role require flexible options to seek information and support. The HMHF program and Carer Gateway can help meet the needs of carers through their free online, interactive sites.

myWAY Employability: Supporting the transition to work for young people on the autism spectrum

The transition from high school into adulthood can be a challenging time for adolescents and especially for adolescents on the autism spectrum—many of whom find it difficult to plan for a future life. This is evidenced by unemployment rates among people on the autism spectrum that are six times higher than people without autism. Of the 44,000 young Australians on the autism spectrum who are aged 14–25 years, about 29,000 are unemployed or under-employed (The Foundation for Young Australians, 2018). Individuals on the spectrum have unique personal strengths and interests, and characteristics associated with their unique perceptions of the physical and social world around them that make them excellent potential employees. When environments are unable to accommodate the physical, emotional or cognitive characteristics of autistic individuals, this can result in disability (den Houting, 2019) manifested as anxiety, social communication difficulties, sensitivities to sensory and physical environments, and difficulties coping with unexpected change. A clear, coordinated approach to transition-planning increases the likelihood of school-leavers on the autism spectrum becoming employed or participating in post-secondary education or vocational training. Occupational therapists are involved in transition planning, but few existing resources for career exploration and goal setting consider the unique abilities and needs of autistic individuals (Murray et al., 2016).

myWAY Employability (www.mywayemployability.com.au) is an online evidence-based and individualised resource to guide young people on the autism spectrum in planning their transition from school to adulthood. The resource is also designed for people who provide formal and informal transition-planning support to young people on the spectrum, such as parents, family and friends; educators; allied health professionals (including occupational therapists); and employment support specialists. myWAY Employability is funded by the Telstra Foundation, and extensive co-production and consultation occurred among the co-creators of myWAY Employability—the Cooperative Research Centre for Living with Autism (Autism CRC) and Dr Marina Ciccarelli from Curtin University, and adolescents and young adults on the autism spectrum. This co-design was to guide the content and design features at all stages of development and ensure the resource is relevant, appropriate, and from the perspectives of autistic individuals—characteristics that are absent in existing career exploration and transition planning resources.

myWAY Employability adopts a strengths-based approach and incorporates the Better Outcomes and Successful Transitions for Autism (BOOST-A) career exploration and goal-setting tool that was developed by occupational therapy researchers at Curtin University in collaboration with young people on the spectrum. The five interrelated employability principles underpinning the BOOST-A are: (i) encourage the adolescent to dream big; (ii) start transition planning early, ideally in Year nine or as soon as possible; (iii) promote adolescent-centred planning; (iv) have a champion on the team; and (v) focus on the big picture of what work offers through real-life experiences such as work experience, part-time work or volunteering. The BOOST-A was evaluated in a national trial of 94 high-school-aged adolescents on the spectrum. The BOOST-A was found to be successful in building self-determination among young autistic people to plan and prepare for what they would do after they leave school (Hatfield et al., 2017).

The adolescent (or young adult) is prompted to provide information about their strengths, interests, sensory preferences, preferred learning styles and preferred working environments. They also identify any life skills they want to develop, such as independent mobility in the community, meal preparation and money management that may support their future employability. This information is used to provide suggestions for potential jobs that match their unique profile, which the adolescent can explore. They are empowered to create a team of supporters and schedule a first meeting to develop specific, measurable, achievable, realistic and timely (SMART) goals and allocate responsibilities. Goals, action plans and progress towards goals are shared electronically with the team and can be downloaded and used as part of NDIS planning for the adolescent. There are resources available providing information on a range of relevant topics including setting up a work experience; managing anxiety when using public transportation; entrance pathways for post-school education or training; applying for jobs; and rights and responsibilities in the workplace. Young people on the spectrum and peer mentors also share their experiences and advice through short videos.

Young people on the autism spectrum are empowered and supported to take an active role in planning their futures through the online activities that are scaffolded to provide a just-right challenge. This digital resource recognises that adolescents may find face-to-face discussions about planning their futures to be challenging and so activities can be completed at their own pace individually or with support if needed. Occupational therapists around Australia can incorporate myWAY Employability into the transition planning services they provide and the resources they share with adolescents on the spectrum and their families, and teachers, to promote self-determination and build potential for future employment.

Immersive extended realities to promote occupational engagement and performance

Extended reality is an umbrella term that includes augmented and virtual realities. Three applications of extended reality in occupational therapy practice and the associated research are described next.

Virtual embodiment therapy in rehabilitation

Assisting people to manage complex and chronic health issues can be challenging. The immersive quality of virtual reality makes it an effective tool in modifying a person's perception. When used to challenge perceptions that make it difficult to progress, virtual reality has the potential to offer radical new therapies to improve quality of life. One of the most exciting and intriguing areas is the use of virtual reality in physical and neurological rehabilitation through virtual embodiment therapy.

Virtual embodiment therapy uses an avatar to retrain the brain using principles of neuroplasticity, pain education, visual augmentation techniques and corrective movement practice. An avatar is a digital representation of the person's body in virtual environments. The avatar provides opportunity for a person to simulate their limb movements in the virtual environment, as shown in Figure 24.3.

Over time, repeated simulation of movement and performing functional activities through an avatar facilitates neuroplasticity to aid with rehabilitation. The immersive multisensory and multimodal qualities of virtual reality facilitate an engaging approach to therapy. Virtual reality training scenarios can be designed to simulate various activities of daily living, such as playing with a (virtual) dog, preparing a meal and shopping in the community. Improved perception of body ownership and reduction in neuropathic pain symptoms were reported by people with spinal cord injuries following interventions that used virtual reality (Pozeg et al., 2017).

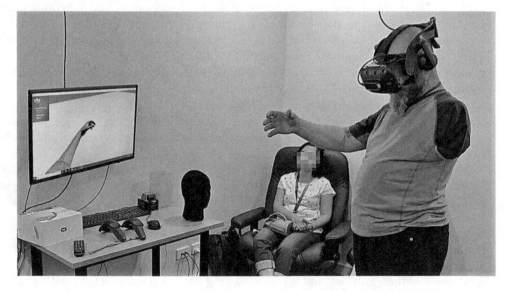

Figure 24.3 Using immersive virtual reality to improve upper limb function following traumatic injury.

Virtual reality uses a wide field of vision and spatial audio input to the user that create a realistic sense of presence in the virtual world. High-quality computer-generated images can immerse the viewer in any scene, including calming environments such as a forest, a waterfall, a beach, or even space. The ability to look around, move and interact with objects in these environments adds to the immersion and sense of presence. The brain has to attend to a stimulus such as pain to perceive it. Virtual reality environments can provide such a degree of visual distraction that it can be beneficial for relaxation and alleviating symptoms of anxiety and pain. Recently, researchers at Cedars Sinai Hospital in New York found that interacting in a virtual reality environment significantly reduced pain among patients (Tashjian et al., 2017), and Ian Cheok, an occupational therapist at LifeWorks Occupational Therapy in Perth, Western Australia, incorporates virtual reality into his pain management program.

Individualised management of anxiety and phobias with virtual reality simulations

Virtual reality has potential therapeutic benefits in mental health interventions. Preliminary studies have identified that virtual reality exposure therapy (VRET) may be useful in helping people manage anxiety and phobias (Botella et al., 2017; Parsons & Rizzo, 2008). Researchers have hypothesised that by gradually exposing an individual to situations that cause distress, they will gradually adapt and learn to cope with the stressors. Virtual reality technology can immerse an individual into simulated environments that they perceive as stressful, such as a crowded public place, revisiting an accident location, being in a high place or speaking in public. The goal of the virtual reality intervention is to reduce avoidance behaviours so that the person is able to resume their daily activities without being limited by anxiety or fear. Clinical trials suggest a reduction in post-traumatic stress disorder symptoms for people who received VRET (Gonçalves et al., 2012). This unique application of virtual reality technology has potential as a useful modality for occupational therapists working in mental health.

An avatar to improve communication skills among carers of people living with dementia

Dementia-specific training has the potential to improve how professional carers provide person-centred care (Elliott et al., 2012) and support staff to manage increasingly complex and demanding roles (Elliott et al., 2013). Training carers in communication with people with dementia is important because improved communication supports the well-being and quality of life of people with dementia (Eggenberger et al., 2013). In Australia, formal carers are trained to communicate with people with dementia using DVDs or traditional classroom activities; however, training that includes active engagement is more effective in developing communication skills (Morris et al., 2018). Using realistic simulation-based training techniques increases the clinical skills of student health professionals more than traditional lectures or computer-based programs (Harder, 2010). Simulation-based training supports students to develop strong links between theoretical information and application in practice contexts (Lateef, 2010). A virtual learning environment developed by researchers at Curtin University (the Curtin University Empathy Simulator—CUES). The CUES features an older male (Jim) living in a clinic environment, and an older couple (Jim and his wife Moira)

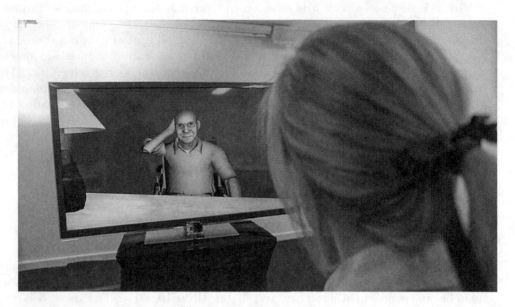

Figure 24.4 The Curtin University Empathy Simulator.
Image credit: J. Beilby, Curtin University & J. Spitalnick, Citrine Technologies

living at home. Jim is a retired farmer who presents with varying levels of dementia (see Figure 24.4). A trained operator controls Jim's 45 verbal and non-verbal responses, allowing real-time communication.

The CUES is effective in improving communication skills among student health professionals (Quail et al., 2016), but less is known about how training with the CUES improves communication in clinical practice. Curtin University occupational therapy and speech pathology researchers evaluated the feasibility of using the CUES for training community-based support workers in how to communicate with people with dementia. Support workers received training that combined an initial interaction with the CUES, small group training, and follow-up interaction with the CUES. Each participant was observed communicating with a person with dementia, and with the CUES before and immediately after the training, and then two months later. The researchers collected information using observations of the support workers' communication skills and a questionnaire about their knowledge of dementia before and after the training, and an interview with the support workers at the two-month follow-up.

Support workers improved in their knowledge, satisfaction, and use of appropriate communication strategies when communicating with the avatar and with people with dementia after the CUES training and at the two-month follow-up, regardless of their prior knowledge of dementia. Some of the support workers found the experience of speaking with an avatar strange and uncomfortable.

More research is needed into the use of augmented reality and avatars for training health professionals, formal carers and family members of people with dementia and other cognitive and communication needs. Implementation of augmented and virtual realities show promise in occupational therapy practice; however, it is not a panacea for all occupational performance issues. More clinical trials and education are required to determine for whom this novel approach to occupational therapy is both safe and effective.

Translating the National Disability Insurance Scheme Housing Policy into an online game space and 3D virtual housing tours

An important role of occupational therapists is to collaborate with people living with disability or chronic health conditions to consider assistive and mainstream technologies, home modifications or accessible housing design (Ainsworth & de Jonge, 2018; Steel et al., 2017; Waldron & Layton, 2008). Specific to environmental controls, occupational therapists have traditionally been involved in assessment and advice on systems for home automation and communication (e.g., to control lights, blinds, doors or intercom systems). However, the emerging mainstream smart home technology retail market is offering additional capability in this area. Movement sensing technologies and artificial intelligence are creating options to identify and learn 'typical' versus 'out of the ordinary' patterns of daily activity. This allows the construct of a range of customised 'if this, then that' responses. These responses may include checking with the user, initiating alerts or contacting a nominated third party in the case of the need for assistance, and are designed to maintain independent living and participation in daily tasks (Brandt et al., 2011). The capacity to retrofit these and other smart technologies—including smart switches, smart lights and automated door or blind openers—into housing means that in place of more expensive base-build cabling, often all that is required is wireless internet capability (Callaway & Tregloan, 2018).

The introduction of Australia's NDIS has included new policies guiding development of coordinated housing, assistive technology and support responses, called Specialist Disability Accommodation (SDA) (Commonwealth of Australia, 2016; Callaway & Tregloan, 2018). Given this policy change, there is a need to assist people with disability, their families, occupational therapists and architects to understand application of NDIS SDA rules and guidelines within built design. To address this need, an interactive website was developed, called My Home Space (www.myhomespace.org). My Home Space was co-designed by an occupational therapist and architect with NDIS participants and their families to ensure relevance for users (Tregloan & Callaway, 2017). Its development was guided by the implementation of Australia's ten-year National Disability Strategy, and evidenced post-occupancy evaluations undertaken (Callaway et al., 2016; Department of Social Services, 2015; Tregloan & Callaway, 2019). My Home Space translates Australia's National Disability Strategy principles and NDIS SDA policy and rules (Commonwealth of Australia, 2016) into 3D interactive housing tours and 2D detailed plan drawings of key considerations within housing, technology, support and community design.

My Home Space presents key findings from research and policy in an accessible 'gamespace' format: the My Home Space tool (see Figure 24.5). This tool (accessed from the main library of the website), and its embedded suite of 3D virtual housing tours, allow the user to select and navigate through different housing types (e.g., apartment, villa/townhouse, house) and NDIS SDA design categories (e.g., improved liveability, robust, fully accessible, high physical support needs) (National Disability Insurance Scheme, 2019). Users can explore the application of NDIS SDA design guidelines, policies and associated rules in these 3D virtual spaces, via embedded text and graphic detail.

Information detail the user explores can be filtered via a 2D plan level entry point to the My Home Space tool. Categories of information include 'assistive technology', 'tenant experience', 'standards' and 'circulation and safety'. Details of specific activity types including cooking, dressing, bathing and socialising can also be filtered in the

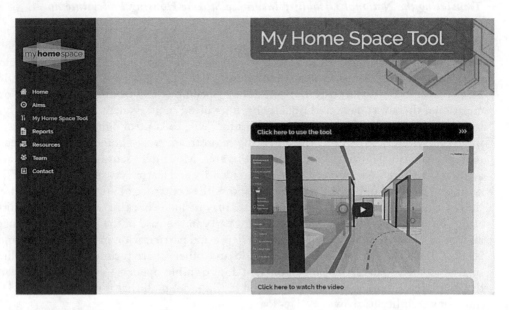

Figure 24.5 Access to the My Home Space tool via the website main library.
Image credit: Libby Callaway

tool. Before they move from the 2D plan view to the 3D navigable spaces, the user's view can be set to their eye height in centimetres. At this point, the user can enter the 3D virtual housing tour. They can navigate through different indoor and outside areas of a virtual home and click on text box information or the 2D detail buttons in each main area (e.g., external areas of the home, the bedroom, bathroom, or kitchen). Users can also explore 2D detail drawings relating to support delivery and use of assistive technology. This allows each user to explore further detail of NDIS SDA design rules and guidance relating to these areas of consideration, applied to their individual context.

The use of technology to develop the online gamespace and 3D virtual housing tours in My Home Space offers innovation, accessible research and policy translation methods. These methods can assist people with disability and their families, occupational therapists, designers and funding bodies to understand and apply government policy regarding housing and technology design in real-world contexts.

Designing with technology to improve participation in occupations

3D printing of upper limb prosthetic devices

Occupational therapists commonly work in interdisciplinary upper limb prosthetic rehabilitation teams and provide input into the design and functional training needed to use the prosthetic device. Prosthetic limbs are typically custom-designed and custom-made for each patient by a qualified prosthetist (Eklund & Sexton, 2017). Properly fabricated prostheses have sockets that closely replicate a residual or incomplete limb or stump, and specially fitted attachments (Therapeutic Goods Administration, 2017). Consumers should also receive training in their use.

The Fourth Industrial Revolution, in which manufacturing technology will soon be in most people's homes, has created an emerging phenomenon of Do–It–Yourself Assistive Technology (DIY-AT). One example is e-NABLE, a bottom-up virtual collection of volunteer engineers, academics, 3D-printing enthusiasts, occupational therapists, designers, parents and teachers. Their goal is to use 3D printing to create affordable prosthetic devices for children and under-served populations with upper limb differences around the world, as only 5 per cent of those needing prosthetic care worldwide have access (World Health Organization, 2017). It is important to note, however, that devices produced by volunteer makers are *not prostheses*, although many makers refer to them as such. The Australian Orthotic Prosthetic Association (AOPA), whilst welcoming new technologies that offer consumers greater choices, highlighted the many real safety, health and emotional risks when providing prosthetic devices without the regulatory frameworks and controls within which qualified prosthetists work (Australian Orthotic Prosthetic Association, 2017).

In 2018, Dr Lisa O'Brien, an Australian occupational therapist and accredited hand therapist, explored the issues of design and delivery of 3D-printed prosthetic hand devices. She met with the AOPA and expert prosthetists, occupational therapists, engineers and designers in Europe and North America. She has strongly discouraged models of practice which involve makers/designers creating prosthetic devices remotely (i.e., without working face-to-face with the consumer and their health care team), responding to evidence that these are not successful. Achieving good socket interface is crucial; however, downloadable designs have inadequate sockets, raising the risk of skin injury and the likelihood of device abandonment. Follow-up care with skilled health practitioners is recommended for re-fitting of devices as required, along with training consumers in how to use the devices to do the activities they want and need to do. Consumer training is clearly an area in which occupational therapists have an important role.

Dr O'Brien subsequently collaborated with an international team of prosthetists, biomechanical engineers and human movement experts to test a new passive adjustable prosthetic hand with Australian consumers. This device—the Self Grasping Hand—was developed at Delft University of Technology in the Netherlands and requires no harness or cable to activate its grasp and release mechanism (see Figure 24.6). It combines a strong and lightweight metal skeleton with a 3D-printed shell fabricated using Selective Laser Sintering (SLS). This method of printing produces smoother, stronger and more precise shapes than the cheaper and more commonly used Fused Deposition Modelling (FDM). A prosthetist fitted the Self Grasping Hand to consumers' existing sockets and an occupational therapist conducted customised training in how to operate the grasp and release function to perform common bimanual tasks (e.g., tying shoelaces). Accelerometers were worn on the intact wrist, the Self Grasping Hand, and usual terminal device (e.g., split hook). After two weeks of using the hand at home and work, participants completed the Orthotics and Prosthetics Users' Survey Function Scale and the Trinity Amputations and Prosthesis Experience Scale. Data from the accelerometers were uploaded into software to calculate percentage of total prosthesis wear-time and identify patterns of bilateral limb use.

Data obtained from consumers and accelerometers showed that the Self Grasping Hand is a promising design for people who currently use a cosmetic hand, but is unlikely to be adopted by long-term users of body powered split hooks who require grips that are more powerful. The team are currently working on more advanced models of the hand that will include easier activation of the grasp and release mechanism.

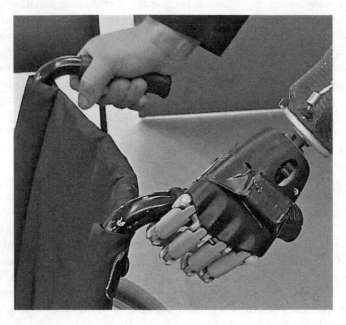

Figure 24.6 The Self Grasping Hand (version 1) being tested by a consumer.
Image credit: Lisa O'Brien

Conclusion

Life in modern Australian society is influenced by constantly evolving social, financial and environmental factors that may affect the occupations of individuals, families and communities and their need for occupational therapy services on a local or global scale. Twenty-first century technologies are emerging rapidly, presenting a digital transformation of occupational therapy practice. Agile occupational therapists see opportunities to combine emergent technologies with other intervention tools. This chapter has outlined examples where occupational therapists have collaborated with other health professionals, technology specialists, consumers and families to create technology-enabled solutions that met an emergent individual or community need. This can further facilitate participation in meaningful occupations, build autonomy among individuals and groups, change how support is received, and offer ability to monitor and respond to health and safety issues in everyday life

VisaAbility's remote orientation and mobility training of vision-impaired people; the Healthy Mothers Healthy Families program supporting at risk mothers; and the online myWAY Employability to support autistic individuals to build capacity to participate in work occupations all offer accessible remote occupational therapy services to communities, regardless of the recipients' geographic location. These services were all co-designed with end users, are delivered to scale, and help reduce inequities in access to services, especially for people living in rural and remote communities. These shared characteristics are hallmarks of successful telehealth services that have become vital in recent times in response to the physical distancing requirements of the global COVID-19 pandemic. The applied immersive virtual and augmented reality technologies in physical rehabilitation, pain management and communication skills training describe 'early adopters' using customisable 'just-right' experiences in low-risk environments to facilitate participation in valued occupations among consumers, for whom existing conventional services have not been effective. Finally, the digital My Home Space and the 3D-printed Self Grasping Hand exemplify how occupational therapists can use technologies for customised design purposes. These technology-enabled solutions allow occupational therapists to collaborate with consumers to provide bespoke and affordable solutions that meet their individual needs.

The lesson from these examples of technology-enabled occupational therapy practices is that occupational therapists can embrace digital transformation and be innovative and prudent in their use of emerging technologies to drive new practice approaches in changing times. Co-design, collaboration and openness to technology-enabled ways of working are characteristics that will underpin future occupational therapy practice that is agile and responsive to the changing and sometimes unpredictable needs of modern society.

Summary

- Occupational therapists in Australia are using emergent technologies to meet the diverse occupational needs of people across the lifespan in contemporary society.
- Responses to recent states of emergency in Australia, including national bushfire disasters and pandemic infectious disease, have placed restrictions on human interactions and access to medical and allied health services. Emergent technologies offer potential solutions for the remote delivery of occupational therapy services to the community.
- Occupational therapists use an individualised approach in the application of emergent technologies to create co-design partnerships, modify environments and empower individuals, groups and communities to achieve active participation in meaningful occupations.
- Re-imagined occupational therapy practice aims to utilise an evidence-based approach to the development and implementation of programs and services.

Review questions

1. Select any three of the examples of re-imagined occupational therapy practice initiatives or programs described in this chapter. Describe the unique community need identified in each area and explain how the technology-based initiative/program complements traditional service delivery to promote participation in a meaningful occupation for the target population.
2. Consider the multicultural nature of contemporary Australian society. How might the practice initiatives/programs described in this chapter be relevant across different socio-demographic groups in the community? What adaptations to the initiatives may be required to increase inclusion?
3. What aspect(s) of occupational performance does the technology-enabled occupational therapy services impact? For example, are there modifications to the environment(s), adaptations to the how occupations are performed, or changes to the person's capacities?

References

Ainsworth, E., & de Jonge, D. (Eds.) (2018). *An occupational therapist's guide to home modification practice* (2nd edn). SLACK Inc.

Australian Institute of Health and Welfare. (2018). *Australia's health 2018.* https://www.aihw.gov.au/reports/australias-health/australias-health-2018/contents/table-of-contents

Australian Orthotic Prosthetic Association. (2017). *Prosthetic inaccuracies reported by the Australian media.* https://www.aopa.org.au/news/prosthetic-inaccuracies-reported-by-the-australian-media

Bishop, L., Ransom, A., & Laverty, M. (2017). *Health care access, mental health, and preventive health: Health priority survey findings for people in the bush.* https://rfds-media.s3.amazonaws.com/files/RN032_Healths_Needs_Survey_Result-no_crop_marks_P3.pdf

Botella, C., Fernández-Álvarez, J., Guillén, V., García-Palacios, A., & Baños, R. (2017). Recent progress in virtual reality exposure therapy for phobias: A systematic review. *Current Psychiatry Reports, 19,* 1–13. https://doi.org/10.1007/s11920-017-0788-4

Bourke-Taylor, H., & Jane, F. (2018). Mothers' experiences of a women's health and empowerment program for mothers of a child with a disability. *Journal of Autism and Developmental Disorders, 48,* 2174–2186. https://doi.org/10.1007/s10803-018-3486-0

Bourke-Taylor, H., Jane, F., & Peat, J. (2019). Healthy Mothers Healthy Families workshop intervention: A preliminary investigation of healthy lifestyle changes for mothers of a child with a disability. *Journal of Autism and Developmental Disorders, 49*(9), 935–949. https://doi.org/10.1007/s10803-018-3789-1

Bourke-Taylor, H., Pallant, J. F., Law, M., & Howie, L. (2012). Predicting mental health among mothers of school-aged children with developmental disabilities: The relative contribution of child, maternal and environmental factors. *Research in Developmental Disabilities, 33*(6), 1732–1740. https://doi.org/10.1016/j.ridd.2012.04.011

Brandt, Å., Samuelsson, K., Töytäri, O., & Salminen, A. L. (2011). Activity and participation, quality of life and user satisfaction outcomes of environmental control systems and smart home technology: A systematic review. *Disability and Rehabilitation: Assistive Technology, 6*(3), 189–206. https://doi.org/10.3109/17483107.2010.532286

Callaway, L., & Tregloan, K. (2018). Government perspectives on housing, technology and support design within Australia's National Disability Strategy. *Australian Journal of Social Issues, 53*(3), 206–222. https://doi.org/10.1002/ajs4.40

Callaway, L., Tregloan, K., Williams, G., & Clark, R. (2016). Evaluating access and mobility within a new model of supported housing for people with neurotrauma: A pilot study. *Brain Impairment, 17*(1), 64–76. https://doi.org/10.1017/BrImp.2016.7

Commonwealth of Australia. (2011). *National Carer Strategy Action Plan (2011–2014).* https://www.dss.gov.au/sites/default/files/documents/10_2012/ncs_action_plan.pdf

Commonwealth of Australia. (2013). *My Aged Care.* https://www.myagedcare.gov.au/

Commonwealth of Australia. (2016). *Federal Register of Legislation: National Disability Insurance Scheme (Specialist Disability Accommodation) Rules 2016.* https://www.legislation.gov.au/Series/F2017L00209/Amendments

den Houting, J. (2019). Neurodiversity: An insider's perspective. *Autism, 23*(2), 271–273. https://doi.org/10.1177/1362361318820762

Department of Health. (2020). *Bushfire information and support.* https://www.health.gov.au/health-topics/emergency-health-management/bushfire-information-and-support

Department of Social Services. (2011). *National Disability Strategy (2010–2020).* https://www.dss.gov.au/our-responsibilities/disability-and-carers/publications-articles/policy-research/national-disability-strategy-2010-2020

Department of Social Services. (2015). *National Disability Strategy Second Implementation Plan: Driving Action 2015–2018.* https://www.dss.gov.au/disability-and-carers/programs-services/government-international/national-disability-strategy-second-implementation-plan

Eklund, A., & Sexton, S. (2017). *WHO standards for prosthetics and orthotics.* World Health Organization. http://www.who.int/rehabilitation/prosthetics-and-orthotics-standards/en/

Eggenberger, E., Heimerl, K., & Bennett, M. I. (2013). Communication skills training in dementia care: A systematic review of effectiveness, training content, and didactic methods in different care settings. *International Psychogeriatrics, 25*(3), 345–358. https://doi.org/10.1017/S1041610212001664

Elliott, K.-E. J., Scott, J. L., Stirling, C., Martin, A. J., & Robinson, A. (2012). Building capacity and resilience in the dementia care workforce: A systematic review of interventions targeting worker and organizational outcomes. *International Psychogeriatrics, 24*(6), 882–894. https://doi.org/10.1017/S1041610211002651

Elliott, K.-E., Stirling, C. M., Martin, A. J., Robinson, A. L., & Scott, J. L. (2013). Perspectives of the community-based dementia care workforce: 'occupational commnion' a key finding from the Work 4 Dementia Project. *International Psychogeriatrics, 25*(5), 765–774. https://doi.org/10.1017/S1041610212002323

Fairthorne, J., Hammond, G., Bourke, J., Jacoby, P., & Leonard, H. (2014). Early mortality and primary causes of death in mothers of children with intellectual disability or Autism Spectrum Disorder: A retrospective cohort study. *PLoS ONE, 9*(12), 1–15. https://doi.org/10.1371/journal.pone.0113430

Gonçalves, R., Pedrozo, A. L., Coutinho, E. S. F., Figueira, I., & Ventura, P. (2012). Efficacy of virtual reality exposure therapy in the treatment of PTSD: A systematic review. *PLoS ONE, 7*(12), e48469. https://doi.org/10.1371/journal.pone.0048469

Harder, B. (2010). Use of simulation in teaching and learning in health sciences: A systematic review. *Journal of Nursing Education, 49*(1), 23–28. https://doi.org/10.3928/01484834-20090828-08

Hatfield, M., Falkmer, M., Falkmer, T., & Ciccarelli, M. (2017). Effectiveness of the BOOST-A online transition planning program for adolescents on the autism spectrum: A quasi-randomized controlled trial. *Child and Adolescent Psychiatry and Mental Health, 11*(54). https://doi.org/10.1186/s13034-017-0191-2

Hinings, B., Gegenhuber, T., & Greenwood, R. (2018). Digital innovation and transformation: An institutional perspective. *Information and Organization, 28*(1), 52–61. https://doi.org/10.1016/j.infoandorg.2018.02.004

Lateef, F. (2010). Simulation-based learning: Just like the real thing. *Journal of Emergencies, Trauma and Shock, 3*(4), 348–352. http://www.onlinejets.org/text.asp?2010/3/4/348/70743

Morris, L., Horne, M., McEvoy, P., & Williamson, T. (2018). Communication training interventions for family and professional carers of people living with dementia: A systematic review of effectiveness, acceptability and conceptual basis. *Aging & Mental Health, 22*(7), 863–880. https://doi.org/10.1080/13607863.2017.1399343

Murray, N., Hatfield, M., Falkmer, M., & Falkmer, T. (2016). Evaluation of career planning tools for use with individuals with autism spectrum disorder: A systematic review. *Research in Autism Spectrum Disorders, 23*, 188–202. https://doi.org/10.1016/j.rasd.2015.12.007

Mynard, L. (2020). Normal life has been disrupted: Managing the disruption caused by COVID-19. https://otaus.com.au/publicassets/af469002-6f6a-ea11-9404-005056be13b5/OT%20Guide%20COVID-19%20March%202020.pdf

National Disability Insurance Scheme. (2019). *Specialist Disability Accommodation overview.* https://www.ndis.gov.au/providers/housing-and-living-supports-and-services/housing/specialist-disability-accommodation

Parsons, T. D., & Rizzo, A. A. (2008). Affective outcomes of virtual reality exposure therapy for anxiety and specific phobias: A meta-analysis. *Journal of Behavior Therapy and Experimental Psychiatry, 39*(3), 250–261. https://doi.org/10.1016/j.jbtep.2007.07.007

Pozeg, P., Palluel, E., Ronchi, R., Solcà, M., Al-Khodairy, A.-W., Jordan, X., Kassouha, A., & Blanke, O. (2017). Virtual reality improves embodiment and neuropathic pain caused by spinal cord injury. *Neurology, 89*(18), 1894–1903. https://doi.org/10.1212/WNL.0000000000004585

Quail, M., Brundage, S., Spitalnick, J., Allen, P. J., & Beilby, J. (2016). Student self-reported communication skills, knowledge and confidence across standardised patient, virtual and traditional clinical learning environments. *BMC Medical Education, 16*, 73. https://doi. org/10.1186/s12909-016-0577-5

Steel, E. J., Buchanan, R., Layton, N., & Wilson, E. (2017). Currency and competence of oc-cupational therapists and consumers with rapidly changing technology. *Occupational Therapy International, 12* (5612843). https://doi.org/10.1155/2017/5612843

Tashjian, V. C., Mosadeghi, S., Howard, A. R., Lopez, M., Dupuy, T., Reid, M., Martinez, B., Ahmed, S., Dailey, F., Robbins, K., Rosen, B., Fuller, G., Danovitch, I., IsHak, W., & Spiegel, B. (2017). Virtual reality for management of pain in hospitalized patients: Results of a controlled trial. *JMIR Mental Health, 4*(1), e9. https://doi.org/10.2196/mental.7387

The Foundation for Young Australians. (2018). *The new work reality*. https://www.fya.org.au/wp-content/uploads/2018/06/FYA_TheNewWorkReality_sml.pdf

Therapeutic Goods Administration. (2017). *Proposed regulatory changes related to personalised and 3D printed medical devices. Consultation paper*. https://www.tga.gov.au/sites/default/files/consultation-proposed-regulatory-changes-related-personalised-and-3d-printed-medical-devices.pdf

Tregloan, K. A., & Callaway, L. (2017). *My Home Space: Interactive information resources for the design of housing, technology, and support within Australia's National Disability Strategy*. www.myhomespace.org

Tregloan, K., & Callaway, L. (2019). *OpenHouse CoLab: Projects*. https://www.openhousecolab.com/colab-projects-1

Waldron, D., & Layton, N. (2008). Hard and soft assistive technologies: Defining roles for clinicians. *Australian Occupational Therapy Journal, 55*(1), 61–64. https://doi.org/10.1111/j.1440-1630.2007.00707.x

Wilcock, A. A. (2006). *An occupational perspective of health* (2nd edn). SLACK Inc.

World Health Organization. (2017). *WHO standards for prosthetics and orthotics*. https://www.who.int/phi/implementation/assistive_technology/prosthetics-and-orthotics/en/

World Health Organization. (2019a). *Coronavirus disease (COVID-19) pandemic*. https://www.who.int/emergencies/diseases/novel-coronavirus-2019

World Health Organization. (2019b). *Coronavirus disease (COVID-19) advice for the public*. https://www.who.int/emergencies/diseases/novel-coronavirus-2019/advice-for-public

25 Occupational therapy assessment

Ted Brown and Helen Bourke-Taylor

Chapter objectives

Upon completion of this chapter, the reader will be able to:

* Provide an overview of the purpose of assessment, approaches to assessment and types of assessment in an occupational therapy context.
* Describe top-down and bottom-up assessments.
* Outline the skills, attributes, areas and domains that occupational therapists typically assess.
* Present a summary of the tests, scales and measures typically used by occupational therapists in their professional practice.

Key terms

assessment; test; scale; measurement; validity; reliability; psychometrics; occupational performance

Introduction

As part of professional practice, occupational therapists must be knowledgeable in their selection, administration, scoring and interpretation of assessments for a broad range of occupational therapy clients. Assessment is one of the most fundamental, yet very complex, aspects of what therapists do in their day-to-day practice. In its broadest sense, assessment assists an occupational therapist to make reasoned and informed decisions about goal setting, therapy planning, intervention provision and re-evaluation. Ultimately, effective assessment permits a therapist to better understand the unique situation and occupational needs of any client and his/her family. Therefore, assessment is a crucial part of a collaborative therapeutic process and intervention. This chapter will provide an introductory overview of the purpose, approaches and types of assessments within an occupational therapy context. Features of 'top-down' and 'bottom-up' assessments plus the occupational performance domains which therapists typically assess will be outlined. Finally, a list of commonly used assessments with children and adults will be provided and assessments authored by Australian occupational therapists will be highlighted.

Purpose of assessment

Assessments are best categorised as having descriptive, discriminative, predictive and evaluative purposes (Brown, 2012). Descriptive assessments can establish an individual's baseline skill set (e.g., cognitive, motor, psychological, social, affective, self-care, play/ leisure, productivity, education, social participation, sleep) and indicate if he/she falls within typically expected score ranges. Descriptive assessments provide a baseline or way of describing functional status to inform goal setting and intervention planning. Discriminative assessments are norm-based tools that aim to distinguish between individuals or groups on some characteristic or underlying dimension (Fawcett, 2007). They determine whether a client is functioning in the specified range of typical development or performance and can classify individuals into groups of different abilities (e.g., above average, average or below average) or discernible traits.

Some assessment scores are used to predict a client's future performance. Specifically, predictive assessments 'classify people onto pre-defined categories of interest in an attempt to predict an event or functional status in another situation' (Fawcett, 2007, p. 99). For example, children's performance on the *Beery Buktenica Developmental Test of Visual Motor Integration* (Beery VMI) (Beery et al., 2010) in kindergarten was found to be predictive of future academic performance and handwriting skills in subsequent grades (Kurdek & Sinclair, 2000; Lee et al., 2016; van Hartingsveldt et al., 2015).

Evaluative assessments or outcome measures detect changes over time. Evaluation tools such as the Goal Attainment Scaling (Kiresuk & Sherman, 1968) or Perceived Efficacy and Goal Setting (Missiuna et al., 2004) may be selected as outcome measures. Evaluative assessments will provide both the occupational therapist and the client with an objective indication of meaningful progress during or following occupational therapy intervention.

Approaches to and types of assessment

Assessments can have various categories or classifications. The two primary classifications are formal and informal (Brown, 2012). Formal assessments have established protocols directing the method of administration, guidelines for standardised use, established validity and reliability, and standardised scores (e.g., percentile rank, standard score, z-score, T-score, stanine score, scaled score), which are generated from raw scores. Informal assessments (also known as dynamic or clinical observations) are less structured and formal in their administration (Neaum, 2016; Shulman, 2013). Often the assessor is less directive and observes the client completing tasks in naturalistic settings. Dynamic observation of a person participating in an important occupation may warrant more formal assessment, or implementation of collaborative goal setting as a part of the occupational therapy process. Dynamic observation also constitutes an example of a descriptive type of assessment.

Assessments can also be clinically and/or research orientated. Professionals use clinical assessments to gather baseline information about a client's diagnosis, functional skills or current status. This data is important in informing and guiding decisions about therapy goal setting and intervention planning. Examples of clinical assessments include the *Peabody Developmental Motor Scales—2nd edition* (Folio & Fewell, 2000) and the *Sensory Processing Measure* (Glennon et al., 2007). Research-orientated assessments are designed for research purposes and aim to gather information to answer research questions.

Assessments usually have concurrent clinical and research purposes. The Movement Assessment Battery for Children—2nd edition (Henderson et al., 2007) and the Beery VMI are often used to clinically assess children suspected of presenting with Developmental Coordination Disorder (DCD) (Blank et al., 2012). The *Movement Assessment Battery for Children—2nd edition* is also frequently used in research to assess and monitor children's motor skills.

Assessment tools vary in how they elicit client perspectives and measure client performance (Hocking, 2001). The perspective or performance of a client may be directly sought and measured (e.g., self-report); a person knowledgeable about the client's perspective or performance may be sought (e.g., third party or proxy report); or the occupational therapist may score, rate or evaluate the client's perspective or performance. Some assessments use ratings of clients' performance, such as the *Test of Gross Motor Skills—3rd edition* (Ulrich, 2019) which assesses children's gross movement skills by having the examining therapist rate children's performance when running, hopping and jumping. Some assessments use client self-report. For example, the *Beck Depression Inventory* (Beck et al., 1996), *Self-Perception Profile* (Harter, 1985) and the *Piers–Harris Self-Concept Scale—3rd edition* (Piers et al., 2018) are completed by the client and scored by the practitioner.

Other assessments use third party proxy report. Children's parents and classroom teachers are often asked to complete standardised questionnaires about children. The *Sensory Processing Measure—Preschool* (Glennon et al., 2010), the *Child Behavior Checklist* (Achenbach & Rescorla, 2001) and the *Children Participation Questionnaire—School* (Rosenberg & Bart, 2015) are examples of proxy report scales.

Standardised tests and scales all have a set of specific characteristics. Tests are designed to measure a defined construct, ability or attribute. The construct is subsequently operationalised into specific items (and related subscales) that are rated, answered or performed by the clients being assessed. For example, self-concept is an overarching construct and its sub-constructs (such as academic self-concept, social self-concept, athletic self-concept and family self-concept) (Butler & Gasson, 2005; Piers et al., 2018) are assessable through items considered to adequately represent the construct. Children's motor skills may be assessed through the completion of a series of standardised motor skills tasks (or items) rated by an experienced examiner using specific criteria.

As stated, standardised tests have a manual or set of instructions describing use, application and interpretation. The manual will typically contain details of how the test was developed, standardised and validated. Test authors complete various psychometric studies that confirm or report on reliability, validity, responsiveness, interpretability and utility features of the test. Types of reliability usually reported about a test include internal consistency, test–retest reliability, intra-/inter-rater reliability, and measurement error (Fawcett, 2007; Mokkink et al., 2010; Shaughnessy et al., 2006). Types of validity traditionally featured in the psychometric development and evaluation of tools include content validity (which includes face validity), criterion validity (which includes concurrent validity and predictive validity) and construct validity (which includes structural validity, hypothesis testing and cross-cultural validity) (Brown, 2012; Mokkink et al., 2010; Shaughnessy et al., 2006). Other types of validity also reported in the literature include convergent validity, divergent validity, ecological validity, internal validity, external validity, known-groups validity, discriminant validity, representation validity (also known as translation validity), statistical conclusion validity and factorial validity (Brown, 2012; Classen & Velozo, 2019; Davidson, 2014).

Authors of standardised tests typically gather a large dataset of scores, known as a normative sample. The normative sample often mirrors a population's traits (e.g., gender, age, ethnicity, socio-economic status, geographical distribution) based on census data. Test authors then use the standardisation sample to generate performance scores to compare test-takers against. Score examples include stanines, z-scores, standard scores, percentile ranks and age equivalents (Kubiszyn & Borich, 2013).

The final trait of a standardised test is its ongoing and iterative refinement and revision. A body of empirical literature is usually established about its measurement properties and its application in different contexts (e.g., with diverse client groups, applied in cross-cultural environments). This evidence is dynamic and continually supplemented by test-users and researchers; subsequently the test constantly evolves. The *Assessment of Motor and Process Skills* (AMPS) (Fisher & Bray Jones, 2010) and the Beery VMI are tests with substantial bodies of empirical work published about their use, application and measurement properties and these tests are used by occupational therapists.

In psychometric theory, the two primary approaches to developing standardised tests are Classical Test Theory (CTT) and Item Response Theory (IRT). Both CTT and IRT generate measures of a standardised test's reliability and validity (Salkind, 2010). CTT is based on the guiding principle that 'observed test scores (TO) are composed of a true score (T) and an error score (E) where the true and the error scores are independent' (Magno, 2009, p. 1) and is represented by the formula TO = T + E. The assumption in CCT is that each individual who completes a test would have a true score if there were no errors in measurement present (Franzen, 2011). However, given that tests and measures are often imprecise, the test scores obtained by respondents are often inaccurate or different from their actual (true) capabilities (Frey, 2017). IRT is a newer branch of psychometric theory and focuses on respondents' chances of answering assessment items correctly or incorrectly given their ability (Reise, 2014). Another component of IRT is that the performance of a test item is related to the amount of the latent trait in a respondent it measures (Thissen & Steinburg, 2009). Hence, IRT is concerned the test item difficulty and the test-taker's ability. When developing new tests, researchers will often use a combined CTT and IRT approach to document evidence of its reliability and validity data (Jabrayilov et al., 2016; Petrillo et al., 2015).

Outcome measurement in occupational therapy

Outcome measurement refers to the practice of objectively determining whether the participant or population has experienced change due to a defined intervention after being exposed to a situation or condition. Baseline assessment provides the initial point from which comparisons can be made and the client's status may be re-assessed against that status at multiple points in the occupational therapy process. Most outcome measures are formal and standardised and have undergone substantial psychometric evaluation to ensure that the test users and scorers can have confidence that the tool is measuring what it purports to measure consistently and accurately. Within all areas of occupational therapy practice, substantial work has been completed developing useful clinical tools that will measure outcomes. For example, the *Canadian Occupational Performance Measure* (COPM) is the most widely used rehabilitation outcome measure in the research literature as the COPM is known to be psychometrically sound (Law et al., 2005). The COPM has a dedicated website with up-to-date research evidence supporting usage (see http://www.thecopm.ca/).

Occupational therapists are increasingly using the COnsensus-based Standards for the selection of health Measurement INstruments (COSMIN) taxonomy to both assist in the selection of sound outcome measures and to psychometrically evaluate assessment tools used in clinical practice and in research. A recent special edition of the *Australian Occupational Therapy Journal* was dedicated to assessment development of occupational therapy measurement tools and noted occupational therapists' uptake of the COSMIN as a guiding framework (Bourke-Taylor et al., 2018).

The COSMIN was rigorously developed through researching the opinions of world experts in outcome development research across the health professions (Mokkink et al., 2010; Mokkink et al., 2018). Multistage Delphi studies were used to reach international consensus on terminology and definition of all measurement properties (e.g., validity, reliability and responsiveness) and how the properties relate to one another (Terwee et al., 2018). The COSMIN has a comprehensive website that includes a checklist for evaluation of assessment tools and systematic reviews about the psychometric properties of outcome measures (see https://www.cosmin.nl/).

The COSMIN specifies that evidence of the following seven types of measurement properties should be reported about health-related instruments: internal consistency, reliability, measurement error, content validity (that includes face validity), construct validity, criterion validity and responsiveness (Mokkink et al., 2018). More specifically, the components of construct validity evidence with regard to health and epidemiological scales that should be reported according to the COSMIN are structural validity, hypothesis testing and cross-cultural validity (Mokkink et al., 2006; Rios & Wells, 2014).

Bottom-up and top-down approaches to assessment

Approaches to assessment can be categorised as being bottom-up or top-down (Chien & Brown, 2017). Bottom-up assessments are common in occupational therapy practice, fit easily within the traditional medical model approach to assessment, and focus on assessing body functions and structures components (Majnemer, 2012). Bottom-up assessments tend to focus on separate components of a client's abilities, rather than the broader occupational perspective. Moreover, items in bottom-up assessments are frequently administered in rigid, contrived, standardised contexts that may not be meaningful to the person's perspective and are often isolated from meaningful daily occupations and real-life environments. Examples of bottom-up assessments often used with clients include the *Test of Visual Perceptual Skills—4th edition* (Martin, 2017), *Purdue Pegboard Test* (Lafayette Instrument Company, 1985) and *Mini–Mental State Examination* (Folstein & Folstein, 2001).

A top-down assessment takes a global perspective and focuses on the client's participation in his/her contexts to determine what is important to the client and his/her family (Cordier et al., 2016). It focuses on assessing activity (limitations), participation (restrictions), and environmental and personal factors (Imms & Green, 2020). The top-down assessment approach fits with a client-centred approach to occupational therapy practice (DeGrace, 2003). Trombly (1993) advised occupational therapists to use top-down assessments that first focus on an individual's occupational performance issues. Examples of top-down assessments include the COPM (Law et al., 2005), *Evaluation of Social Interaction* (Fisher & Griswold, 2010) and *School Setting Interview* (Hoffman et al., 2005).

What skills, attributes and domains do occupational therapists assess?

Occupational therapists focus on and assess the occupational performance of clients. Occupational performance has been defined as 'the ability to carry out activities of daily life, including basic activities of daily living (BADL) and instrumental activities of daily living (IADL), education, work, play, leisure, and social participation' (AOTA 2002, p. 617). Law and Baum considered occupational performance to be 'the point when the person, the environment, and the person's occupation intersect to support the tasks, activities, and roles that define that person as an individual' (Law & Baum, 2005, p. 7).

Occupational therapists assess a variety of skills, traits, features, roles and occupations of the clients that they service. Types of occupations that typically are assessed include self-care (e.g., drinking, dressing, toileting, combing hair, brushing teeth, bathing), productivity (e.g., paid employment, volunteer work, meal planning, preparation and other home-making), education (e.g., going to school, role as a student), play and leisure, social participation, sleep and rest (Law et al., 2005). These skills may be grouped together under the categories of instrumental activities of daily living, personal activities of daily living, community activities of daily living and domestic activities of daily living. Often therapists will also assess the body function and structure level skills such as a person's motor, perceptual, cognitive, social, communication and sensory skills (Chien & Brown, 2017) to gather more information about factors that may be affecting a client's occupational performance. Further, therapists may also assess a client's time use, life roles, habits, values, beliefs, rituals and routines to further gather understanding of a client's unique perspective and performance. Meaningful occupational therapy assessment must include consideration of aspects of the context and environment including cultural, personal, physical, social, temporal and virtual features as well (AOTA, 2008). Occupational therapy assessment measures must be valid, reliable, clinically relevant, culturally appropriate, easy to use and occupation-focused.

Examples of tests and measures that occupational therapists administer

Occupational therapists use a wide range of tests and measures and some of the more commonly known or used assessments are listed in Table 25.1.

Table 25.1 Assessment tools used by occupational therapists in clinical practice

Children	Adults and older adults
Motor	**Motor**
• Peabody Developmental Motor Scales—2nd edition (PDMS-2) • Bruininks-Oseretsky Test of Motor Proficiency—2nd edition (BOT-2) • Movement Assessment Battery for Children—2nd edition (MABC-2) • Developmental Coordination Disorder Questionnaire (DCDQ)	• Wide Range Assessment of Visual Motor Abilities (WRAVA) • Crawford Small Parts Dexterity Test • Nine-Hole Peg Test • O'Connor Finger Dexterity Test • Bruininks Motor Ability Test (BMAT) • O'Connor Tweezer Dexterity Test • Clinical Observations of Motor and Postural Skills (COMPS)

Children	Adults and older adults

Children

- Erhardt Developmental Prehension Assessment
- Gross Motor Function Measure (GMFM)
- Test of Gross Motor Development—3rd edition (TGMD-3)
- Test of Infant Motor Development (TIMD)
- Toddler and Infant Motor Evaluation (TIME)
- Alberta Infant Motor Scale (AIMS)
- Quick Neurological Screening Test—II (QNST-II)
- Sensory Integration and Praxis Tests (SIPTS)
- *DeGangi-Berk Test of Sensory Integration* (TSI)
- Melbourne Assessment 2 (MA2): A test of quality of unilateral upper limb function [a]

Cognitive

- *Cognitive Assessment of Young Children (CAYC)*
- Behavioural Assessment of the Dysexecutive Syndrome in Children (BADS-C)
- Dynamic Occupational Therapy Cognitive Assessment for Children (DOTCA-Ch)
- Behaviour Rating Inventory of Executive Functioning (BRIEF)

Developmental

- Denver Developmental Screening Test (Denver II)
- FirstSTEP Screening Test for Evaluating Preschoolers
- Hawaii Early Learning Profile (HELP)
- Miller Assessment of Preschoolers (MAP)
- Ages and Stages Questionnaire
- Batelle Developmental Inventory
- Bayley Scales of Infant and Toddler Development—3rd edition (Bayley-III Screening Test)
- Pediatric Evaluation of Disability Inventory (PEDI)
- Vulpe Assessment Battery—Revised
- Vineland Adaptive Behavior Scale (VABS)
- Crawford Small Parts Dexterity Test (CSPDT)
- Jebsen-Taylor Hand Function Test
- Purdue Pegboard Test
- Disabilities of the Arm, Shoulder and Hand Questionnaire

Human occupation

- Canadian Occupational Performance Measure (COPM)
- Model of Human Occupation Screening Tool (MOHOST)
- Occupational Circumstances Assessment Interview Rating Scale (OCAIRS)
- Occupational Performance History Interview—II (OPHI-II)
- Occupational Self Assessment (OSA)
- Volitional Questionnaire (VQ)
- Occupational Questionnaire (OQ)
- Occupational Role History (ORH)
- Model of Human Occupation Exploratory Level Outcome Ratings (*MOHO-ExpLOR*)
- Self-Discovery Tapestry
- Personal Projects Analysis (PPA)
- Personal Projects Analysis (PPA)

Cognitive

- Chessington Occupational Therapy Neurological Assessment Battery (COTNAB)
- *Rowland Universal Dementia Assessment Scale (RUDAS)*
- Clock Face Test
- Rivermead Perceptual Assessment Battery (RPAB)
- Dynamic Lowenstein Occupational Therapy Cognitive Assessment (DLOTCA)
- Dynamic Lowenstein Occupational Therapy Cognitive Assessment—Geriatric (DLOTCA-G)
- Allen Cognitive Level Screen 5 (ACLS-5)
- Allen Diagnostic Module—2nd edition (ADM-2)
- Cognitive Assessment of Minnesota (CAM)
- Developmental Profile—III
- Adaptive Behavior Assessment System (ABAS)
- Developmental Assessment of Young Children—2nd edition (DAYC-2)
- Child Development Inventory (CDI)

Play and playfulness

- Knox Preschool Play Scale—Revised
- Transdisciplinary Play-Based Assessment
- Pediatric Volitional Questionnaire (PVQ)

(Continued)

Children	*Adults and older adults*

Children

- Play History
- Test of Playfulness [a] (ToP)
- Children's Leisure Assessment Scale (CLASS)
- McDonald Play Inventory (MPI)
- Child-Initiated Pretend Play Assessment [a] (ChIPPA)
- Play Skills Self-Report Questionnaire [a] (PSSRQ)
- Children's Playfulness Scale (CPS)
- Children's Behaviors Inventory of Playfulness (CBI)

Sensory

- Sensory Processing Measure/Sensory Processing Measure—Preschool (SPM/SPM-P)
- Sensory Profile 2: Infant, Toddler, Child, Short, and School Companion
- Erhardt Developmental Vision Assessment
- Infant/Toddler Sensory Profile (ITSP)
- Test of Sensory Function in Infants (TSFI)

Activity participation

- Functional Independence Measure for Children (WeeFIM)
- Children's Assessment of Participation and Enjoyment/Preferences for Activities (CAPE/PAC)
- Assessment of Life Habits Scale
- Miller Function and Participation Scales (M-FUN-P)
- Participation and Environment Measure for Children and Youth (PEM-CY)
- Activities Scale for Kids (ASK)
- Pediatric Activity Card Sort (PACS)
- Pediatric Interest Profiles (PIP)
- Child Occupational Self Assessment (COSA)
- Mini Mental State Examination—2nd edition (MMSE-2)
- Montreal Cognitive Assessment (MoCA)
- Neurobehavioral Cognitive Status Screening Examination (Cognistat)
- Scales of Cognitive Ability for Traumatic Brain Injury (SCATBI)
- Test of Everyday Attention (TEA)
- Toglia Category Assessment
- Arnadottir OT-ADL Neurobehavioral Evaluation (A-ONE)
- Cognitive Performance Test (CPT)
- Addenbrooke's Cognitive Examination Revised (ACE-R)

Activities of daily living

- Functional Independence Measure (FIM)
- Klein-Bell Activities of Daily Living Scale
- Kohlman Evaluation of Living Skills
- Barthel Index of ADL (Barthel)
- Bay Area Functional Performance Evaluation (BaFPE)
- Katz Index of Activities of Daily Living
- Milwaukee Evaluation of Daily Living Skills (MEDLS)
- Nottingham Extended Activities of Daily Living Scale
- Personal Care Participation Assessment and Resource Tool (PC-PART)
- Bristol Activities of Daily Living Scale

Activity participation

- Work Environment Impact Scale (WEIS)
- Activity Card Sort—2nd edition (ACS-2)
- Activity Card Sort—Australia [a] (ACS-Aus)
- Community Integration Measure (CIM)
- Community Integration Questionnaire (CIQ)
- Assessment of Motor and Process Skills (AMPS)
- Interest Checklist

Leisure and playfulness

- Leisure Competence Measure (LCM)
- Leisure Satisfaction Scale (LSS)
- Leisure Activity Profile (LAP)
- Leisure Diagnostic Battery
- Leisure Aptitude Measure (LAM)
- Perceived Efficacy and Goal Setting System (PEGS)
- Child Helping Out: Responsibilities, Expectations and Supports (CHORES)
- Child Health Questionnaire (CHQ)
- Short Child Occupational Profile (SCOPE)
- Do-Eat
- Assessment of Preschool Children's Participation (APCP)
- Assistance to Participate Scale (APS)
- Children Participation Questionnaire—School
- Perceived Meaning of Occupation Questionnaire (PMOQ)
- Child and Adolescent Scale of Participation (CASP)

Children	*Adults and older adults*

Perception

- Beery Buktenica Developmental Test of Visual Motor Integration (Beery VMI)
- Developmental Test of Visual Perception—3rd edition (DTVP-3)
- Test of Visual-Motor Skills—4th edition (TVMS-4)
- Jordan Left–Right Reversal Test—3rd edition (JLRT-3)
- Motor-free Visual Perception Test—3rd edition (MVPT-3)
- Motor-free Visual Perception Test—3rd edition (MVPT-3)
- Test of Visual Perceptual Skills—4th edition (TVPS-4)

School function

- Minnesota Handwriting Assessment (MHA)
- Evaluation Tool of Children's Handwriting (ETCH)
- School Assessment of Motor and Process Skills (School AMPS)
- School Setting Interview (SSI)
- Educational Assessment of School Youth for Occupational Therapists (EASY-OT)
- School Function Assessment (SFA)
- Test of Handwriting Skills—Revised (THS-R)
- Children's Handwriting Evaluation Scale (CHES)
- Detailed Assessment of Speed of *Handwriting* (DASH)
- 'Here's How I Write' handwriting assessment
- Adolescent Playfulness Scale
- Young-Adult Playfulness Scale
- Older-Adult Playfulness Scale
- Leisure Bordom Scale (LBS)
- Leisure Interest Measure (LIM)
- Leisure Motivation Scale (LMS)
- Leisure Interest Profile for Adults
- Leisure Interest Profile for Seniors
- Other-directed, Lighthearted, Intellectual, and Whimsical (OLIW) scale for playfulness

Sensory/perceptual

- Adolescent/Adult Sensory Profile (AASP)
- Developmental Test of Visual Perception—Adolescent and Adult (DTVP-A)
- Occupational Therapy Adult Perceptual Screening Test [a] (OT-APST)

Psychosocial/behavioural

- Beck Depression Inventory—II (BDI-II)
- Beck Anxiety Inventory (BAI)
- Adult Self-Perception Profile (ASPP)
- Rosenberg Self-Esteem Scale (RSES)
- Tennessee Self-Concept Scale (TSCS)
- Coping Inventory
- Parenting Stress Index (PSI)
- Ways of Coping Questionnaire
- Interpersonal Style Inventory (ISI)
- Social Support Inventory for People with Disabilities (SSIPD)
- Interview Schedule for Social Interaction (ISSI)

Habits, roles and time use

- Role Checklist
- Time Use Diary
- National Institutes of Health Activity Record (NIH Activity Record)

Psychosocial/behavioural

- Childhood Autism Rating Scale (CARS)
- Children's Depression Rating Scale—Revised (CDRS-R)
- Culture Free Self-Esteem Inventories—3rd edition (CFSEI-III)
- Piers-Harris Self-Concept Scale—3rd edition (Piers-Harris III)
- Connors' Rating Scales—Revised
- Revised Children's Manifest Anxiety Scale
- Infant Toddler Social and Emotional Assessment (ITSEA)
- Self-Perception Profile for Children/Self-Perception Profile for Adolescents
- Childhood Autism Rating Scale—2nd edition (CARS-2)
- Coping Inventory for Children/Early Coping Inventory
- Child's Challenging Behaviour Scale
- Evaluation of Social Interaction (ESI)

Environment

- Children's Physical Environments Rating Scale
- Home Observation for Measurement of the Environment (HOME)
- Test of Environmental Supportiveness [a] (TOES)
- Environmental Restriction Questionnaire (ERQ)

(Continued)

Children	*Adults and older adults*

Other

- Health Promoting Activities Scale a (HPAS)
- Assistance to Participate Scale a
- Child's Challenging Behaviour Scale version 2 [a]
- Pragmatics Observational Measure [a]
- Functional Behavior Profile
- Life Habits Assessment (LHA)
- Craig Handicap Assessment and Reporting Technique (CHART)

Falls

- Falls Efficacy Scale (FES)
- Home Falls and Accidents Screening Tool (HFAST)
- Westmead Home Safety Assessment (WHSA)
- Falls Behavioral Scale for Older People

Work

- Worker Role Interview (WRI)
- Valpar Component Work Samples

Adults and older adults

- Assessment of Work Performance (AWP)
- Work Environment Scale (WES)

Other

- Health Assessment Questionnaire (HAQ)
- Craig Hospital Inventory of Environmental Factors (CHIEF)
- Measure of Quality of the Environment (MQE)
- Assessment of Communication and Interaction Skills (ACIS)
- DriveSafe Driveaware [a]
- Occupational Therapy Driver Off Road Assessment Battery [a] (OT-DORA)
- Australian Therapy Outcome Measures for Occupational Therapy [a] (AusTOMs—OT)
- In-Home Occupational Performance Evaluation (I-HOPE)
- Dimensions of Home Measure (DOHM)

Note: [a] refers to assessments developed and published by Australian occupational therapists.

Conclusion

Assessment is a vital part of the occupational therapy process. In professional practice with clients and families, occupational therapists use a wide range of tests and measures. A variety of factors impact a therapist's choice of what assessment(s) to select, including the reason for referral; client diagnosis and age; social and cultural history of the client; assessment availability and cost; specialised training required to administer, score and interpret the assessment; organisation/individual funding the occupational therapy services; therapists' skills and expertise with the test; and the time constraints in administering the assessments. Assessments can be relatively brief, informal, detailed or standardised to administer and score.

Assessment is a key professional competency for occupational therapists and it is important for therapists to stay informed about new assessments and revisions of existing ones. Assessment results, therapists' clinical reasoning and judgement, plus the client's occupational profile, all provide the foundation of successful goal setting and intervention planning and implementation. Occupational therapists in Australia use a number of assessments that have been developed and standardised in other countries. This needs to be taken into consideration when generating standard test scores (that are based on standardisation samples from other countries). However, a growing number of assessments are being authored by Australian occupational therapists and standardised using Australian population samples which is encouraging.

Summary

- All occupational therapists engage in some form of assessment with all clients.
- Assessment assists with establishing a baseline of clients' strengths, challenges and interests; collaborative goal setting and monitoring changes in clients' occupational performance.
- Assessments can be categorised as formal or informal, standardised or non-standardised, top-down or bottom-up, and self-report, performance-based or proxy report.
- Occupational therapists typically assess clients' skills, interests, participation and performance abilities in the areas of self-care, productivity, leisure/play, social participation, rest and sleep.

Review questions

1. What is the purpose of occupational therapists completing an assessment with a client?
2. What is an outcome measure and why do occupational therapists commonly use such assessments?
3. What are two primary differences between top-down and bottom-up assessments?
4. What are four categories of occupations that occupational therapists typically assess?
5. Name four tests that occupational therapists commonly administer.

References

Achenbach, T. M., & Rescorla, L. A. (2001). *Manual for the ASEBA School-Age Forms & Profiles*. University of Vermont, Research Centre for Children, Youth & Families.

American Occupational Therapy Association (AOTA). (2002). Occupational Therapy Practice Framework: Domain and Process. *American Journal of Occupational Therapy, 56*(6), 609–639. https://doi.org/10.5014/ajot.56.6.609

American Occupational Therapy Association (AOTA). (2008). *Occupational Therapy Practice Framework: Domain and Process* (2nd edn). American Occupational Therapy Association.

Beck, A. T., Steer, R. A., & Brown, G. K. (1996) *Manual for the Beck Depression Inventory-II*. Psychological Corporation.

Beery, K. E., Buktenica, N. A., & Beery, N. A. (2010). *Beery Buktenica Developmental Test of Visual Motor Integration* (6th edn). Pearson.

Blank, R., Smits-Engelsman, B., Polatajko, H., & Wilson, P. (2012). European Academy for Childhood Disability (EACD): Recommendations on the definition, diagnosis and intervention of developmental coordination disorder (long version). *Developmental Medicine and Child Neurology, 54(1)*, 54–93. https://doi:10.1111/j.1469-8749.2011.04171.x

Bourke-Taylor, H. M., Brown, T., & Cordier, R. (2018). Special Issue: Innovations in occupational therapy measurement (editorial). *Australian Occupational Therapy Journal, 65*(5), 343–345. https://doi.org/10.1111/1440-1630.12521

Brown, T. (2012). Assessment, measurement, and evaluation/Why can't I do what everyone expects me to do? In S. J. Lane & A. C. Bundy (Eds.), *Kids can be kids: A childhood occupations approach* (pp. 320–348). F.A. Davis Co.

Butler, R. J., & Gasson, S. L. (2005). Self esteem/self concept scales for children and adolescents: A review. *Child and Adolescent Mental Health, 10*(4), 190–201. https://doi.org/10.1111/j.1475-3588.2005.00368.x

Chien, C. W., & Brown, T. (2017). Assessing children's occupations and participation. In S. Roger & A. Kennedy-Behr (Eds.), *Occupation-centred practice with children: A practical guide for occupational therapists* (2nd edn, pp. 133–163). Wiley Blackwell.

Classen, S., & Velozo, C. A. (2019). Critiquing assessments. In B. A. Boyt Schell & G. Gillen (Eds.), *Willard & Spackman's occupational therapy* (13th edn, pp. 390–412). Wolters Kluwer.

Cordier, R., Chen, Y.-W., Speyer, R., Totino, R., Doma, K., Leicht, A., Brown, N., & Cuomo, B. (2016). Child-report measures of occupational performance: A systematic review. *PLoS ONE, 11*(1), e0147751. https://doi.org/10.1371/journal.pone.0147751

Davidson, M. (2014). Known-groups validity. In A. C. Michalos (Ed.), *Encyclopedia of quality of life and well-being research* (pp. 3481–3482). Springer.

DeGrace, B. W. (2003). Occupation-based and family-centered care: A challenge for current practice. *American Journal of Occupational Therapy, 57*(3), 347–350. https://doi.org/10.5014/ajot.57.3.347

Fawcett, A. L. (2007). *Principles of assessment and outcome measurement for occupational therapists and physiotherapists: Theory, skills and application.* Wiley and Sons Ltd.

Fisher, A. G., & Bray Jones, K. (2010). *Assessment of Motor and Process Skills, vol. 2: User manual* (7th edn). Three Star Press.

Fisher, A. G., & Griswold, L. A. (2010). *Evaluation of Social Interaction* (2nd edn). Three Star Press.

Folio, M. R., & Fewell, R. R. (2000). *Peabody Developmental Motor Scales: Examiner's manual* (2nd edn). Pro-Ed.

Folstein, M., & Folstein, S. (2001). *Mini-Mental State Examination (MMSE).* Psychological Assessment Resources, Inc.

Franzen, M. D. (2011). Classical test theory. In J. S. Kreutzer, J. DeLuca, & B. Caplan (Eds.), *Encyclopedia of clinical neuropsychology* (pp. 586–587). Springer.

Frey, F. (2017). Test theory, classical test theory. In J. Matthes, C. S. Davis, & R. F. Potter (Eds.), *The international encyclopedia of communication research methods* (pp. 1–2). Wiley.

Glennon, T., Miller-Kuhaneck, H., Henry, D. A., Parham, L. D., & Ecker, C. (2007). *Sensory Processing Measure manual.* Western Psychological Services.

Glennon, T., Miller-Kuhaneck, H., Henry, D. A., Parham, L. D., & Ecker, C. (2010). *Sensory Processing Measure—Preschool manual.* Western Psychological Services.

Harter, S. (1985). *Manual for the Self-Perception Profile for Children.* University of Denver.

Henderson, S. E., Sugden, D. A., & Barnett, A. L. (2007). *Movement Assessment Battery for Children—2 examiner's manual.* Harcourt Assessment.

Hocking, C. (2001). Implementing occupation-based assessment. *American Journal of Occupational Therapy, 55*(4), 463–469. https://doi.org/10.5014/ajot.55.4.463

Hoffman, O. R., Hemmingsson, H., & Kielhofner, G. (2005). *A user's manual for the School Setting Interview Version 3.0.* University of Illinois at Chicago.

Imms, C., & Green, D. (2020) *Participation: Optimising outcomes in childhood-onset neurodisability.* Mac Keith Press.

Jabrayilov, R., Emons, W. H. M., & Sijtsma, K. (2016). Comparison of classical test theory and item response theory in individual change assessment. *Applied Psychological Measurement, 40*(8), 559–572. https://doi.org/10.1177/0146621616664046

Kiresuk, T. J., & Sherman, R. E. (1968). Goal attainment scaling: A general method for evaluating comprehensive community mental health programs. *Community Mental Health Journal, 4*(6), 443–453. https://doi.org/10.1007/BF01530764

Kubiszyn, T., & Borich, G. (2013). *Educational testing and measurement: Classroom application and practice* (10th edn). Wiley & Sons Inc.

Kurdek, L. A., & Sinclair, R. J. (2000). Psychological, family, and peer predictors of academic outcomes in first- through fifth-grade children. *Journal of Educational Psychology, 92*(3), 449–457. https://doi.org/10.1037/0022-0663.92.3.449

Lafayette Instrument Company. (1985). *Instructions and normative data for Model 32020.* LIC.

Law, M., Baptiste, S., Carswell, S., McColl, A., Polatajko, H., & Pollock, N. (2005). *Canadian Occupational Performance Measure* (4th edn). CAOT Publications.

Law, M., & Baum, C. (2005). Measurement in occupational therapy. In M. Law, C. Baum, & W. Dunn (Eds.), *Measuring occupational performance: Supporting best practice in occupational therapy* 2nd edn, pp. 3–20). SLACK Inc.

Lee, T-I., Howe, T. H., Chen, H. L., & Wang, T. N. (2016). Predicting handwriting legibility in Taiwanese elementary school children. *American Journal of Occupational Therapy, 70*(6), 7006220020p1–7006220020p9. https://doi.org/10.5014/ajot.2016.016865

Magno, C. (2009). Demonstrating the difference between classical test theory and item response theory using derived test data. *The International Journal of Educational and Psychological Assessment, 1*(1), 1–11. https://files.eric.ed.gov/fulltext/ED506058.pdf

Majnemer, A. (2012). *Measures of children with developmental disabilities: An ICF-CY approach.* Mac Keith Press.

Martin, N. A. (2017). *Test of Visual Perceptual Skills* (4th edn). Academic Therapy Publications.

Missiuna, C., Pollock, N., & Law, M. C. (2004). *Perceived Efficacy and Goal Setting System (PEGS).* Pearson Education Inc.

Mokkink, L. B., de Wet, H. C. W., Prinsen, C. A. C., Patrick, D. L., Alonso, J., Bouter, L. M., & Terwee, C. B. (2018). COSMIN risk of bias checklist for systematic reviews of patient-reported outcome measures. *Quality of Life Research, 27*(5), 1171–1179. https://doi.org/10.1007/s11136-017-1765-4

Mokkink, L. B., Terwee, C. B., Knol, D. L., Stratford, P. W., Alonso, J., Patrick, D. L., Bouter, L. M., & de Wet, H. C. W. (2006). Protocol of the COSMIN study: COnsensus-based Standards for the selection of health Measurement INstruments. *BMC Medical Research Methodology, 6*(1), 2. https://doi.org/10.1186/1471-2288-6-2

Mokkink, L. B., Terwee, C. B., Patrick, D. L., Alonso, J., Stratford, P. W., Knol, D. L., Bouter, L. M., & de Wet, H. C. W. (2010). The COSMIN Study reached international consensus on taxonomy, terminology, and definitions of measurement properties for health-related patient-reported outcomes. *Journal of Clinical Epidemiology, 63*(7), 737–745. https://doi.org.10.1016/j.jclinepi.2010.02.006

Neaum, S. (2016). *Child development for early years students and practitioners.* Sage.

Petrillo, J., Cano, S. J., McLeod, L. D., & Coon, C. D. (2015). Using classical test theory, item response theory, and Rasch measurement theory to evaluate patient-reported outcome measures: A comparison of worked examples. *Value in Health, 18*(1), 25–34. https://doi.org/10.1016/j.jval.2014.10.005

Piers, E. V., Shemmassian, S. K., & Herzberg, D. S. (2018). *Piers-Harris Self-Concept Scale, Third Edition (Piers-Harris 3).* Western Psychological Services.

Reise, S. P. (2014). Item response theory. In R. L. Cautin & S. O. Lilienfeld (Eds.), *The encyclopedia of clinical psychology* (pp. 1–10). Wiley and Sons Ltd.

Rios, W., & Wells, C. (2014). Validity evidence based on internal structure. *Psicothema, 26*(1), 108–116. https://doi.org/10.7334/psicothema2013.260

Rosenberg, L., & Bart, O. (2015). Development and initial validation of the Children Participation Questionnaire–School (CPQ–School). *IJOT: Israeli Journal of Occupational Therapy, 24,* E70–E87. http://www.isot.org.il/Uploads/Attachments/37255/cpq_school.pdf

Salkind, N. J. (2010). *Encyclopedia of research design (Vols. 1–0).* Sage Publications, Inc.

Shaughnessy, J. J., Zechmeister, E. B., & Zechmeister, J. S. (2006). *Research methods in psychology* (7th edn). McGraw-Hill.

Shulman, C. (2013). Informal assessment. In F. R. Volkmar (Ed.), *Encyclopedia of autism spectrum disorders* (n.p.). Springer. https://doi.org/10.1007/978$$1$$4419$$1698$$3

Terwee, C. B., Prinsen, C. A. C., Chiarotto, A., Westerman, M. J., Patrick, D. L., Alonso, J., Bouter, L. M., de Vet, H. C. W., & Mokkink, L. B. (2018). COSMIN methodology for evaluating the content validity of patient-reported outcome measures: A Delphi study. *Quality of Life Research, 27,* 1159–1170. https://doi.org/10.1007/s11136-018-1829-0

Thissen, D., & Steinburg, L. (2009). Item response theory. In R. E. Millsap & A. Maydeu-Olivares (Eds.). *The SAGE handbook of quantitative methods in psychology* (pp. 148–177). Sage.

Trombly, C. (1993). Anticipating the future: Assessment of occupational function. *American Journal of Occupational Therapy, 47*(3), 253–257. https://doi.org/10.5014/ajot.47.3.253

Ulrich, D. A. (2019). *Test of gross motor development—third edition*. Pro-Ed.

van Hartingsveldt, M. J., Cup, E. H. C., Hendriks, J. C., de Vries, L., de Groot, I. J., & Nijhuis-van der Sanden, M. W. (2015). Predictive validity of kindergarten assessments on handwriting readiness. *Research in Developmental Disabilities, 36C*, 114–124. https://doi.org/10.1016/j.ridd.2014.08.014

World Health Organization. (2001). *International Classification of Functioning, Disability and Health*. https://www.who.int/classifications/icf/en/

26 The role of occupational therapy in primary health care in Australia

Annette Peart, Emma George, Kylie Vogt and Tahnee Elliot

Chapter objectives

Upon completion of this chapter, the reader will be able to:

*   Introduce primary health care as a model and a field of practice for occupational therapy.
*   Explain the link between occupational therapy and primary health care.
*   Highlight three examples of primary health care in Australia.

Key terms

primary health care; equity; empowerment; social justice; social determinants of health; community

Introduction

Primary health care is both a model and a field of practice. Principles of primary health care strongly reflect occupational therapy principles of client–centred practice and participation in meaningful occupation. Occupational therapists can apply primary health care principles in all settings and when working with people, families, communities and populations. Occupational therapists in primary health care bring a focus on meaningful occupation when providing services to promote health and prevent illness. This chapter outlines primary health care as a model and discusses its principles of equity, empowerment and social justice. It introduces the 'Upstream, Midstream, Downstream' model as a tool for planning and practice. Three examples of primary health care are provided to highlight the role and opportunities for occupational therapy in the primary health care context in Australia.

Primary health care emerged as a model of community-based health service delivery following the World Health Organization's (WHO) Declaration of Alma-Ata (WHO, 1978). Representatives from 134 nations agreed and supported the WHO's definition of health as a 'state of complete physical, mental and social well-being and not merely the absence of disease or infirmity' (WHO, 1948). This recognised health as a human right and an important worldwide goal that deserved the attention of health and other sectors. The Declaration of Alma Ata (WHO, 1978) documented that health is impacted by inequalities and inequities present between and within countries and communities. It highlighted the presence of the social gradient in health where disadvantaged people have worse health. In 2018, the Global Conference on Primary Health Care endorsed a new declaration, reaffirming the Declaration of Alma-Ata, to strengthen primary health care and achieve universal health coverage (WHO, 2018).

As outlined in the Declaration of Alma-Ata (WHO, 1978), primary health care as a field of practice promotes individual and community participation in prevention, curative and rehabilitative services. This includes but is not limited to education, nutrition, access to clean water and sanitation, maternal and child health, family planning, immunisation, disease control, treatment and the provision of essential drugs. The Declaration of Alma Ata emphasises the need for an international commitment to health, more responsible use of the world's resources, and peace.

In Australia, primary health care is provided predominantly through community health services, Aboriginal community-controlled health services, and specialist health services, for example, targeting women, mental health and youth.

Primary care vs primary health care

Primary health care was designed and has always strived to be more than primary care and yet there remains confusion and debate about the context and definition of primary health care in practice. Primary care refers to the first point of call when people seek help for health concerns. Primary care services within this structure should be basic, accessible, affordable and essential (Baum, 2015). But primary health care is more than primary care. Primary health care should be integrated and coordinated to address the social determinants of health (Baum, 2015). These are the circumstances in which people are born, grow, live, work and age (Commission on Social Determinants of Health, 2008). The social determinants of health are shaped by power and money at local, national and global levels. Therefore, primary health care has a holistic approach to health that considers the context of social determinants of health for people, families, communities and populations.

Key principles of primary health care

Equity, empowerment and social justice are the three principles of primary health care (Talbot & Verrinder, 2014). Together these principles create a foundation for addressing health and the social determinants that impact people and populations.

Equity

Equity is about fairness. Equity is an ethical concept and can be defined as the absence of disparities in health, and is connected to advantage and disadvantage (Braveman & Gruskin, 2003). If equity is about fairness, then equality can be described as sameness. Health equity focuses on the fair distribution of resources so people who need the most support have access to it. Achieving equality in service provision but providing the same services to all people does not necessarily translate to equity, because some people need more services or different services. For example, in Figure 26.1, if all four people were provided with equal services (the same size bike), participation would remain unequal. However, when an adapted bike is provided for the person who uses a wheelchair, and suitable sized bikes are provided for other people, resources are equitable, and all people can participate.

Importantly, not all health disparity is unfair. It is expected that younger adults will be healthier than elderly adults, or men will have prostate problems and women will

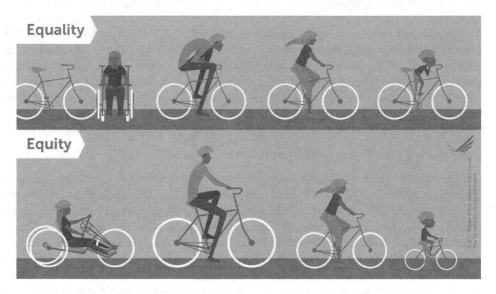

Figure 26.1 Equality and equity.
Source: rwjf.org/en/library/infographics/visualizing-health-equity.html

not (Braveman & Gruskin, 2003). These disparities are not unfair. A disparity that is unfair, or inequitable, is avoidable. A commitment to health equity demonstrates a commitment to fair and just policies and service provision for people and communities who need it the most.

Empowerment

Empowerment is a process that seeks to redress the inequalities in health and promote participation to bring about personal, social and political change (Keleher & MacDougall, 2016; Laverack, 2006). Empowerment requires partnership with people, families and communities on issues of importance to that community and determined by the community. A commitment to empowerment involves supporting people to participate and goes beyond tokenistic consultation or collaboration towards decision-making and community ownership (Talbot & Verrinder, 2014). Participation in health supports people to build trust and rapport, develop belonging and relationships within a community, focus on strengths, and foster partnership (Laverack, 2006). Working in health always involves some power relationships between different stakeholders, especially between health professionals, who may be regarded as the experts, and their clients or communities with whom they work. The challenge for health professionals is to provide opportunities for people to gain greater control over decision-making processes and access to resources to address disparities in social determinants of health (Keleher & MacDougall, 2016).

Social justice

Social justice is an ethical concept based on human rights, fairness and equity in society (Keleher & MacDougall, 2016). In occupational therapy, there is an increased focus on global connection and addressing issues of social injustice, as well as closing the gap in health status caused by health disparities (Braveman & Bass-Haugen, 2009). A commitment to social justice is reflected in the People's Health Movement's (2000) definition of health as a 'social, economic and political issue and above all a fundamental human right'. When human rights are violated, health suffers; when human rights are promoted, vulnerability to ill health is reduced (Talbot & Verrinder, 2014). Therefore, socially just approaches to health reflect the ethical concept of equity and a commitment to empowerment.

Comprehensive vs selective primary health care

Comprehensive primary health care reflects a commitment to addressing social determinants of health. Medical care is only one aspect of this approach. Intervention that remains focused on treating illness is described as selective primary health care (Baum, 2015). Examples of selective primary health care are immunisation or health screening. Both services are essential in promoting health but a more comprehensive approach would also consider structural factors that might prevent access to or use of such services. For example, Aboriginal Community Controlled Health Organisations are structured to respond to community need and therefore more comprehensive in their approach than medical care-focused health services (National Aboriginal Community Controlled Health Organisation, 2020). Baum (2015) explains how comprehensive primary health care draws on community development strategies in addition to clinical work. For example, 'working with local environmental action groups or with public housing tenants, providing nutrition education and advice that is sensitive to the constraints imposed by poverty' (p. 496). Comprehensive primary health care can be provided by a range of sectors, including:

- Private fee-for-service practitioners including medical and allied health professionals;
- Community health centres;
- Not-for-profit organisations who may receive government funding (e.g., family planning associations); and
- Community-led organisations and volunteer communities.

Upstream, midstream, downstream model

Examples of primary health care can be seen through the 'upstream, midstream, downstream' model, part of a broader conceptual framework to identify relationships between social determinants and health (Turrell & Mathers, 2000). In this model, the main components are grouped into upstream (macro), midstream (intermediate) or downstream (micro) factors. Each factor has an associated approach to primary health care. For example, upstream factors include education, employment, income and housing determinants. Upstream approaches are focused on keeping people healthy in the first place and often focus on public policy and the environment (Orleans, 2000), which is consistent with comprehensive primary health care. Midstream factors include psychosocial processes and health behaviours. Midstream approaches address behaviour to prevent illness or limit risk factors. Midstream approaches focus on perceived individual choices but target communities and groups. Downstream factors primarily involve the functioning of various body systems. Downstream approaches treat illness and provide rehabilitation for individual people, representing a selective primary health care approach.

Primary health care and occupational therapy

The principles of equity, empowerment and social justice are aligned with occupational therapy's commitment to client-centred practice and participation in meaningful occupation (Galheigo, 2005; Tse et al., 2003). Occupational therapists work *with* people, individually or in groups or communities, and promote participation in meaningful occupation in physical, social, cultural, attitudinal and legislative environments (World Federation of Occupational Therapists, 2012). Occupational therapists in Australia work as clinicians, educators, supervisors, administrators, managers, project officers, consultants, coordinators, program directors, researchers, advocates, support staff and more.

The importance of engaging in meaningful occupation is directly linked to empowerment. When people and communities participate in occupations that have meaning for them, health will improve. Occupational therapists bring an occupational perspective to primary health care practice and can demonstrate leadership within this field.

Example 1: Normanton student-led placement program

The remote community of Normanton, in the Gulf of Carpentaria, is located on the traditional country of the Gkuthaarn, Kukatj and Kurtijar people. In the 2016 Australian census, 1,210 people were living in Normanton. Aboriginal and/or Torres Strait Islander people make up 61.7 per cent of the population (Australian Bureau of Statistics, 2017).

James Cook University (JCU) Mount Isa Centre for Rural and Remote Health (CRRH) is a University Department of Rural Health located in remote north-west Queensland. The JCU Mount Isa CRRH works with local communities, health professionals and service providers to identify and develop solutions to address Indigenous health challenges and health inequity (Centre for Rural and Remote Health, 2020). Some of the challenges experienced include access to culturally appropriate health care services; recruitment and retention of staff; and irregular outreach clinics for services such as allied health, ear and hearing health, and paediatric health care services.

The Australian Government funded the Rural Health Multidisciplinary Training, focused on addressing health inequity through high-quality and regionally based opportunities in rural and remote Australia (Australian Government Department of Health, 2020). The program is an example of an upstream approach, where universities have been able to cultivate local solutions and develop service learning teams, led by allied health professionals (Going Rural Health, 2020). The team at JCU Mount Isa CRRH works to promote local workforce development and community capacity building through the co-design and delivery of high-quality, inter-professional allied health placements. For example, occupational therapy students on placement provide blocks of intensive intervention to children who require regular and ongoing allied health services within a school setting. This upstream approach involves partnering across sectors with Aboriginal Community Controlled Health Organisations, education, health, local community groups, and non-government organisations.

A midstream approach to this example is the collaboration between JCU Mount Isa CRRH and Gulf Christian College (GCC) in Normanton. The GCC is an independent school for children from grade prep to year 9, and enrolment aims to reflect that of the Normanton community population. In 2016, the JCU Mount Isa CRRH completed a needs assessment, where it was identified that Normanton had no primary health care services in the community and minimal visiting outreach services on an annual basis. Together with community and service representatives, Normanton was identified as a priority site for service learning placements. From this, the principal of GCC expressed interest in collaborating with the JCU Mount Isa CRRH to host service learning placements to provide occupational therapy services to the GCC. In 2017 a pilot placement was established for third- and fourth-year occupational therapy students in the school. The collaboration provides the basis for a primary health care approach to health care delivery, where students participate in a placement using an interdisciplinary supervision model. An essential foundation for this type of placement is cultural orientation at JCU Mount Isa before travelling to Normanton. In Normanton, students are involved in regular activities exposing them to Aboriginal culture, including yarning with elders, visits to the Old Reserve and fishing.

Occupational therapy services for students at GCC reflect a downstream approach. Service provision occurs at the individual, group and whole class levels. For example, individual interventions can focus on handwriting, sensory-based activities and managing behaviours in the classroom. The students also provide services at a whole school level, including professional development for staff about medical conditions, disability and principles of occupational therapy practice. At a broader community level, students on service learning placements also participate in existing community events, raising awareness of occupational therapy and how to make a referral to the service. This model demonstrates movement between the downstrea, and midstream approaches.

In 2019, recognising the success of the service learning placements, GCC employed an occupational therapist to manage the program and continue to work collaboratively with the CRRH to host service learning placements. This meets the need of the community and aligns with the aims of the JCU Mount Isa CRRH to build a health workforce in, and for, the region.

Example 2: Falls prevention

Falls prevention is one intervention contributing to the maintenance of health and function for older people in Australia. It is estimated that one in three Australians living in the community aged over 65 years will have a fall each year. Of those falls, it is estimated that 50 per cent occur in the person's home. There is a general under-reporting of non-injurious falls, with fewer than half of the total number of falls being reported to a health care professional (Australian Commission on Safety and Quality in Health Care, 2009)

Falls and injuries sustained during a fall are a leading cause of morbidity and mortality in older Australians. More than 80 per cent of injury-related hospital admissions in people aged 65 years and over are due to falls and falls-related injuries (Kannus et al., 2006).

Falls prevention is often a part of daily professional practice for occupational therapists providing services for older people. Falls and injuries sustained from falls can impact a person's confidence, their physical and psychological function, and subsequently their ability to engage in daily occupations. Falls prevention interventions offered by occupational therapists can be applied at various points in the health care continuum, and as such align with the 'Upstream, Midstream and Downstream Model' of primary health care.

Upstream approaches to falls prevention have increased in recent times. The Australian Commission on Safety and Quality in Health Care released the 'Best Practice Guidelines for Preventing Falls and Harm from Falls in Older People' in 2009. These guidelines support best practice falls prevention in a variety of different settings including the community, hospitals and residential aged care facilities. The development of a set of clear guidelines enables best practice of care to be applied on population and nationwide levels. Occupational therapists are able to use these guidelines to assist in determining appropriate assessments for clients who may be at risk of falls.

Another 'upstream' approach applied to falls prevention within Australia is the implementation of 'April Falls Month', a national initiative designed to raise awareness of falls and falls injury prevention. Service providers are encouraged to develop promotional displays and provide resources to clients and the general community to facilitate better falls prevention awareness, and to reduce the incidence of falls in older adults.

Midstream approaches to falls prevention generally target the 'at-risk' population, such as people who may have had a recent fall, or who are demonstrating physical or cognitive decline which could increase the likelihood of them falling. Occupational therapists can be involved in risk screening and assessment and assist to identify 'falls risk factors', in both community and inpatient care settings. Interventions address the identified risk factors and may include recommendations for home modifications or equipment to enable a person to engage in daily occupations with a reduced risk of falling. Strength and balance-based exercise programs also fit the midstream approach to falls prevention.

As part of the screening and assessment process, occupational therapists are also involved in identifying the need for other health professional input in a person's care. For example, an older person with poorly fitting footwear, in conjunction with peripheral neuropathy, may benefit from advice to see a podiatrist. The podiatrist can then provide recommendations to ensure adequate foot care and guidelines regarding safe and appropriate footwear to prevent falls.

One example of a specific falls prevention program is Stepping On, a group-based seven-week program used across Australia and the United States, aiming to improve falls self-efficacy, encourage behaviour change and reduce falls. Stepping On is effective for community-living older people in reducing falls (Clemson et al., 2004).

Downstream falls prevention generally targets those already hospitalised due to a fall or related injury. Addressing the consequences of the fall can be the occupational therapist's role. This role may include providing rehabilitation, for example following a hip fracture sustained in a fall. In these instances, the focus is on education, safety and intervention to prevent further falls, to enable a return to occupational performance for the injured person.

Example 3: South Australia's Health in All Policies

'Health in All Policies' (HiAP) is a global strategy that supports a whole-government systems approach to tackle health inequities (WHO, 2020). This approach recognises that action to address health problems must come from within and outside the health sector, including housing, education, employment and transport (Southgate Institute for

Health, Society & Equity, n.d.). As stated in the WHO's Helsinki Statement on Health in All Policies:

> Policies made in all sectors can have a profound effect on population health and health equity. In our interconnected world, health is shaped by many powerful forces, especially demographic change, rapid urbanization, climate change and globalization. While some diseases are disappearing as living conditions improve, many diseases of poverty still persist in developing countries. In many countries lifestyles and living and working environments are influenced by unrestrained marketing and subject to unsustainable production and consumption patterns. The health of the people is not only a health sector responsibility, it also embraces wider political issues such as trade and foreign policy. Tackling this requires political will to engage the whole of government in health.
>
> (WHO, 2013, p. 1)

In South Australia, the HiAP initiative was introduced in 2007 as an approach to work across government departments to consider the potential health and well-being implications of policies as they are conceptualised, developed and implemented (SA Health, 2012). This upstream approach built upon a commitment to work collaboratively and in partnership across agencies. The HiAP approach has been applied to transport, water management, migration, sustainable developments, digital technologies, Indigenous well-being, education and training, and healthy ageing (Delany et al., 2014).

One example of a midstream approach within HiAP is the Healthy Kids Menu Initiative. Australian families are eating out more and spending more household income on food and dining out (SA Health, n.d.). This food is often of poorer nutritional quality, and children's menus offer limited choices. In response, SA Health collaborated with parents, local restaurants, cafés, hotels and the health sector to develop the Healthy Kids Menu.

Families and children are encouraged to look for the Healthy Kids Menu when they are eating out to make it easier for families to make healthy choices. Participating businesses are required to ensure at least half of the options on children's menus are healthy, and water should be free and readily accessible. Importantly, there are 43 venues registered and they are spread out across the metropolitan area and one in the far north of SA. These businesses are located within a range of socio-economic regions both north and south of Adelaide, SA.

A criticism of this initiative is that it only reaches families and children who can afford to eat in participating restaurants and those with time to eat out together. For these children, they will have opportunities to make healthy choices but it could be argued this initiative may not be accessible to other children in more marginalised or disadvantaged communities, where the occupation of eating outside of the home may be unfamiliar. Alternative and complementary programs to coincide with this type of initiative could include education programs in schools for cooking and nutrition, along with the school or community vegetable gardens.

A downstream approach that aligns with HiAP would respond to illness or social problems that impact health. For example, in the education sector, a child may present at school hungry, inattentive and under- or overweight. If a child has no food at school, schools often can provide a sandwich for lunch. This meets an immediate need and is an appropriate downstream approach. A common response from a school would be a referral to other health services, a catalyst for a school breakfast program, or promoting free fruit from local supermarkets, moving the response to more midstream approaches.

An occupational focus can be embedded within upstream, midstream and downstream approaches consistent with HiAP. Strategies at all levels promote participation in meaningful activity for people, families, communities and society. Occupational therapists bring a holistic understanding of health, founded on the importance of occupation, and therefore are advocates for the promotion of health in all sectors.

Conclusion

There are many opportunities for occupational therapy in primary health care, and for occupational therapists to demonstrate principles of equity, empowerment and social justice in occupational therapy service provision. The challenge for occupational therapy is to take a leadership role to promote health and well-being for people, families, communities and populations.

Summary

- Primary health care is both a model and a field of practice.
- Primary health care addresses the social determinants of health.
- Principles of primary health care are equity, empowerment and social justice.
- Client-centred practice and participation in meaningful occupation reflect principles of primary health care.
- Occupational therapists who work in primary health care demonstrate commitment to equity, empowerment and social justice.

Review questions

1. What is the difference between selective and comprehensive primary health care?
2. How does a commitment to client-centred practice demonstrate a commitment to equity?
3. Describe the different ways that occupational therapists work in upstream, midstream and downstream areas of practice.

References

Australian Bureau of Statistics. (2017). *2016 Census community profile (Normanton).* https://quickstats. censusdata.abs.gov.au/census_services/getproduct/census/2016/communityprofile/ UCL321086?opendocument

Australian Commission on Safety and Quality in Health Care. (2009). *Preventing falls and harm from falls in older people: Best practice guidelines for Australian community care.* https://www.safetyandquality. gov.au/publications-and-resources/resource-library/preventing-falls-and-harm-falls-older-people-best-practice-guidelines-australian-community-care

Australian Government Department of Health. (2020). *Rural health multidisciplinary training program.* https://www1.health.gov.au/internet/main/publishing.nsf/Content/rural-health-multidisciplinary-training

Baum, F. (2015). *The new public health* (4th edn). Oxford University Press.

Braveman, B., & Bass-Haugen, J. D. (2009). Social justice and health disparities: An evolving discourse in occupational therapy research and intervention. *American Journal of Occupational Therapy, 63*(1), 7–12. https://doi.org/10.5014/ajot.63.1.7

Braveman, P., & Gruskin, S. (2003). Defining equity in health. *Journal of Epidemiology and Community Health, 57*(4), 254–258. http://dx.doi.org/10.1136/jech.57.4.254

Centre for Rural and Remote Health. (2020). *About us.* https://www.crrh.jcu.edu.au/about-us/

Clemson, L., Cumming, R. G., Kendig, H., Swann, M., Heard, R., & Taylor, K. (2004). The effectiveness of a community-based program for reducing the incidence of falls in the elderly: A randomized trial. *Journal of the American Geriatrics Society, 52*(9), 1487–1494. https://doi.org/10.1111/j.1532-5415.2004.52411.x

Commission on Social Determinants of Health. (2008). Closing the gap in a generation: Health equity through action on the social determinants of health. In *Final report of the Commission on Social Determinants of Health.* World Health Organization. https://www.who.int/social_determinants/thecommission/finalreport/en/

Delany, T., Harris, P., Williams, C., Harris, E., Baum, F., Lawless, A., Wildgoose, D., Haigh, F., MacDougall, C., Broderick, D., & Kickbusch, I. (2014). Health impact assessment in New South Wales & Health in All Policies in South Australia: Differences, similarities and connections. *BMC Public Health, 14*, art. 699. https://doi.org/10.1186/1471-2458-14-699

Galheigo, S. M. (2005). Occupational therapy and the social field. In F. Kronenburg (Ed.), *Occupational therapy without borders: Learning from the spirit of survivors* (pp. 87–98). Churchill Livingstone.

Going Rural Health. (2020). *Service learning placements.* https://goingruralhealth.com.au/student-information/service-learning-placements/

Kannus, P., Khan, K. M., & Lord, S. R. (2006). Preventing falls among elderly people in the hospital environment. *Medical Journal of Australia, 184*(8), 372–373. https://doi.org/10.5694/j.1326-5377.2006.tb00283.x

Keleher, H., & MacDougall, C. (2016). *Understanding health* (4th edn). Oxford University Press.

Laverack, G. (2006). Improving health outcomes through community empowerment: A review of the literature. *Journal of Health Population and Nutrition, 24*(1), 113–120. https://www.jstor.org/stable/23499274

National Aboriginal Community Controlled Health Organisation (NACCHO). (2020). *About NACCHO.* https://www.naccho.org.au/about/

Orleans, T. C. (2000). Promoting the maintenance of health behavior change: Recommendations for the next generation of research and practice. *Health Psychology, 19*(1), 76–83. https://doi.org/10.1037/0278-6133.19.Suppl1.76

People's Health Movement. (2000). *People's charter for health.* https://www.phmovement.org/sites/www.phmovement.org/files/phm-pch-english.pdf

SA Health. (n.d.). *Healthy Kids Menu initiative.* https://www.sahealth.sa.gov.au/wps/wcm/connect/public+content/sa+health+internet/about+us/about+sa+health/health+in+all+policies/healthy+childrens+menus+initiative

SA Health. (2012). *Health in All Policies.* https://www.sahealth.sa.gov.au/wps/wcm/connect/public+content/sa+health+internet/about+us/about+sa+health/health+in+all+policies

Southgate Institute for Health, Society & Equity (n.d.). *Policy brief: Does a Health in All Policies approach improve health, wellbeing and equity in South Australia?* https://www.flinders.edu.au/content/dam/documents/research/southgate-institute/hiap-policy-brief.pdf

Talbot, L., & Verrinder, G. (2014). *Promoting health: The primary health care approach* (5th edn). Elsevier Australia.

Tse, S., Penman, M., & Simms, F. (2003) Literature review: Occupational therapy and primary health care. *New Zealand Journal of Occupational Therapy, 50*(2), 17–23. file:///C:/Users/gtbro/Downloads/Volume-50-Issue-02.pdf

Turrell, G., & Mathers, C. D. (2000). Socioeconomic status and health in Australia. *Medical Journal of Australia, 172*(9), 434–438. https://doi.org/10.5694/j.1326-5377.2000.tb124041.x

World Federation of Occupational Therapists. (2012). *Definition of occupational therapy.* https://www.wfot.org/about

World Health Organization (WHO). (1948). *World Health Organization Constitution. (Online).* https://www.who.int/about/who-we-are/constitution

World Health Organization (WHO) (1978). *Declaration of Alma-Ata.* http://www.who.int/publications/almaata_declaration_en.pdf

World Health Organization (WHO). (2013). *The Helsinki statement on Health in All Policies.* https://www.who.int/healthpromotion/conferences/8gchp/8gchp_helsinki_statement.pdf?ua=1

World Health Organization (WHO). (2018). *Declaration of Astana.* https://www.who.int/docs/default-source/primary-health/declaration/gcphc-declaration.pdf?ua=1

World Health Organization (WHO). (2020). *Health in All Policies.* http://www.euro.who.int/en/health-topics/health-determinants/social-determinants/policy/entry-points-for-addressing-socially-determined-health-inequities/health-in-all-policies-hiap

27 Occupational therapy practice in regional, rural and remote Australia

Monica Moran, Carol McKinstry and Michael Curtin

Chapter objectives

Upon completion of this chapter, the reader will be able to:

- Describe characteristics of populations in regional, rural and remote Australia.
- Identify two commonly used remoteness classification systems.
- Recognise the contexts of health care service relevant to regional, rural and remote occupational therapy practice.
- Grasp the diversity of occupational therapy roles in regional, rural and remote Australia.
- Identify strategies for successful occupational therapy practice in regional, rural and remote locations.
- Understand options for rural and remote student placement.

Key terms

regional, rural and remote practice; occupational therapy; workforce; rural service delivery

Introduction

'Regional, rural and remote Australia' is an umbrella term that encompasses non-metropolitan geographical, political, economic, cultural and spiritual contexts across this continent. This term may conjure up different visions for different individuals, depending on their experiences. In this chapter some of the contextual variations of regional, rural and remote locations will be explored along with how those variations impact on the provision of occupational therapy and other health services.

Regional, rural and remote Australia—a big place

Australia is a large country (7,672,024 km^2) with a small population of 25 million people and a much lower population density in comparison to most other developed countries (Australian Bureau of Statistics [ABS], 2019a; 2019b). Australia's population is mainly concentrated along the eastern and south-eastern coastline. Less than 20 per cent of Australians live more than 50 kilometres from the coastal areas where most towns and cities are located; however, there are more than 1,500 communities across Australia classified as rural or remote.

Classifying remoteness

It is common to refer to all areas outside Australia's major cities as 'rural', with little recognition that there are considerable differences between regional, rural and remote locations, as well as differences within each of these geographical areas. To assist with distinguishing the different locations, remoteness classification systems have been developed. The purpose of these classification systems is to provide an understanding of the impact of living in different locations in Australia, which in turn can influence the development and implementation of Federal, State and Territory government policies and priorities, and resource allocation.

The 2018 Australian health report (Australian Institute of Health and Welfare [AIHW], 2018) indicates that the more remote a population the higher the rates of:

- Health risk factors (e.g., smoking, alcohol consumption, physical inactivity, and being overweight);
- Burden of disease as measured by the health impact of disease on a population in a given year in terms of dying and living with disease and injury—this is referred to as Disability-Adjusted Life Years (DALYs);
- Mortality;
- Potentially avoidable death—that is, deaths among people under 75 years considered to be preventable due to individual or primary health/hospital care; and
- Potentially preventable hospitalisations.

The AIHW (2018) Report suggests that the poorer health outcomes may be a result of factors such 'disadvantage in education, employment opportunities, income and access to services' (AIHW, 2018, p. 259). The Report concludes that the 'challenges of geographic spread, low population density, limited infrastructure, as well as the higher costs of delivering rural and remote health care, can affect access to health care' (p. 265). In part, this access to health care is due to a significant decline in the number of health care professionals, or hours of health professionals' service, as remoteness increases. Hence, systems to classify location are an important way to assess the health and workforce needs, and the resources needed to meet those needs (Services for Australian Rural and Remote Allied Health [SARRAH], n.d.). It should be noted that although the AIHW report indicates poorer health outcomes the more remote a person lives, studies indicate that people living in rural communities experience higher levels of social participation and inclusion than people living in metropolitan settings (McIntosh et al., 2019; Wilkins, 2015).

There are two commonly accepted approaches to classifying remoteness in Australia: Australian Standard Geographical Classification—Remoteness Areas (ASGC-RA) and the Modified Monash Model (MMM) (SARRAH, n.d.)

Australian Standard Geographical Classification—Remoteness Areas

The ASGC-RA is employed by the Australian Bureau of Statistics (ABS, 2016). This classification system defines remoteness into five categories of relative remoteness across Australia (Table 27.1).

Relative remoteness is measured using the Accessibility and Remoteness Index (ARIA+) developed by the Hugo Centre for Migration and Population Research, University of Adelaide. ARIA+ is a continuous varying index with values ranging from

0 (high accessibility) to 15 (high remoteness). The calculated ARIA+ for a location is based on road distance of the location from the five nearest service centres of different population sizes. The five different service centre population sizes used to calculate the ARIA+ score for a location are listed in Table 27.2 (Hugo Centre for Migration and Population Research, n.d.).

This ASCG-RA classification system is based on the assumption that any locality with a population greater than 1,000 people will have a basic level of health and education services, and shops. The larger the population in a locality, the greater the level of service provision. A map of the 2016 Remoteness Areas for Australia can be seen in Figure 27.1.

Modified Monash Model

The Modified Monash Model (MMM) was developed by the Department of Health to identify the disparities in access to health services across Australia (Department of Health, n.d.). The MMM uses the five categories of the ASGS-RA classification system as its basis and further subdivides geographical remoteness based on the size of local towns or cities. This recognises that there can be significant differences between towns, even if they have the same population and share the same ASGC-RA classification. There are seven location categories in the MMM (Department of Health, n.d.). These are listed in Table 27.3. Figure 27.2 illustrates the location of the MMM categories on a map of Australia.

The MMM has been used to determine financial incentives to attract and retain health professionals to offer services in rural and remote areas. For example, some employers may offer subsidised housing and other allowances to assist health professionals to live and practice in MMM regions 4–7.

Table 27.1 Classes of relative remoteness with ARIA+ ranges

Categories of relative remoteness	ARIA+ value ranges
Major cities (RA1)	0 to 0.2
Inner regional (RA2)	> 0.2 and ≤ 2.4
Outer regional (RA3)	> 2.4 and ≤ 5.92
Remote (RA4)	> 5.92 and ≤ 10.53
Very remote (RA5)	> 10.53

Table 27.2 Service centre categories

Service centre category	Urban centre population
A	250,000 persons or more
B	48,000–249,999 persons
C	18,000–47,999 persons
D	5,000–17,999 persons
E	1,000–4,999 persons

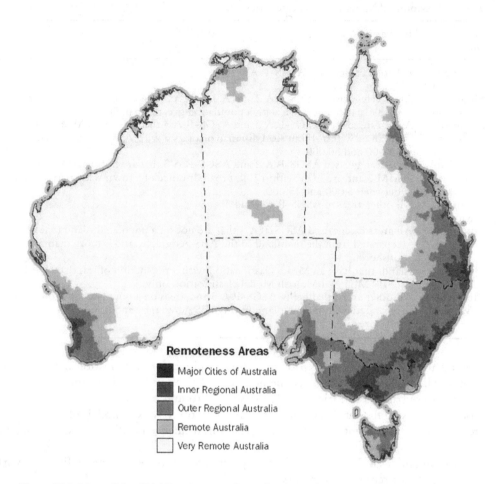

Figure 27.1 Map of the 2016 Remoteness Areas for Australia.

Source: Creative Commons Attribution-ShareAlike 2.5 Licence http://creativecommons.org/licenses/by-nc-sa/2.5/au/
https://www.abs.gov.au/ausstats/abs@.nsf/Latestproducts/1270.0.55.005Main%20Features 5July%202016?opendocument&tabname=Summary&prodno=1270.0.55.005&issue=July%20 2016&num=&view=

Life in regional, rural and remote areas

Communities in regional, rural and remote areas of Australia differ quite significantly to urban communities. Whilst people of many backgrounds live outside urban areas, and these communities are heterogeneous and diverse, there are some marked variations in population distribution. Fewer people who were born overseas are living in regional areas (14 per cent), rural areas (13 per cent) and very remote areas (8 per cent), in comparison to those born overseas and living in the major cities (31 per cent) (Baxter et al., 2011). On the other hand, Aboriginal and Torres Strait Islander peoples are more heavily represented in regional, rural and remote communities. They comprise approximately 1 per cent of the population in major cities 15 per cent in rural areas and up to 50 per cent in very remote areas (Baxter et al., 2011).

A common stereotype is that the lives of rural dwelling Australians revolve around agriculture and jobs associated with the land. However, heavy industries are major employers

Table 27.3 Modified Monash Model categories

MMM category	Brief description
Modified Monash 1	All areas categorised ASGS-RA1.
Modified Monash 2	Areas categorised ASGS-RA 2 and ASGS-RA 3 that are in or within 20km road distance of a town with a population greater than 50,000.
Modified Monash 3	Areas categorised ASGS-RA 2 and ASGS-RA 3 that are not in MM 2 and are in or within 15km road distance of a town with a population between 15,000 and 50,000.
Modified Monash 4	Areas categorised ASGS-RA 2 and ASGS-RA 3 that are not in MM 2 or MM 3 and are in or within 10km road distance of a town with a population between 5,000 and 15,000.
Modified Monash 5	All other areas in ASGS-RA 2 and 3.
Modified Monash 6	All areas categorised ASGS-RA 4 that are not on a populated island that is separated from the mainland in the ABS geography and is more than 5km offshore. Islands that have an MM 5 classification with a population of less than 1,000 (2019 Modified Monash Model classification only).
Modified Monash 7	All other areas; that being ASGS-RA 5 and areas on a populated island that is separated from the mainland in the ABS geography and is more than 5km offshore.

in rural and remote locations. In these sectors employment participation may fluctuate widely. The cyclical boom and decline pattern of the resources and mining industries in particular contributes to major population shifts into and out of regional, rural and remote areas. Fly in fly out (FIFO) and drive in drive out (DIDO) models of employment are also factors. Transient employment populations influence rural social issues such as:

- housing prices inflated by lack of supply—it can be more expensive to live and work in a rural or remote community;
- less social connectedness for families with workers commuting long distances to outer regional or remote locations on rotating work schedules; and
- high turnover of workforce.

Although it is recognised that people living in regional, rural and remote parts of Australia 'make a profound contribution to the economic and social fabric of the nation', there is 'significant maldistribution of many health professions in Australia including allied health providers, which results in much poorer access to services for rural people, negatively impacting their health, wellbeing and economic participation' (National Rural Health Commissioner [NRHC], 2019, p. 5). The limitations of service provision contribute to poorer population health outcomes across a number of indicators. In addition, the lack of availability of health services can mean that many people need to travel to towns and cities that are regional hubs, as well as to major cities in order to access specialised health services and resources.

Occupational therapy workforce distribution

There were 23,655 registered occupational therapists in Australia as at 31 December 2019 (Occupational Therapy Board of Australia, 2019). Although there has been an

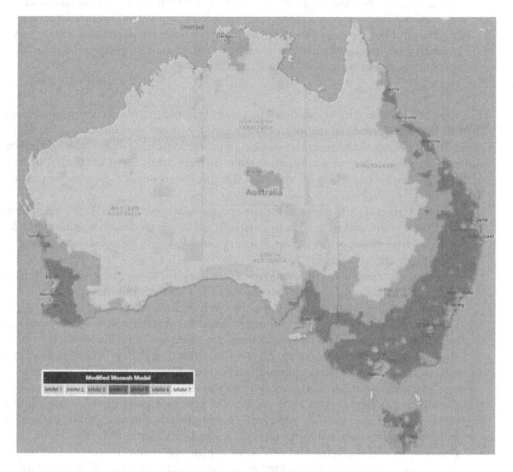

Figure 27.2 Map of the Modified Monash Model regions.
Source: Creative Commons Attribution-ShareAlike 2.5 Licence http://creativecommons.org/licenses/by-nc-sa/2.5/au/
https://blog.coviu.com/2019/01/08/what-is-the-modified-monash-model-and-why-is-it-important/

increase in the numbers of occupational therapists in Australia, the demand for their services as part of a rural health workforce is anticipated to grow as the populations in rural areas become older, rates of chronic diseases continue to increase and team-based service delivery models evolve (Drabsch, 2015; Humphreys et al., 2010).

Occupational therapy practice in regional, rural and remote settings

Health professionals, including occupational therapists, in regional, rural and remote areas generally work:

Across a broad scope of practice, large geographic catchments, visiting multiple communities, with fewer resources and higher [client] to therapist ratios and less infrastructure than their counterparts in urban areas. They require a broad range of skills including paediatrics, culturally appropriate practice, chronic diseases, health

promotion and prevention, primary health, and health service management knowledge in delivering appropriate services to diverse population groups across the age
spectrum. There are not enough practitioners to service population need. Service
prioritisation and rationalisation therefore occurs based on the providers available,
their skills, population need and infrastructure.

(NRHC, 2019, p. 6)

The unique issues faced by occupational therapists practising in regional, rural and remote
areas of Australia have been the subject of research for some time (Devine, 2006; Merritt
et al., 2013). Occupational therapists working in these locations require a broad skill base
and well-developed caseload prioritisation skills (Lannin & Longland, 2003, p. 186). Some
of the unique issues impacting occupational therapists working in these locations include:

- Caseload diversity and the need for the occupational therapist to have a broad range
  of clinical skills, and to quickly understand and develop competence in operational
  skills such as intake prioritisation, waiting list management, case conferencing and
  inter-professional practice.
- Sole therapists may have difficulty accessing back-fill (temporary cover or replace-
  ment) and might need to temporarily cease their services in order to take leave and
  deal with a substantial caseload upon their return to work.
- Lengthy travel times are common in occupational therapy practice in regional, rural and remote areas. It is not uncommon for therapists to be employed by a public
  community health service with a hub in one town, and have to travel to provide
  outreach services to clients in numerous surrounding communities, some of which
  can be hundreds of kilometres away from the service hub.
- Occupational therapists in both public and private sectors in these communities
  work with populations that experience poorer health outcomes, have higher rates
  of hospital admission and lower rates of hospital procedures (AIHW, 2018).
- Perceptions of geographic and professional isolation, reduced access to continuing
  professional development, concerns about future career paths and opportunities.
- Social complexities of living and working among regional communities.

Allied health professionals working in regional, rural and remote areas can develop expertise to become an allied health rural generalist. This role involves:

Delivering services that responds to the broad range of health care needs of a regional, rural or remote community. This includes delivering services to people
with a wide range of clinical presentations, from across the age spectrum, and in a
variety of clinical settings (inpatient, ambulatory care and community).

(NRHC, 2019, p. 11)

To be an effective allied health rural generalist the NRHC (2019) state that allied health
professional needs to be:

- Comfortable with their professional and discipline identity;
- Willing to embrace an extended scope of practice way of working, including skill
  sharing;
- Able to work effectively with, and delegate work to, support workers;

- Competently use telehealth services; and
- **Able to develop collaborative partnerships across agencies and sectors.**

Factors influencing workforce retention in rural and remote areas

O'Toole et al. (2010) explored why allied health professionals (AHPs) in rural Victoria left their jobs. Lincoln et al. (2014) carried out a similar study examining the challenges faced by AHPs working in the disability sector in rural and remote locations. Both studies reported that a combination of organisational, professional and/or personal experiences impacted on their decisions to stay in their position or leave. Factors that contributed to AHPs leaving included variations in pay between service providers and insecure employment arrangements, long waiting lists, the burden of travel between remote sites and heavy administrative loads. A range of factors considered to positively influence rural and remote AHP retention is listed by Services for Australian Rural and Remote Allied Health (SARRAH, 2015) including:

- Being part of a collaborative work team;
- Participation in a peer and professional support network;
- Having regular opportunities for professional and career development;
- Access to adequate administrative and technological resources;
- Receiving appropriate recognition, rewards and remuneration; and
- An existing workplace culture that enables life role balance.

Strategies to enhance rural practice

One strategy to equip occupational therapists to manage the unique demands of working in regional, rural and remote locations is to prepare them during their pre-registration university programs. This involves designing a curriculum to prepare graduates with appropriate skills for rural practice and providing them with access to quality rural placements. A number of Australian universities have established occupational therapy courses in regional areas while some courses require students to undertake at least one placement in a regional or rural area.

A second strategy is to advocate for and utilise innovative health workforce models that support the development of a sustainable workforce through providing support for career development. Recently the Allied Health Rural Generalist (AHRG) Pathway was introduced to address issues relating to recruitment and retention (https://sarrah. org.au/ahrgp). The pathway aims to provide support to employ new graduates and early career therapists, ensuring that the graduates have intensive support and formal training to continue their learning and professional development. New graduates are provided with time during work to undertake online study modules and receive regular supervision from an experienced occupational therapist. Some Government funding is available for public health services and not-for-profit organisations to support employers to utilise the AHRG pathway. Support is also available for therapists to receive financial assistance for ongoing education such as attending conferences through funding from the state branches of Rural Health Workforce Australia (http://www.rhwa.org. au/ruralworkforceagencies).

A third strategy for supporting therapists in managing their rural caseload is the introduction of telehealth services. Telehealth is defined as the 'use of telecommunication techniques for the purpose of providing telemedicine, health education and medical education over a distance' (Australian Government Department of Health, 2015). Tele-health has the capacity to reduce costs and save travel time for consumers and therapists in rural areas and is increasingly used in public sector organisations (Lepard et al., 2015; Wade et al., 2012). The COVID-19 pandemic resulted in a surge of telehealth resources including practice guidelines for occupational therapy (Occupational Therapy Australia, 2020; World Federation of Occupational Therapists, 2014). As communication technologies become more sophisticated and the National Broadband Network reaches into more remote areas, the opportunities to use telehealth for occupational therapy service delivery will continue to expand.

Developing and managing oneself in rural practice

Working in regional, rural and remote locations requires a different skill set than working in a metropolitan area, due to caseload diversity and the prevalence of clients with complex, chronic conditions such as diabetes, arthritis and mental illness (AIHW, 2018). Statistics indicate that higher frequencies of injury occur in regional areas, and death rates from injury are higher in regional and remote areas (National Rural Health Alliance, 2009). This may be related to higher levels of participation in dangerous occupations such as farming, fishing, road transportation and forestry (National Rural Health Alliance, 2009).

The broad-based, unique and specialised rural practice skills required to meet the needs of rural populations means that occupational therapists require diverse continuing professional development, focusing on both the variety and complexity of clinical presentations, as well as administrative competencies. Accessing continuing professional development can be a significant ongoing challenge. Relevant training often involves travel and accommodation away from the workplace and therapists need to strongly advocate for their continuing professional development needs to be met.

Opportunities are increasing for rural therapists to undertake continuing professional development, supervision and mentoring relevant to the characteristics of their work context via online platforms. Regular participation in training opportunities is an essential characteristic of successful rural practice. Membership of professional associations enables rural therapists to develop their professional networks, take on leadership roles and access evidence-based online professional development.

Studies from overseas and within Australia have suggested that building relationships with community leaders including Aboriginal and Torres Strait Islander Elders, and

> *"It hard to realise the impact of limited access to services on rural people e.g.*
>
> *having to fly to a city three hours away for a test. "*
>
> *"Getting aids and appliances e.g. wheelchair could take months. Local people say*
>
> *that's all we have access to so we just have to make it work."*

Reflection from occupational therapy student on remote placement

Figure 27.3 Preparing the rural health workforce of the future.

developing skills in culturally appropriate practice, enable rural therapists to appreciate the strengths of the community in which they work (Chipp et al., 2011). Participating in the community via informal interactions, sports, leisure and cultural events are strategies to prevent social isolation and establish networks (Chipp et al., 2011). These strategies for connection can contribute positively to self-management and self-care by increasing personal and professional support networks.

Preparing the rural health workforce of the future

There is strong evidence that completing a regional, rural and/or remote placement as part of occupational therapy pre-registration training increases the likelihood of students returning to work in these locations after graduation (Playford et al., 2020). However, many metropolitan students are hesitant about completing a regional, rural and/or remote placement. Fear of the unknown, financial worries and concerns about the quality of learning that would be available to them can all impact on students' readiness for these types of placements.

In order to increase the number of allied health students (including occupational therapy students) experiencing regional, rural and remote placements, the Commonwealth Government has over the past 20 years developed and funded 16 University Departments of Rural Health (UDRH). The functions of the UDRH are listed in Box 27.1.

Box 27.1 Functions of University Departments of Rural Health

- Increase and improve rural experiences for undergraduate students in the health professions, including training to encourage cultural awareness and sensitivity to Indigenous health issues, for undergraduate students in the health professions;
- Expand educational opportunities relevant to rural and remote practice, in particular in relation to existing rural and remote health professionals and Indigenous students;
- Undertake research into rural and remote health issues, including publication of papers and reports and applying for research grants and consultancies;
- Provide training and support for rural health professionals (including mentors, supervisors and preceptors), consumers and communities, including Indigenous communities;
- Contribute to innovation in education, research and service development through collaborations with universities, health services and professional and community organisations, including Indigenous communities;
- Embrace a strong public or population health focus; and contribute to the development of innovative service delivery models in rural and remote health; and
- Endeavour to progress the rural health agenda within the medical and other health sciences faculties or departments to maximise the efficient use of resources provided for a range of rural health programs.

Source: RCS-UDRH (2008)

> *"I currently have four staff members in my team who completed a UDRH rural placement in the region. Completing a placement gives students an understanding of our rural context and they make social connections here, so their willingness to apply for roles in our region is increased."*

Rural Director of Community Health Service

Figure 27.4 Completing a placement

Students who complete practice placements in regional, rural or remote locations across the Australia via the UDRH network participate in clinical, community and service learning placements arranged by and in some cases supervised by a team of expert health professional educators. Where students are not directly supervised by UDRH educators, the organisation provides training, mentoring and support to regional, rural and remote clinicians in their supervision role. The critical long-term outcome of this work is to help build the regional, rural and remote health workforce.

Increasingly, virtual networks provide for e-learning back to the metropolitan and regional campuses allowing students to engage in campus-based opportunities from rural and remote sites. This is opening up the possibility for longer placements so that students can become more embedded in regional, rural and remote communities. The UDRH model is designed to provide a safe and supported learning environment that goes beyond academic and clinical support to include practical help with provision of comfortable and secure accommodation, transport, social support and cultural orientation.

Regional, rural and remote placements provide students with exposure to the significant health and social challenges experienced by communities in these locations. They experience work in environments that demand innovation and creative clinical reasoning, often with fewer resources and more distributed service delivery models. Conversely students are exposed to the benefits of regional, rural and remote practice, with smaller close-knit multidisciplinary teams, supportive communities and opportunities to extend their learning.

Completing a regional, rural or remote placement also introduces students to service providers and employers keen to recruit new professionals to their teams. Many students who complete placements in their final years of university return to take up professional roles in regional, rural and remote locations.

Building resilience in the next generation of rural occupational therapists

The concept of resilience, the ability to successfully adapt to life's demands, can be enhanced over time and via a series of learning experiences. It is identified as an important outcome for the successful transition into practice and maintenance of health professionals. There is widespread inclusion of learning opportunities for students in UDRHs to work together in supported inter-professional teams, develop cross cultural skills and have practical support as they learn. These immersive learning experiences in a supportive environment contribute to building resilience in health professional students. The exposure to regional, rural and remote communities further strengthens students' resilience and sense of security regarding a future career in similar locations. It is no surprise that many of the health professionals currently practising in regional, rural and remote locations in Australia have passed through a UDRH as a student.

> Having students on placement was a very rewarding experience for us. At the end of their placement they were offered short term contracts because I saw them in action and felt satisfied they had the right qualifications, skills and personality for our organisation. Without the UDRH providing these opportunities for rural and remote placements, many metropolitan based students wouldn't get the rich learning experiences that come with these placements, which ultimately encourage these students to apply for positions in these regions upon graduation.
>
> (Rural Director of Mental Health Services)

Case study

Michael was camping on the Murray River during his summer holidays with his friends when a branch from a gum tree fell on his tent, causing a spinal injury and fracturing his 12th thoracic vertebrae. Michael lives in Robinvale and was in his third year of a plumbing apprenticeship when his accident happened. He spent over six months in hospital and inpatient rehabilitation in Melbourne and was then transferred to Bendigo for further inpatient rehabilitation. Often people living in regional, rural and remote settings need to travel to cities for specialist care, putting a strain on the individual and their family.

Suzie was Michael's occupational therapist in Bendigo, two hours north of Melbourne. Suzie had been working on the rehab ward for 12 months since graduating. She works on this ward with another more experienced occupational therapist, Chloe, who is her supervisor. Suzie is fortunate to have a more experienced therapist as her supervisor, particularly as Chloe has lived and worked in Bendigo for many years. She also works closely with two physiotherapists, a speech pathologist, a social worker, a dietician, an exercise physiologist, a clinical psychologist and a rehabilitation physician. Suzie had never worked with someone with spinal injuries; however, Michael's physiotherapist had a lot of experience. In regional, rural and remote settings occupational therapists often have to be able to work with a diverse range of clients, because there is usually not as many clients with a similar condition attending rehabilitation as there is in metropolitan centres. This diversity of caseload is often considered an advantage when working regionally, rurally and remotely. Initially Suzie was feeling quite overwhelmed with the range of occupational issues Michael reported. However, she had fortnightly supervision sessions with Chloe, frequent informal catch-ups, and worked in a supportive team, and so received the guidance that she required. Michael was very keen to return home to Robinvale where he lived with his girlfriend, and where his parents and brothers also live.

Suzie was working with Michael to further improve his ability to do self-care occupations. Michael needed assistance with showering but could dress himself. Suzie needed to work closely with the social worker to submit a NDIS application to arrange for Michael's home and car modifications, as well as obtain the necessary personal care assistance he needed. She also worked closely with Maddy, the occupational therapist in Robinvale.

Maddy is one of only two occupational therapists working in Robinvale. Robinvale is a town with 3,300 people situated on the New South Wales and Victorian border, five hours from Melbourne. Maddy had been at Robinvale for six months when she first met Michael and was working in Mildura for the previous 12 months after she graduated. She was attracted to working in Robinvale because of the varied caseload. Maddy covers all the inpatient services including the acute ward and maternity ward, as well as people having renal dialysis and the aged care residential service. She provides services to people in their homes and community. The other occupational therapist works with children and families.

Michael was on weekend leave at his parents' house when Maddy first met him. He had travelled for nearly four hours to Robinvale on the Friday and was quite exhausted when he met Maddy and the community nurses at his parents' home. Maddy had some temporary equipment for the home and worked closely with the community nurses to problem-solve the issues that Michael, his girlfriend and parents had identified. Maddy had met Suzie when they were both involved in professional development at a recent regional allied health conference in Bendigo and talked to Suzie via teleconference about Michael's ongoing rehabilitation.

Michael successfully gained an NDIS package to have his home and car modifications funded and moved back to Robinvale. He needed to travel back to Bendigo for driving rehabilitation because there was no occupational therapist qualified to conduct his driving assessment in the Robinvale area. Maddy continued working with Michael, continuing his rehabilitation in his home, working on leisure and vocational goals, particularly a return to study. Maddy and her employer had taken up the Allied Health Rural Generalist Pathway and Maddy had completed two online study modules while also receiving weekly supervision from the other occupational therapist in Robinvale. Maddy had also made contact with the occupational therapists who had worked with Michael as an inpatient in Melbourne, using telehealth technology to ask questions related to Michael's rehabilitation. As Michael was unable to receive all the health services he required in Robinvale or Bendigo, he still needed to attend some specialist appointments in Melbourne.

Conclusion

Practice in regional, rural and remote areas offers many opportunities, rewards and challenges for occupational therapists. Understanding the geographical, social and cultural contexts for practice is essential for therapists to successfully participate in the regional, rural and remote health workforce. Implementing a variety of evidence-based strategies that assist them to manage these unique challenges is critical for personal and professional development and sustainability.

Summary

- The majority of the population of Australia live in urban areas on the eastern coast of the country; only about 20 per cent of the population live in regions classified as regional, rural and remote.

- There are a number of potential challenges associated with practising as an occupational therapist in a regional, rural and/or remote location, but there are also numerous rewards.
- Understanding the geographical, social and cultural contexts for regional, rural and remote practice is essential for occupational therapists to support their practice.
- Support networks exist for occupational therapy students to complete professional placements in regional, rural and remote locations.

Review questions

1. Describe the influence of level of remoteness on occupational therapy workforce distribution.
2. How can new graduates working in regional, rural and remote locations sustain their professional development needs?
3. Explain the benefits and challenges associated with providing occupational therapy services in regional, rural and remote settings.
4. Read the case study. What interests you about these therapists' experiences?
5. Can you see yourself practising in rural and remote health, and if so how you would seek out more information?

References

Australian Bureau of Statistics. (2016). *Defining remoteness areas.* https://www.abs.gov.au/ausstats/abs@.nsf/Latestproducts/1270.0.55.005Main%20Features15July%202016?opendocument&tabname=Summary&prodno=1270.0.55.005&issue=July%202016&num=&view

Australian Bureau of Statistics. (2019a). *Defining remoteness areas.* https://www.abs.gov.au/ausstats/abs@.nsf/Latestproducts/3218.0Main%20Features102018-19?opendocument&tabname=Summary&prodno=3218.0&issue=2018-19&num=&view=

Australian Bureau of Statistics. (2019b). *Australian demographic statistics.* https://www.abs.gov.au/AUSSTATS/abs@.nsf/mf/3101.0

Australian Government Department of Health. (2015). *Telehealth.* http://www.health.gov.au/internet/main/publishing.nsf/content/e-health-telehealth

Australian Institute of Health and Welfare. (2018). *Rural, regional and remote health: Indicators of health system performance.* https://www.aihw.gov.au/reports/rural-health/rural-regional-and-remote-health-indicators-of-health-system-performance/contents/table-of-contents

Baxter, J., Gray, M., & Hayes, A. (2011). *Families in regional, rural and remote Australia.* Australian Institute of Family Studies. https://aifs.gov.au/sites/default/files/publication-documents/fs201103.pdf

Chipp, C, Dewane, S., Brems, C., Johnson, M. E., Warner, T. D., & Roberts, L. W. (2011). 'If only someone had told me …': Lessons from rural providers. *The Journal of Rural Health, 27*(1), 122–130. https://doi.org/10.1111/j.1748-0361.2010.00314.x

Department of Health. (n.d.). *Modified Monash Model.* https://www.health.gov.au/health-workforce/health-workforce-classifications/modified-monash-model

Devine, S. (2006). Perceptions of occupational therapists practising in rural Australia: A graduate perspective. *Australian Occupational Therapy Journal, 53*(3), 205–210. https://doi.org/10.1111/j.1440-1630.2006.00561.x

Drabsch, T. (2015). Rural collaborative guideline implementation: Evaluation of a hub and spoke multidisciplinary team model of care for orthogeriatric inpatients—a before and after study of adherence to clinical practice guidelines. *Australian Journal of Rural Health, 23(2)*, 80–86. https://doi.org/10.1111/ajr.12139

Hugo Centre for Migration and Population Research. (n.d.). *Accessibility/Remoteness Index of Australia (ARIA)*. https://www.adelaide.edu.au/hugo-centre/services/aria#aria-methodology

Humphreys, J., Chisholm, M., & Russell, D. (2010). *Rural allied health workforce retention in Victoria: Modelling the benefits of increased length of stay and reduced staff turnover*. Monash University School of Rural Health.

Lannin, N., & Longland, S. (2003). Critical shortage of occupational therapists in rural Australia: Changing our long-held beliefs provides a solution. *Australian Occupational Therapy Journal, 50(3)*, 184–187. https://doi.org/10.1046/j.1440-1630.2003.00394.x

Lepard, M. G., Joseph, A. L., Agne, A. A., & Cherrington, A. L. (2015). Diabetes self-management interventions for adults with type 2 diabetes living in rural areas: A systematic literature review. *Current Diabetes Reports, 15(6)*, 1–12. https://doi.org/10.1007/s11892-015-0608-3

Lincoln, M., Gallego, G., Dew, A., Bulkeley, K., Veitch, C., Bundy, A., Brentnall, J., Chedid, R. J., & Griffiths, S. (2014). Recruitment and retention of allied health professionals in the disability sector in rural and remote New South Wales, Australia. *Journal of Intellectual and Developmental Disability, 39(1)*, 86–97. https://doi.org/10.3109/13668250.2013.861393

McIntosh, K., Kenny, A., Masood, M., & Dickson-Swift, V. (2019). Social inclusion as a tool to improve rural health. *Australian Journal of Primary Health, 25(2)*, 137–145. https://doi.org/10.1071/PY17185

Merritt, J., Perkins, D., & Boreland, F. (2013). Regional and remote occupational therapy: A preliminary exploration of private occupational therapy practice. *Australian Occupational Therapy Journal, 60(4)*, 276–287. https://doi.org/10.1111/1440-1630.12042

National Rural Health Alliance. (2009). *The state of rural health*. http://ruralhealth.org.au/sites/default/files/fact-sheets/fact-sheet-09-the%20state%20of%20rural%20health_0.pdf

National Rural Health Commissioner. (2019). *Rural allied health quality, access and distribution*. https://ahpa.com.au/wp-content/uploads/2019/08/190816-Rural-Remote-Discussion-Paper-response-FINAL.pdf

Occupational Therapy Australia. (2020). *Telehealth guidelines*. https://otaus.com.au/publicassets/553c6eae-ad6c-ea11-9404-005056be13b5/OTA%20Telehealth%20Guidelines%202020.pdf

Occupational Therapy Board of Australia. (2019). *Registrant data October 2019 to December 2019*. https://www.occupationaltherapyboard.gov.au/About/Statistics.aspx

O'Toole, K., Schoo, A., & Hernan, A. (2010). Why did they leave and what can they tell us? Allied health professionals leaving rural settings. *Australian Health Review, 34(1)*, 66–72. https://doi.org/10.1071/AH09711

Playford, D., Moran, M. C., & Thompson, S. (2020). Factors associated with rural work for nursing and allied health graduates 15–17 years after an undergraduate rural placement through the University of Rural Health programme. *Rural and Remote Health, 20*, 5334. https://doi.org/10.22605/RRH5334

RCS-UDRH. (2008). *RCS-UDRH Final Report: Rural Clinical Schools Program*. https://www1.health.gov.au/internet/main/publishing.nsf/content/A3760E61F341B7F5CA257BF0001D73AB/$File/udrhcon.pdf

Services for Australian Rural and Remote Allied Health (SARRAH). (2015). *Defining remote and rural context*. http://www.sarrah.org.au

Wade, V. A., Eliott, J. A, & Hiller, J. E. (2012). A qualitative study of ethical, medico-legal and clinical governance matters in Australian telehealth services. *Journal of Telemedicine and Telecare, 18(2)*, 109–114. https://doi.org/10.1258/jtt.2011.110808

Wilkins, R. (2015). *The household, income and labour dynamics in Australia survey: Selected findings from waves 1 to 12*. Melbourne Institute of Applied Economic and Social Research.

World Federation of Occupational Therapists. (2014). Position statement on telehealth. *International Journal of Telerehabilitation, 6(1)*, 37–39. https://doi.org/10.5195/ijt.2014.6153

28 Population and community occupational therapy practice and project management in Australia

Lisa Knightbridge, Susan Gilbert-Hunt and Nerida Hyett

Chapter objectives

Upon completion of this chapter, the reader will be able to:

- Describe how population-centred and community-centred occupational therapy is delivered in Australia.
- Describe the contribution of the Alma-Ata declaration to occupational therapy practice.
- Discuss the similarities and differences of individual-centred, population-centred and community-centred practices.
- Explain the key steps involved in a project approach as used by occupational therapists in population and community level practice roles.
- Advise how this approach can be applied to practice across a range of occupational challenges, populations and settings.

Key terms

population approaches to health; population-centred practice; community-centred practice; project management; occupational justice

Introduction

A population approach to health is concerned with the health outcomes of a group of individuals, community or population with particular attention to the distribution of the outcomes within the group (Kindig & Stoddart, 2003). Occupational therapists are able to use occupation to promote health and well-being with populations and address disparities that may exist (Commission on Education, 2011). The majority of occupational therapists, however, practise with individual clients because of system and funding structures (such as Medicare) and due to the dominant historical discourse of individualism that underpins occupational therapy practice models (Gerlach et al., 2017). Increasingly, key occupational therapy authors in Australia and internationally call for a paradigm shift, to extend occupational therapy practice beyond an individual focus, to populations and communities (Gerlach et al., 2017; Hyett et al., 2016). This practice shift requires guidance on how to apply occupational therapy practice processes at population and community levels, and the development and incorporation of new practices that respond to occupational injustices and contribute to societal change

(Whiteford et al., 2018). Such a shift requires occupational therapists to learn additional skills. Practice with populations and communities can often take on the form of projects that address specific occupational participation and engagement issues, for example social isolation. Therefore, project management is an essential skill (Gilbert Hunt et al., 2017).

This chapter provides an overview of population and community-centred occupational therapy practice including key elements and practice processes. A project management approach is outlined, informed by the five essential elements of occupation-based practice (Townsend & Polatajko, 2013, p. 207) and the Canadian Practice Process Framework (Townsend & Polatajko, 2013, p. 233). Four case studies are presented to illustrate population-centred and community-centred practice incorporating project management and enablement strategies.

Population and community occupational therapy practice: Background and influences

The realisation that disease-focused, episodic, acute care intervention was not effective in managing chronic diseases or the disparities in health status across population groups led to the development of the Alma-Ata declaration in 1978, which signalled the need for action by all governments to promote the health of all citizens and not just address issues of ill health (World Health Organization [WHO], 1978). In the years leading up to this conference, hospital-based care and specialist medical treatments were proving to be increasingly expensive, resource-intensive and out of reach of those most in need. Moreover, the requirement to adopt the principles of universal and equitable access to community-based services and the move beyond the biomedical make-up of the individual were necessary.

Importantly, environmental, social and economic factors were recognised as playing key roles in the determinants of health and well-being. Through the Ottawa Charter, health was reframed as no longer being merely the absence of disease, but also a state of complete physical, mental and social well-being (WHO, 1986). It also acknowledged many sectors, such as education, housing and transport, as well as the economic sector, play a role in health (WHO, 1986). The practice of health professionals, including occupational therapists, has evolved to encompass community-based settings, health and well-being as intervention outcomes, and environmental and social determinants among the health issues targeted.

Influences in occupational therapy

In Australia, Ann Wilcock was a strong advocate for the occupational therapy profession to embrace the underlying principles of the Alma-Ata. Wilcock argued that the profession's understanding of the relationship between people's engagement in occupation and health positioned occupational therapists to provide expertise in developing and providing public or population health-based practice (Wilcock, 1998). In the United States, Gail Fidler (2000) urged the occupational therapy profession to shift to underpinning principles more consistent with this approach to health: 'I am advocating that we find the courage to shift our priorities from the acute short-term hospital of today to environments that will make it possible for society and systems to benefit from the practice of authentic occupational therapy' (p. 99).

This shift has been pervasive as reflected in the World Federation of Occupational Therapists (WFOT) Occupational Therapy and Community-Centred Practice position statement (WFOT, 2019) and Standard 3 of the Australian Occupational Therapy Competency Standards, which states 'An occupational therapist's practice acknowledges the relationship between health, wellbeing and human occupation, and their practice is client-centred for individuals, groups, communities and populations' (Occupational Therapy Board of Australia, 2018). Australian registration standards recognise that occupational therapists might not be employed in positions which identify them as occupational therapists, and this is particularly relevant in population and community level positions. Occupational therapists' practice at the population and community levels extends beyond direct clinical care and includes non-clinical relationships with a range of clients and roles in management, community education, policy development and research (Occupational Therapy Board of Australia, 2018).

Occupational therapy incorporates health, well-being and inclusion as fundamental outcomes for interventions targeting complex, systemic and environmental determinants at a population level:

> Occupational therapy is the art and science of enabling engagement in everyday living, through occupation; of enabling people to perform the occupations that foster health and well-being; and of enabling a just and inclusive society so that all people may participate to their potential in the daily occupations of life.
>
> (Townsend & Polatajko, 2013, p. 380)

Occupation-based concepts, models and frameworks are being developed to guide occupational therapists with population-centred and community-centred practice. Key concepts such as *occupational justice*, occupational deprivation and occupational alienation are valuable for enabling occupational therapists to identify and address environmental determinants of occupational performance issues in populations and communities (Malfitano et al., 2016). An occupational injustice is when 'where people are prevented from equitable participation in society' (Occupational Therapy Australia, 2016, p. 4). Identifying occupational injustices enables the development of actions and interventions that increase people's access to resources or opportunities needed for engagement in occupations and for social inclusion (Whiteford et al., 2018).

Whereas individual occupational therapy approaches seek to address specific occupational challenges for an individual or a small group of clients, often with a specific diagnosis, population-centred approaches generally target groups of people whose occupational challenges are positively or negatively determined by common physical, social, economic and/or environmental determinants. *Population-centred practice* in occupational therapy is focused on designing and implementing interventions that improve health and well-being for a targeted group of people through enabling occupation or through addressing occupational injustice. The population shares one or more common elements such as geographic boundaries, health and well-being issues, social group attributes, and personal attributes. *Community-centred practice* involves collaborative practices that occupational therapists undertake in partnership with communities to plan and facilitate health and well-being interventions that can enable communities to achieve an occupational goal (WFOT, 2019). The next section considers population- and community-centred occupational therapy practice, essential elements and a practice process.

Population-centred and community-centred occupational therapy practice: Essential elements

According to Townsend and Polatajko (2013) there are five essential elements of occupation-based practice:

1. presence of an occupational challenge;
2. need for occupational enablement and possibility of solutions;
3. population- or community-specific goals, challenges and solutions;
4. a multidisciplinary knowledge base; and
5. a reasoning process that can deal with complexity.

These elements unify the occupational therapy profession across a wide range of practice settings and approaches, including population-centred and community-centred practice. The first step is to identify the challenge that limits or prevents the client (in this instance a population or community) from participating in occupations through an assessment and information gathering process. Following this, solutions can be developed that draw on occupational reasoning and the multidisciplinary knowledge base. A wide range of population-centred and community-centred interventions exist; however, the use of a project management approach has been selected to illustrate one potential evidence-based approach in-depth.

Occupational challenges in populations and communities

Occupational challenges are due to transactions and interactions that occur between people, occupational factors and environment determinants including social and political. Determining occupational challenges at a population or community-level requires analytical skills that extend to multiple and diverse sources of information and data, and views and perspectives. Occupational challenges might be identified for populations via statistical data or surveys. Community-centred practice requires identification of occupational challenges through collaboration and partnership with community members and understanding and prioritising issues in ways that centralise their strengths, experiences and needs (Gilbert Hunt et al., 2017; Hyett et al., 2018; WFOT, 2019).

Occupational models should be used to identify occupational challenges in a population or with a community. Models such as the Canadian Model of Occupational Performance-Engagement (CMOP-E) (Townsend & Polatajko, 2013) and the Person–Environment–Occupation (PEO) model (Law et al., 1996) can be helpful for analysing and understanding people, environment and occupation interactions. However, these models were developed for individual-focused practice which limits their capacity to explain the complex interactions that occur in populations and communities. The Kawa model, an occupational model developed for use with collectives, might be helpful to formulate this analysis (Iwama et al., 2009). Alternatively, the Participatory Occupational Justice Framework can be used to identify occupational challenges caused by social and political environmental determinants (Whiteford et al., 2018).

A multidisciplinary knowledge base

The profession has always drawn on knowledge from outside and within the field, as is relevant to the identified occupational challenge (Kielhofner, 2004). Research findings from occupational therapy and occupational science that demonstrate the links between occupation and health will underpin the design and facilitation of all solutions. In addition, knowledge sources from outside the field can guide the development of population-centred and community-centred practice processes and interventions. Such sources include community development, community-based rehabilitation, human rights, health promotion, public health, project management, socio-ecological and systems theory, trans-theoretical and organisational change models, leadership models as well as program evaluation.

A reasoning process that can deal with complexity

Occupational therapy takes place in a complex and unpredictable open system which acknowledges the dynamic interaction between people and their environments. This understanding underpins occupational therapy practice models. Within population-centred and community-centred practice the impact of environmental factors increases the complexity of occupational therapy practice. The health care setting for occupational therapists is now being described by some as super complex, acknowledging the political adeptness and problem-solving acumen required to be effective (Fortune et al., 2013). This complexity results in less predictability and no right or wrong answer, requiring an approach that allows for the consideration of multiple solutions. This requires a form of reasoning referred to by Townsend and Polatajko (2013) as 'abductive reasoning' which is suitable for complex situations and multiple solutions. Abductive reasoning entails inductive processes where observations, problem-solving and intuitive processes lead to the best possible explanation.

This complexity also means that when working with populations and communities, prescribed off-the-shelf assessment and treatment approaches that were designed for use with individuals can be ineffective in guiding practice. As a result, occupational therapists are trialling and evaluating different therapeutic processes and strategies to build evidence for practice at population and community levels. Examples of these include appreciative enquiry (Clarke & Thornton, 2014), community development (Galvaan & Peters, 2014; Leclair et al., 2019), community-centred practice framework (Hyett et al., 2018), social occupational therapy (Malfitano et al., 2014), participatory action research (Taylor et al., 2004), project management (Gilbert Hunt et al., 2017; Knightbridge, 2014), school-based practice and universal design (Camden et al., 2015; Wegner et al., 2014), and socially inclusive occupational therapy using CORE (Pereira et al., 2020).

Project management approach

A *project management* approach can assist in managing the challenges associated with the complexity of population-centred practice as it allows a defined goal to be addressed within a time-limited manner (Scaffa & Reitz, 2014). Project management occurs sequentially across three broad stages: i) information gathering; ii) outcomes and operational planning; and iii) project implementation and evaluation (Dwyer et al., 2019). As such, project management closely mirrors the occupational therapy practice process stages outlined in the *Canadian Practice Process Framework*: enter/initiate, set the stage, assess/evaluate, agree—objectives and plan, implement plan, monitor/modify, evaluate outcome and conclude/exit (Townsend & Polatajko, 2013, p. 233).

Community-centred practice can involve applying the project management approach with a community. Adaptations should be made to emphasise collaboration and partnership at all stages of the process. The project must be focused on an occupational challenge or goal identified and prioritised by the community, and processes used to develop solutions must be co-produced and tailored to community context and centralise community strengths, experiences and needs (Hyett et al., 2018; WFOT, 2019).

Information gathering

In project management, information gathering is often described as a 'situation profile' or 'needs assessment'. This starts broadly, focused on the project context and can include: policies concerning the issue; organisational and service system vision statements; and perspectives of key stakeholders. Information gathering methods are rigorous and can include policy review; focus groups; epidemiological and demographic data analysis; participant observations; stakeholder mapping; partnership analysis; and best practice review (Gilbert Hunt et al., 2017; Knightbridge, 2014). Information gathered gradually becomes more focused, drilling down to the most salient PEO elements impacting on the issues being targeted.

The PEO elements are broad and take account of geographic regions, social attributes, personal attributes, economic factors, culture/cultures and determinants of health. Existing Australian Bureau of Statistics (ABS) demographic and epidemiological data (ABS, 2011), as well as empirical literature and government reports, can be accessed to help understand the population. Information can also be gathered first-hand from population stakeholders or representatives using methods such as narratives, focus groups and semi-structured interviews. Ethical principles as outlined in the National Statement on Ethical Conduct in Human Research (NHMRC, 2018a) and the guidelines for Ethical Conduct in Research with Aboriginal and Torres Strait Islander Peoples and Communities (NHMRC, 2018b) are valuable for designing ethical project processes and need to be adhered to.

As with individual approaches, environmental elements of concern will include built and natural physical environments such as public transport and the availability of and access to natural spaces. However, they should also include complex, systemic environmental determinants, i.e., social, economic, cultural and institutional factors, and consider the interactions between these factors at the population level. Systems theory such as Bronfenbrenner's socio-ecological model provides explanation as to foundational models that address such complexity (Bronfenbrenner, 1979).

Agree—on objectives and plan

Project planning begins with an outcomes plan which is underpinned by a rationale informed by the extensive information gathering stage. The outcomes plan is developed through collaboration with key stakeholders and begins with longer-term goals for the population or community targeting health and well-being through occupational engagement that align with objectives targeting relevant environmental determinants. Specific, measurable and achievable project objectives are linked directly to one or more occupational enablement strategies, for example, adapt, advocate, coach, collaborate, consult, coordinate, design/build, educate, engage and specialise (Townsend & Polatajko, 2013). Enablement strategies with communities can also include community capacity building, leadership development, partnership development and leveraging, and use of social media (Hyett et al., 2017).

This final step in the project action planning sequence entails breaking down these strategies into activities and the resources needed and detailing plans for managing time, quality and risks (Dwyer et al., 2019). Responsible professional practice is embedded though the addition of specific plans for ethical practice, collaborative communication and project review evaluation.

Project implementation and evaluation

In the project implementation stage, the quality of the operations (e.g., timelines, resources, risks) are monitored and controlled; communications and relationships are managed; strategies are delivered and immediate objectives are met (Dwyer et al., 2019). At the conclusion of the time limited project, the outcomes and processes are evaluated, conclusions drawn, recommendations made, and information disseminated.

Case studies

Four case studies are presented in brief in the next section to illustrate population-centred and community-centred occupational therapy practice. All cases are real, although some identifying features have been altered.

Case study 1: Positive child and infant health through strong relationships

This project was undertaken to address the occupational challenges associated with parenting in collaboration with a state government program aimed at supporting families with children from birth to four years so that parents are more involved in their children's learning to develop strong parent–child relationships. While the program was effective in supporting those families who attended the program, marginalised and more at-risk families in the community were not always reached. Using the enablement strategies of coach, collaborate, engage and design/build, two occupational therapy students worked with families using the service to develop a resource titled 'Building Blocks: Helping to build stronger relationships between parent and child'. This booklet offered key tips about how to nurture the relationship with one's child from the pregnancy stage through to the pre-school years (Hill & Learhinan, 2008). By working directly with the families to develop the resource, the format was more closely matched with the literacy levels of the target client group and offered visual cues and messages from the parent and child perspective as well as prompts for self-reflection. Within the organisation, the resource is now provided to all pregnant mothers as part of their overall support package.

Case study 2: A culturally accessible community garden

The project was undertaken to address the occupational challenges of community and social participation. The setting for this project was a community health centre in a low-income area where the population included newly arrived and settled refugees. The refugees were not engaged with the community centre. Community gardening provides an occupation that is inclusive of different cultures and levels of ability. There are broad benefits for public health and well-being and for addressing health priorities such as food security. It also provides the opportunity for participation in meaningful occupations and social connection. Secondary data gathering summarised research around occupational deprivation experienced by refugees and practice guidelines (e.g., Kinébanian & Stomph, 2010). Primary data gathered using first-hand narratives from the refugee community provided a deeper understanding of the impacts of preclusion from those meaningful everyday occupations. Utilising enablement strategies of advocate, collaborate, engage and design/build, the project managers worked with representatives of this community to establish a culturally accessible community garden that increased participation of the refugee population.

Case study 3: Environmental influences on the occupational engagement of children with disability

This project was undertaken to address the occupational challenge of restricted occupational performance due to an unsupportive environment. The population group in this project was children under eighteen years of age who attended government-funded children's respite facilities. Initial information gathering findings indicated that factors contributing to children demonstrating behaviours-of-concern within these purpose-built respite facilities included limited access to meaningful occupational participation, and poorly designed physical environments in terms of sensory input and functionality. A lack of understanding of these issues by government planners, policy makers and funders had resulted in poor 'fit for purpose' respite facilities being built. Ultimately, such issues were contributing indirectly to service users (children) demonstrating behaviours-of-concern. Using the enablement skills of design/build, specialise, advocate and consult, the project managers compiled and documented design principles that enabled occupational participation within such respite facilities. The recommendations led directly to changed government policy in this area.

Case study 4: Community safety

This project was undertaken to address the occupational challenge of community safety at night-time in public spaces. An occupational therapist working in a community-based alcohol and other drug service was providing case management and counselling services for a caseload of up to 30 adolescents who presented with similar substance use issues and health risks and harms. Seeing the pattern of issues within the community, the occupational therapist realised that a proportion of the problems experienced by the young people they see in their clinical work were caused by community-level social, cultural, political, economic and environmental determinants. The occupational therapist approached their manager to advocate for expanding their individual-focused service to include a community-centred approach. This involved the occupational therapist collaborating and developing partnerships with local young people, schools, sports clubs, businesses and organisations, and working with them to explore and assess community-level issues and barriers, and to develop community-level goals and strategies for intervention that can be implemented through collaboration. It was important to consult to understand different youth perspectives and needs to make sure strategies were tailored to context and were acceptable and practical for addressing the problem. Young people felt a culture of risky drinking and intoxication and violence was affecting their ability to go out with their friends at night-time, and this was made more difficult by a lack of taxis or safe places to wait for taxis or ride-sharing services. As a group, one strategy they designed and built was a safe taxi rank facility to improve safety at night-time for young people visiting pubs and clubs.

Conclusion

This chapter provided an overview of population-centred and community-centred occupational therapy practice. Occupational therapists are increasingly involved in population and community health, well-being and inclusion projects as part of their professional practice. Additional skills and knowledge are needed to enable occupational therapists to expand their practice beyond traditional individual-focused service provision. Occupational therapists can adopt population-centred and community-centred approaches underpinned by the five essential elements of occupation-based practice, which includes identifying an occupational challenge and developing solutions that draw on occupational reasoning and the multi-disciplinary knowledge base. A project management approach informed by the Canadian Practice Process Framework is recommended.

Summary

- Population-centred and community-centred occupational therapy is becoming more prevalent in Australia and internationally.
- Practice at a population or community level aims to address social injustices and environmental determinants that impede occupational engagement and lead to health inequality or disparity.
- Population-centred and community-centred occupational therapy practice incorporates the five essential elements of authentic occupation-based practice.
- Population-centred and community-centred occupational therapy practice is a process approach to occupational therapy practice which can combine a project management approach with occupational therapy practice models.

- Population-centred and community-centred occupational therapy practice relies on clearly identified goals and objectives and is based on a rationale drawn from a thorough and rigorous information gathering stage.

Review questions

1. List some of the occupational challenges being experienced by people in your community; how are these being determined by social and environmental factors?
2. Compare and contrast individual-centred, population-centred and community-centred occupational therapy practice approaches and skills needed.
3. Outline the sequential steps followed in the project management approach for working with populations.
4. Identify the occupational enablement strategies utilised in each of the case studies.

References

Australian Bureau of Statistics (ABS). (2011). *Census of population and housing: Estimating homelessness.* https://www.abs.gov.au/AUSSTATS/abs@.nsf/DetailsPage/2049.02011

Bronfenbrenner, U. (1979). *The ecology of human development: Experiments by nature and design.* Harvard University Press.

Camden, C., Leger, F., Morel, J., & Missiuna, C. (2015). A service delivery model for children with DCD based on principles of best practice. *Physical & Occupational Therapy in Pediatrics, 35*(4), 412–425. https://doi.org/10.3109/01942638.2014.978932

Clarke, M., & Thornton, J. (2014). Using appreciative inquiry to explore the potential of enhanced practice education opportunities. *British Journal of Occupational Therapy, 77*(9), 475–478. https://doi.org/10.4276/030802214X14098207541153

Commission on Education. (2011). The philosophical base of occupational therapy. *American Journal of Occupational Therapy, 65,* S65. https://doi.org/10.5014/ajot.2011.65S65

Dwyer, J. A., Zhanming, L., & Thiessen, V. (2019). *Project management in health and community services: Getting good ideas to work* (3rd edn). Allen & Unwin.

Fidler, G. S. (2000). Beyond the therapy model: Building our future. *American Journal of Occupational Therapy, 54*(1), 99–101. https://doi.org/10.5014/ajot.54.1.99

Fortune, T., Ryan, S., & Adamson, L. (2013). Transition to practice in supercomplex environments: Are occupational therapy graduates adequately prepared? *Australian Occupational Therapy Journal, 60*(3), 217–220. https://doi.org/10.1111/1440-1630.12010

Galvaan, R., & Peters, L. (2014). *Occupation-based community development framework.* University of Cape Town. https://open.uct.ac.za/handle/11427/6651

Gerlach, A. J., Teachman, G., Laliberte-Rudman, D., Aldrich, R. M., & Huot, S. (2017). Expanding beyond individualism: Engaging critical perspectives on occupation. *Scandinavian Journal of Occupational Therapy, 25*(1), 35–43. https://doi.org/10.1080/11038128.2017.1327616

Gilbert Hunt, S., Sellar, B., Berndt, A., George, E., Thomas, K., & Foley, K. M. (2017). From rhetoric to reality: Community development in occupational therapy curriculum. In D. Sakellariou & N. Pollard (Eds.) *Occupational therapies without borders: Integrating justice with practice* (2nd edn, pp. 561–573). Elsevier Ltd.

Hill, K., & Learhinan, K. (2008). *Building Blocks.* Unpublished student report. University of South Australia, School of Health Sciences.

Hyett, N., Kenny, A., & Dickson-Swift, V. (2017). Approaches for building community participation: A qualitative case study of Canadian food security programs. *OTJR: Occupation, Participation and Health, 37*(4), 199–209. https://doi.org/10.1177/1539449217727117

Hyett, N., Kenny, A., & Dickson-Swift, V. (2018). Re-imagining occupational therapy clients as communities: Presenting the community-centred practice framework. *Scandinavian Journal of Occupational Therapy, 26*(4), 246–260. https://doi.org/10.1080/11038128.2017.1423374

Hyett, N., McKinstry, C., Kenny, A., & Dickson-Swift, V. (2016). Community-centred practice: Occupational therapists improving the health and wellbeing of populations. *Australian Occupational Therapy Journal, 63*(1), 5–8. https://doi.org/10.1111/1440-1630.12222

Iwama, M. K., Thomson, N. A., & Macdonald, R. M. (2009). The Kawa model: The power of culturally responsive occupational therapy. *Disability and Rehabilitation, 31*(14), 1125–1135. https://doi.org/10.1080/09638280902773711

Kielhofner, G. (2004). *Conceptual foundations of occupational therapy practice* (3rd edn). F. A. Davis Co.

Kindig, D., & Stoddart, G. (2003). What is population health? *American Journal of Public Health, 93*(3), 380–383. https://doi.org/10.2105/AJPH.93.3.380

Kinébanian, A., & Stomph, M. (2010). Diversity matters: Guiding principles on diversity and culture. A challenge for occupational therapists working in practice, education or research and for WFOT member organisations. *WFOT Bulletin, 61*(1), 5–13. https://doi.org/10.1179/otb.2010.61.1.002

Knightbridge, L. (2014). Experiential learning on an alternative practice education placement: Student reflections on entry-level competency, personal growth, and future practice. *British Journal of Occupational Therapy, 77*(9), 438–446. https://doi.org/10.4276/030802214X14098207540956

Law, M., Cooper, B., Strong, S., Stewart, D., Rigby, P., & Letts, L. (1996). The Person–Environment–Occupation model: A transactive approach to occupational performance. *Canadian Journal of Occupational Therapy, 63*(1), 9–23. https://doi.org/10.1177/000841749606300103

Leclair, L. L., Lauckner, H., & Yamamoto, C. (2019). An occupational therapy community development practice process. *Canadian Journal of Occupational Therapy, 86*(5), 345–356. https://doi.org/10.1177/0008417419832457

Malfitano, A. P. S., Esquerdo Lopes, R., Magalhaes, L., & Townsend, E. A. (2014). Social occupational therapy: Conversations about a Brazilian experience. *Canadian Journal of Occupational Therapy, 81*(5), 298–307. https://doi.org/10.1177/0008417414536712

Malfitano, A. P. S., Gomes da Mota de Souza, R., & Esquerdo Lopes, R. (2016). Occupational justice and its related concepts: An historical and thematic scoping review. *OTJR: Occupation, Participation and Health, 36*(4), 167–178. https://doi.org/10.1177/1539449216669133

National Health and Medical Research Council. (2018a). *National Health and Medical Research Council 2007—Updated 2018, National statement on ethical conduct in human research.* https://www.nhmrc.gov.au/about-us/publications/national-statement-ethical-conduct-human-research-2007-updated-2018

National Health and Medical Research Council. (2018b). *Ethical conduct in research with Aboriginal and Torres Strait Islander Peoples and communities: Guidelines for researchers and stakeholders.* https://www.nhmrc.gov.au/about-us/resources/ethical-conduct-research-aboriginal-and-torres-strait-islander-peoples-and-communities

Occupational Therapy Australia. (2016) *Position paper: Occupational deprivation.* https://otaus.com.au/publicassets/5e5829df-2503-e911-a2c2-b75c2fd918c5/Occupational%20Deprivation%20(April%202016).pdf

Occupational Therapy Board of Australia. (2018). *Australian occupational therapy competency standards.* https://www.occupationaltherapyboard.gov.au/codes-guidelines/competencies.aspx

Pereira, R. B., Whiteford, G., Hyett, N., Weekes, G., Di Tommaso, A., & Naismith, J. (2020). Capabilities, Opportunities, Resources and Environments (CORE): Using the CORE approach for inclusive, occupation-centred practice. *Australian Occupational Therapy Journal, 67*(2), 162–171. https://doi.org/10.1111/1440-1630.12642

Scaffa, M. E., & Reitz, S. M. (2014). *Occupational therapy in community-based practice settings* (2nd edn). F. A. Davis Co.

Taylor, R. R., Braveman, B., & Hammel, J. (2004). Developing and evaluating community-based services through participatory action research: Two case examples. *American Journal of Occupational Therapy, 58*(1), 73–82. https://doi.org/10.5014/ajot.58.1.73

Townsend, E., & Polatajko, H. (2013). *Enabling occupation II: Advancing occupational therapy vision for health, well-being and justice through occupation* (2nd edn). CAOT Publications ACE.

Wegner, L., Caldwell, L. L., & Smith, E. A. (2014). A public health perspective of occupational therapy: Promoting adolescent health in school settings. *African Journal for Physical, Health Education, Recreation and Dance, 20*(2), 480–491. http://www.ajol.info/.../105520

Whiteford, G. E., Jones, K., Rahal, C., & Suleman, A. (2018). The Participatory Occupational Justice Framework as a tool for change: Three contrasting case narratives. *Journal of Occupational Science, 25*(4), 497–508. https://doi.org/10.1080/14427591.2018.1504607

Wilcock, A. A. (1998). *An occupational perspective of health.* SLACK Inc.

World Federation of Occupational Therapists. (2019). *Occupational therapy and community-centred practice.* https://www.wfot.org/resources/occupational-therapy-and-community-centred-practice

World Health Organization (WHO). (1978). *Declaration of Alma-Ata.* http://www.who.int/publications/almaata_declaration_en.pdf

World Health Organization. (1986). *The Ottawa Charter for Health Promotion.* http://www.who.int/healthpromotion/conferences/previous/ottawa/en/

29 Advocacy, promotion, leadership and entrepreneurship in the occupational therapy profession in Australia

Michelle Bissett and Sylvia Rodger (first edition); updated by Michelle Bissett, Dave Parsons, Angus Buchanan and Angela Berndt (second edition)

Chapter objectives

Upon completion of this chapter, the reader will be able to:

* Define the terms advocacy, promotion leadership and entrepreneurship.
* Understand the relevance of these terms in the practice of occupational therapists.
* Appreciate the importance of these concepts for the occupational therapy profession.

Key terms

profession; leadership; advocacy; promotion; entrepreneurship

Introduction

This chapter provides a brief overview of the concepts of advocacy and promotion, leadership and entrepreneurship within the occupational therapy profession, with a focus on the Australian context. Each of the terms will be defined and their importance within the occupational profession explained. Each section provides examples to further illustrate how these concepts are embedded within occupational therapy practice in Australia. The importance of these concepts for both individual therapists and the profession, as a whole, is addressed.

Advocacy and promotion

Historically, advocacy has been associated with human and civil rights movements and reflected an approach of standing up for people prejudiced by any type of discrimination. Health professionals are often required to advocate for disadvantaged or vulnerable individuals or groups. This includes, but is not limited to, people with disabilities, older adults, Indigenous groups and clients with mental health conditions (Tannous, 2000).

Occupational therapists view advocacy as a part of their routine professional work (Aguilar et al., 2012; Dhillon et al., 2010; King & Curtin, 2014). Occupational therapy professional bodies, including Occupational Therapy Australia (OTA) (2012) and the Canadian Association of Occupational Therapists (CAOT) (2012), state that therapists will engage in advocacy activities as part of their professional work, congruent with therapist's expectations of their role. Advocacy is also embedded as a core aspect of occupational therapy practice within theoretical practice frameworks including the Occupational Therapy Practice Framework (Roley et al., 2008) and the Canadian Model of Client-Centred Enablement (Townsend et al., 2013). In practice, this role enactment typically translates to ensuring that clients are enabled to participate in chosen and meaningful occupations. Advocacy can take different forms, is purposeful, is inherently a political act, must address power relationships and the potential for unintended disempowerment, and requires skills to be effective (Talbot & Verrinder, 2014). It can include advocating for individual clients on specific issues, activation at an organisational level for changes to practices, and action at a community level for changes in legislation and public awareness of professional issues (Stergiou-Kita et al., 2010).

Advocacy and lobbying work together. Advocacy occurs when a person in authority or with negotiating power represents the views or needs of a person, group or community in order to change a situation to improve their lives. Lobbying is the process and activities that occur to create the change in policy or services (Talbot & Verrinder, 2014). Talbot and Verrinder (2014) use the example of the issue of youth safety and participation in occupations reliant on public transport. Advocacy may include working with youth to raise awareness of the risks of assault and other harms due to the lack of safe late-night transport; whereas lobbying might involve targeting the bus service administration or the city council to effect immediate change to accessibility.

The previous examples describe direct advocacy approaches taken by occupational therapists but advocacy can also be indirect. In these scenarios, therapists act on behalf of a community or client group or may include building the skills or working alongside people, in order to foster the capacity for people to advocate directly for themselves. In this way, advocacy reflects occupational therapy, both practices and values. King and Curtin (2014) interviewed therapists who worked with rehabilitation clients post brain injuries. The therapists described the need to advocate for clients to receive funding from government organisations which would support their engagement in activities of daily living. In addition, these therapists also used their professional skills to educate and enable their clients to become self-advocates for their own needs.

At an organisational level, the Koori Occupational Therapy Scheme has advocated for the needs of First Australians. They have done this by increasing the number of First Australian occupational therapists, improving the understanding of health issues for First Australians in occupational therapy services, and educating policy makers on the profile of occupational therapy and its potential application to Aboriginal Health Services (Paluch et al., 2011).

Lastly, professional associations can lobby to influence governments about health care provision (Welchman & Griener, 2005) and policies that affect people's engagement with occupations. In doing so, these organisations advocate for services that meet the needs of the particular client groups. Occupational Therapy Australia employs an advocacy and lobbying expert to provide consultation on health reforms that impact the clients with whom occupational therapists work across all sectors. Examples include the implementation of the National Disability Insurance Scheme (NDIS), services for veterans, submissions to Royal Commissions and other Government inquiries (see the Occupational Therapy Australia website for other examples—https://otaus.com.au). Primarily, advocacy purpose is to mobilise resources, change opinions, catalyse change and cause action (Talbot & Verrinder, 2014).

Promotion is defined by the *Oxford English Dictionary* (2015) as activity that supports or encourages a cause or venture, or endorses a particular view. In this chapter, we conceptualise promotion as being the politicising and advancement of occupational therapy.

Promotion of the profession, and the work of occupational therapists, is critical to professional survival and growth. Health professions need to be actively promoting their services to a range of audiences, including clients, other health care professionals and the general public (Kagan et al., 2015). By doing so, they are able to influence the perception of the services they can offer, and enhance an understanding of their contribution towards health care provision (Kagan et al., 2015). Professional promotion is typically enacted through individual or collective approaches. Individually, occupational therapists should routinely describe and keenly promote their work in their practice with clients (Jacobs, 2012). This can be done in practice, for example, by therapists providing clear communication about the focus of occupational therapy in neurological rehabilitation or by discussing evidence for a planned falls prevention program.

Furthermore, occupational therapists need to promote their work to other health professionals, policy makers, funders and stakeholders. For example, therapists could promote the potential contribution occupational therapy could have in a new interprofessional clinic being established in (a) a hospital, or (b) a new multicultural service in their local government area designed to support refugees and asylum seekers. In these scenarios, occupational therapists could promote their potential contribution based on their unique understanding of the relationship between occupation and health. Alternatively, therapists could disseminate their skills to teachers by informing them about the services they can provide for children with special needs in classroom environments. Throughout the history of the profession, there have been calls to action for occupational therapists encouraging them to incorporate professional promotion in their practice. Jacobs (2012) highlighted this point by stating 'we, as occupational therapy practitioners and students, are the ones best equipped to promote occupational therapy... each of us should take responsibility for the promotion of occupational therapy and also learn strategies for promoting occupational therapy from one another' (p. 668). More recently, Pattison et al. (2018) proposed 'every occupational therapist needs to be an activist in promoting our profession's core values at every opportunity' (p. 241).

Professional associations or collectives, such as Occupational Therapy Australia, also play a key role in the promotion of occupational therapy. In Australia, Occupational Therapy Australia engages in regular promotional activities targeted at the broader community, federal government, funding bodies, key stakeholders and potential occupational therapists. At a professional level, they promote the benefits of engaging in the occupational therapy profession as well as the benefits of working with an occupational therapist (Occupational Therapy Australia, 2020). It is now difficult to imagine occupational therapists being excluded from opportunity to offer mental health services under the Medicare primary care items; however, that was almost the case. Occupational Therapy Australia promoted occupational therapists to government for inclusion as health professionals accessible under a mental health care plan. This work resulted in the inclusion of occupational therapists as listed mental health specialists and, consequently, people are now able to access Medicare-funded occupational therapy to support their mental health. A further example of their promotional activities is the consumer website called 'About Occupational Therapy' (http://aboutoccupationaltherapy. com.au/), which provides clear information to potential clients, carers and facilities about occupational therapy practice. Occupational Therapy Australia also represents occupational therapists at career days and conferences/expo events where promotional material is shared with a range of stakeholders. In recent times, occupational therapy professional associations, nationally and internationally, have increased their utilisation of social media platforms (including Facebook, Twitter and LinkedIn) (Hamilton et al., 2016). Through these mediums, it has been, and is possible, to promote individual occupational therapy organisations, promote the profession to a range of local and international audiences (Hamilton et al., 2016) and demonstrate the scope of occupational therapy and current advocacy activities (Occupational Therapy Australia, 2020).

Leadership

Leadership has been described as the process of an individual influencing a group or team to achieve a united goal (Northouse, 2015). Leadership skills are vital for occupational therapists as they give individuals the ability to positively influence change for themselves and their careers, their clients and, more broadly, the profession and society. Rodger (2011) interviewed emerging occupational therapy leaders and identified that leaders reported the following key characteristics: inspiring others, listening, facilitating change, having a vision and strategic thinking. Rodger (2012) considered that everyone has the capacity to demonstrate leadership abilities and challenged occupational therapists to see themselves as leaders. This may be within work teams, in occupational therapy departments, non–governmental organisations, voluntary boards or within the wider profession.

While management and leadership are often cited synonymously, there are significant differences between the two skill sets that are worth noting (Kotterman, 2006). Management sets about coping with complexity, providing order, stability, consistency and predictability to otherwise turbulent situations. Leadership, on the other hand, is about setting a vision and coping with rapid change (Kotter, 2008). Management involves planning, budgeting, organising and problem solving while leadership involves setting direction, aligning team members and motivating people (Kotter, 2008).

Occupational therapists can demonstrate leadership on a variety of levels. An easy way to help think about leadership is the concept of 'Big L' leadership and 'Little l' leadership. 'Big L' leadership refers to the leaders with defined roles and positions that inherently give them leadership responsibilities (Kotter, 2008). Examples include heads of departments, program directors within universities, and coordinators of services such as rehabilitation units or community mental health facilities. They are responsible for establishing a vision, developing a team culture based on shared values and leading a group of individuals (either occupational therapists or other professionals) towards that vision. Additionally, these leaders often undertake the management and supervision of staff and budgets, administrative duties associated with the health/education or community organisation, oversight of workplace health and safety, discrimination and other workplace policies.

'Little l' leadership can be described as the traits and behaviours that individuals exhibit where others perceive them to be 'good' leaders (Kotter, 2008). Examples of this type of leadership are having the courage to speak up when they see a conflict in their values, exhibiting high emotional intelligence to resolve conflict, advocating for their patients or clients within a multidisciplinary team, suggesting that their team consider a journal discussion group, undertaking a display for World Occupational Therapy Week, reviewing the discharge assessment and reporting template used on the ward, and then coordinating the effort or taking the lead to make these initiatives eventuate. There are many opportunities to proactively see a need, take some action, and lead people to make a change.

Kotter (2008) challenges the commonly held belief that leadership is an innate set of skills comprised of charisma and vision that cannot be learnt. Leadership skills *can* be developed throughout one's career. Occupational therapists have the opportunity to develop leadership skills by supervising students completing practice education placements, taking on additional tasks/duties, becoming a senior clinician who supervises and mentors other therapists, and undertaking further workplace training in leadership, performance management of employees or teamwork. As an occupational therapy student, there are many opportunities in which leadership can be demonstrated and developed, for example, participation in student associations, workgroups on assignments or other academic tasks, or undertaking supervised practice on placements.

Entrepreneurship

Entrepreneurship is both the mindset and process of creating, launching and managing a business, usually often with considerable initiative and risk. The idea is often new, innovative and can challenge the current ways of doing business. The person who does this, referred to as an entrepreneur, undertakes a series of tasks such as developing a business plan and acquiring the personnel and other resources required for the business (Bridge & O'Neill, 2012). Baron (2004, p. 30) states, 'entrepreneurs may or may not be innovators, but they are always experimenters; they are individuals able to recognize opportunities and willing to take the risks necessary to develop those opportunities'. The expressed qualities are also very similar to those held by successful occupational therapists. It is, therefore, no surprise that there are many occupational therapists who through using their entrepreneurial skills have developed successful and profitable businesses. There are many examples of occupational therapy entrepreneurs, the most common being those who set up and work in their own private practices.

While entrepreneurship is often viewed through the lens of commercial business development, there is a growing focus on the value of social entrepreneurship. This is an approach to develop, fund and implement solutions to social, cultural or environmental issues with a strong focus on outcomes and rather than financial profits. Social entrepreneurship in modern society offers an altruistic form of entrepreneurship that focuses on the benefits that society may gain often working in areas such as poverty alleviation, health care and community development (Tan et al., 2005). An example could be developing community-based employment enterprises for people with disabilities or leading the development of micro funding cooperatives to support refugee women develop their own small businesses.

Entrepreneurialism is increasingly being associated with a disruptive innovation that creates a product and service and eventually disrupts an existing way of working, often replacing existing services (Ab Rahman et al., 2017). Opportunities for entrepreneurial activity are often found in areas that are being reformed such as the disability, mental health and aged care sectors. Occupational therapists can leverage their skills and entrepreneurial spirit to further the profession and improve outcomes for their patients, clients and customers. Occupational therapists are perfectly poised to do this based on our understanding of how technology and the environment can impact the health and well-being of our clients. Examples of where there is current scope for development include virtual and augmented reality, 3D printing, using big data, wearable technologies and telehealth delivery. While providing therapeutic skills, most occupational therapy courses will not necessarily provide students with the level of business skills that may be required to successfully engage in entrepreneurial ventures. Occupational therapists ideally should undertake a self-assessment to determine their skill set and identify whether these are skills they need to develop through training and experience, seek professional advice and engage in partnerships.

Conclusion

This chapter has defined the concepts of promotion, advocacy, leadership and entrepreneurship, and provided examples of these concepts within the context of Australian occupational therapy practice. Occupational therapists use these skills in daily practice in order to live occupational therapists' values and advance the participation of clients at an individual, group, community and population level. The chapter has highlighted how occupational therapy students and new graduates can develop these skills to use them effectively in their professional practice.

Summary

- Leadership, advocacy, entrepreneurship and promotion are all concepts that are part of daily occupational therapy practice.
- Occupational therapists have skill sets that enable them to actively pursue leadership, advocacy, entrepreneurship and promotion.
- Development of these skills can commence during university training and be enhanced in the workplace.

Review questions

1. Why is advocacy and promotion important for health professions and health professionals?
2. What are some examples of advocacy that have recently been actioned by Occupational Therapy Australia?
3. Why do professions need to have good leaders?
4. What strategies can student and new graduate occupational therapists employ to develop their own leadership skills?
5. What are some skills that a therapist might need to become a successful entrepreneur?
6. What are the characteristics of social entrepreneurship and occupational therapy principles that complement each other in practice?

References

Ab Rahman, A., Hamid, U. Z. A., & Chin, T. A. (2017). Emerging technologies with disruptive effects: A review. *Perintis e-Journal*, 7(2), 111–128. https://perintis.org.my/ejournal/wp-content/uploads/2018/11/Paper-4-Vol.-7-No.-2-pp.-111-128.pdf

Aguilar, A., Stupans, I., Scutter, S., & King, S. (2012). Exploring professionalism: The professional values of Australian occupational therapists. *Australian Occupational Therapy Journal*, 59(3), 209–217. https://doi.org/10.1111/j.1440-1630.2012.00996.x

Baron, R. C. (2004). *Pioneers and plodders: The American entrepreneurial spirit*. Fulcrum Publishing.

Bridge, S., & O'Neill, K. (2012). *Understanding enterprise: Entrepreneurship and small business*. Macmillan International Higher Education.

Canadian Association of Occupational Therapists. (2012). *Profile of practice of occupational therapists in Canada*. http://www.caot.ca/pdfs/2012otprofile.pdf

Dhillon, S. K., Wilkins, S., Law, M. C., Stewart, D. A., & Tremblay, M. (2010). Advocacy in occupational therapy: Exploring clinicians' reasons and experiences of advocacy. *Canadian Journal of Occupational Therapy, 77*(4), 241–248. https://doi.org/10.2182/cjot.2010.77.4.6

Hamilton, A. L., Burwash, S. C., Penman, M., Jacobs, K., Hook, A., Bodell, S., Legherd, R., & Pattison, M. (2016). Making connections and promoting the profession: Social media use by World Federation of Occupational Therapists member organisations. *Digital Health, 2*, 1–15. https://doi.org/10.1177/2055207616653844

Jacobs, K. (2012). PromOTing occupational therapy: Words, images, and actions. *American Journal of Occupational Therapy, 66*(6), 652–671. https://doi.org/10.5014/ajot.2012.666001

Kagan, I., Biran, E., Telem, L., Steinovitz, N., Alboer, D., Ovadia, K., & Melnikov, S. (2015). Promotion or marketing of the nursing profession by nurses. *International Nursing Review, 62*(3), 368–376. https://doi.org/10.1111/inr.12178

King, D., & Curtin, M. (2014). Occupational therapists' use of advocacy in brain injury rehabilitation settings. *Australian Occupational Therapy Journal, 61*(6), 446–457. https://doi.org/10.1111/1440-1630.12149

Kotter, J. P. (2008). *Force for change: How leadership differs from management*. Simon & Schuster.

Kotterman, J. (2006). Leadership versus management: what's the difference? *Journal for Quality and Participation, 29*(2), 13–17. http://sfxhosted.exlibrisgroup.com.ezproxy.liv.ac.uk/lpu?title=journal+for+quality+%26+participation&volume=29&issue=2&spage=13&date=2006

Northouse, P. G. (2015). *Leadership: Theory and practice*. Sage Publications.

Occupational Therapy Australia. (2020). *Media and advocacy*. https://otaus.com.au/media-and-advocacy/advocacy

Oxford English Dictionary. (2015). *Promotion*. https://www.oxfordlearnersdictionaries.com/us/definition/english/promotion

Paluch, T., Allen, R., McIntosh, K., & Oke, L. (2011). Koori Occupational Therapy Scheme: Contributing to First Australian health through professional reflection, advocacy and action. *Australian Occupational Therapy Journal, 58*(1), 50–53. https://doi.org/10.1111/j.1440-1630.2010.00913.x

Pattison, M., Baptiste, S., & McKinstry, C. (2018). A vision splendid: Visioning for the future of occupational therapy. *Australian Occupational Therapy Journal, 65*(3), 238–242. https://doi.org/10.1111/1440-1630.12490

Rodger, S. (2011). *Final report: Building capacity among emerging occupational therapy academic leaders in curriculum renewal and evaluation at UQ and nationally*. Australian Learning and Teaching Council. https://altf.org/wp-content/uploads/2016/08/Rodger_S_TF_Final-Report_UQ_2011.pdf

Rodger, S. (2012). Leadership through an occupational lens: Celebrating our territory. *Australian Occupational Therapy Journal, 59*(3), 172–179. https://doi.org/10.1111/j.1440-1630.2012.00995.x

Roley, S. S., DeLany, J. V., Barrows, C. J., Brownrigg, S., Honaker, D., Sava, D. I., Talley, V., Voelkerding, K., Amini, D. A., Smith, E., Toto, P., King, S., Lieberman, D., Baum, M. C., Cohen, E. S., Moyers Cleveland, P. A., & Youngstrom, M. J. (2008). Occupational Therapy Practice Framework: Domain & process 2nd edition. *American Journal of Occupational Therapy, 62*(6), 625–683. https://doi.org/10.5014/ajot.62.6.625

Stergiou-Kita, M., Moll, S., Walsh, A., & Gewurtz, R. (2010). Health professionals, advocacy and return to work: Taking up the challenge. *Work: A Journal of Prevention, Assessment and Rehabilitation, 37*(2), 217–223. https://doi.org/10.3233/WOR-2010-1073

Talbot, L, & Verrinder, G. (2014). *Promoting health: The primary health care approach* (5th edn). Churchill Livingstone Elsevier.

Tan, W.-L., Williams, J. N., & Tan, T.-M. (2005). Defining the 'social' in 'social entrepreneurship': Altruism and entrepreneurship. *The International Entrepreneurship and Management Journal, 1*(3), 353–365. https://ink.library.smu.edu.sg/lkcsb_research/1380

Tannous, C. (2000). Therapists as advocates for their clients with disabilities: A conflict of roles? *Australian Occupational Therapy Journal, 47*(1), 41–46. https://doi.org/10.1046/j.1440-1630.2000.00204.x

Townsend, E. A., Beagan, B., Kumas-Tan, Z., Versnel, J., Iwama, M., Landry, J., Stewart, D., & Brown, J. (2013). Enabling: Occupational therapy's core competency. In E. A. Townsend & H. J. Polatajko (Eds.), *Enabling occupation II: Advancing an occupational therapy vision for health, well-being and justice through occupation* (2nd edn, pp. 87–133). CAOT Publications ACE.

Welchman, J., & Griener, G. G. (2005). Patient advocacy and professional associations: Individual and collective responsibilities. *Nursing Ethics, 12*(3), 296–304. https://doi.org/10.1191/0969733005ne791oa

30 Looking forward

Occupational therapy in Australia's future

Ted Brown, Helen Bourke-Taylor, Stephen Isbel, Reinie Cordier and Louise Gustafsson

Chapter objectives

Upon completion of this chapter, the reader will be able to:

* Review the accomplishments of Australian occupational therapists as an indicator and motivator to future success.
* Outline potential future areas of occupational therapy practice.
* Reflect and plan your future career as an occupational therapist.
* Reflect on ways you can contribute to strengthen the profession.

Key terms

occupational therapy; Australia; accomplishments; career planning; future practice

Introduction

Australia is a vast, diverse country with a rich and varied landscape from tropical rainforests to arid deserts and rugged coastlines. Australia is also home to citizens from a wide range of cultural backgrounds including Indigenous Australians and more recent migrants from overseas. The Australian landscape no doubt has an impact on the daily occupations its citizens engage in and, similarly, has shaped the development of the occupational therapy profession. Similarly, when disease and disability have impacted Australians, such as the polio epidemic in the 1930s and the COVID-19 pandemic in 2020, the occupational therapy profession has responded and grown to meet the occupational needs of people directly or indirectly affected. Occupational therapy in the Australian context is still a relatively young profession, first appearing in the health care arena formally in the mid-1930s. Reflecting on the past provides insights into the possibilities for an innovative future for the profession in Australia.

Since the inception of the profession in Australia, occupational therapists have had a growing and significant impact on the profession internationally. For example, OT Australia was one of the founding nations to become a member of the World Federation of Occupational Therapists (WFOT) at its inaugural meetings in 1951–1952. Over the decades, several Australians have held key positions, such as secretary and president, within the WFOT. Marilyn Pattison from South Australia is the current president of the WFOT, having held this position since 2016. Australia has also hosted two WFOT congresses: the 10th WFOT Congress, 2–6 April 1990, Melbourne, Victoria; and the 14th WFOT Congress, 23–28 June 2006, Sydney, NSW (WFOT, 2014a).

As of 2020, there are 24 university campuses that offer entry to practise occupational therapy education at the undergraduate and/or graduate-entry master's level with over 9,000 students enrolled (Occupational Therapy Board of Australia/AHPRA, 2020). All occupational therapy education programs are accredited by the Occupational Therapy Council of Australia (OTC), which in turn ensures that the courses meet the WFOT Minimum Standards for the Education of Occupational Therapists (2002) (Hocking & Ness, 2004; WFOT, 2014b). Over 200 occupational therapists in Australia currently have doctoral level qualifications while another 1,500 have completed post-professional master's level postgraduate education. The profession has flourished in Australia, with so many choosing to enter the profession and many others becoming highly skilled researchers who both solidify the scientific foundations of the profession and spearhead future practice areas.

In 2006, the formation of the Occupational Therapy Board of Australia under the umbrella of the Australian Health Practitioner Regulation Agency, led to national registration of occupational therapists. National registration was a benchmark in professional identity and recognition as only three states—Queensland, South Australia and Western Australia—had achieved recognition previously. Registration means that the Occupational Therapy Board of Australia is charged with the responsibility to protect and represent the rights of the public. Further, the board identifies standards that the public can expect when receiving services from occupational therapists and thereby influences what criteria occupational therapists must meet to achieve and maintain registration. Occupational Therapy Australia represents the profession at the national and international level with state level offices representing the field on the local level.

When the profession formed a national body with an association and the national board, occupational therapy gained considerable strength and solidarity in advocacy and professional issues. Activities such as Occupational Therapy Australia's release of a set of national competencies, known as Australian Minimum Competency Standards for New Graduate Occupational Therapists (OTA, 2018), served to unite and strengthen the identity of members in the profession. Importantly, the new competency standards highlight the essential nature of embedding indigenous perspectives and ways of working alongside communities to refocus occupational therapists towards the health and well-being of indigenous Australians as a priority in the years to come. The occupational therapy profession stands firm in its commitment to Indigenous persons. Indeed, similar to any group in the Australian community where health disparity exists and the opportunity to participate in meaningful occupations is jeopardised, occupational therapists must be compelled to level inequalities and close the gap completely.

Celebrating the profession's recent past

The recent past reveals significant consolidation of the profession, providing evidence that progress is likely to be far-reaching as new occupational therapists enter the profession. The profession has national approaches to education and research developments. An example includes the fieldwork evaluation tool that is used by all accredited occupational therapy education programs: *Student Practice Evaluation Form—Revised Edition* (SPEF-R) (Division of Occupational Therapy, University of Queensland, 2008). Other professional developments added to the profession's success, such as the *Australian Occupational Therapy Journal*, started in 1952 and some 60 years later it is now one of the top peer-reviewed occupational therapy journals in the field internationally. Further,

Table 30.1 Assessments developed by occupational therapists from Australia

- Assessment of Children's Hand Skills (ACHS) (Chien et al., 2012)
- Child Initiated Pretend Play Assessment (ChIPPA) (Stagnitti, 2007)
- Children's Play Skills Self-Report Questionnaire (PSSRQ) (Sturgess & Ziviani, 1996)
- Melbourne Assessment 2: A Test of Unilateral Upper Limb Function (MA2) (Randall et al., 2012)
- Test of Playfulness (ToP) (Skard & Bundy, 2008)
- Test of Environmental Supportiveness (ToES) (Bronson & Bundy, 2001)
- Handwriting Speed Test (HST) (Wallen, 1996)
- Occupational Therapy Adult Perceptual Screening Test (OT-APST) (Cooke et al., 2005)
- Activity Card Sort—Australia (ACS-Aus) (Packer et al., 2008)
- Activity Card Sort—Australia (18–64) [ACS-Aus (18–64)] (Gustafsson et al., 2014)
- OT–DORA Battery: Occupational Therapy Driver Off-Road Assessment Battery (Unsworth, 2012)
- Australian Therapy Outcome Measures for Occupational Therapy (AusTOMs—OT) (Unsworth & Duncombe, 2014)
- Drive Safe and Drive Aware (Kay et al., 2009)
- Health Promoting Activities Scale (Bourke-Taylor et al., 2012)
- Assistance to Participate Scale (Bourke-Taylor & Pallant, 2013)
- Child's Challenging Behaviour Scale version 2 (Bourke-Taylor et al., 2014)
- Pragmatics Observational Measure-2 (Cordier et al., 2014; Cordier et al., 2019)
- Personal Care Participation Assessment and Resource Tool (PC-PART) (Darzins et al., 2016)
- Dimensions of Home Measure (DOHM) (Aplin et al., 2016)

OTseeker, designed, launched and maintained by Australian occupational therapists, remains one of the most extensively used evidence-based practice tools to inform occupational therapists around the world (OTseeker, 2015).

Australian occupational therapists have developed and published a number of assessment tools that are now used in professional practice (see Table 30.1). Many of these assessments are used by occupational therapists as part of their daily clinical practice in Australia and internationally.

Moreover, occupational therapists in Australia have also published books that are being used as key reference texts within the profession (see Table 30.2). There is substantial evidence that Australian occupational therapists have made and continue to make great contributions to the professional body of knowledge and evidence nationally and internationally. Occupational therapy graduates who have been educated in Australia are also well respected internationally for their high skill level and professionalism.

In a relatively short period of time, Australian occupational therapists have made significant contributions to their unique body of knowledge and become a recognised, regulated health care profession. We are moving from traditional arenas of practice to role emerging areas. While we still have significant contributions to make to the acute care and sub-acute sector, occupational therapists are making headway in the areas of health promotion, disease and illness prevention, population health, lifestyle redesign; we are engaging with private industry, occupational health and safety, environmental health, and the creative and inventive use of technology to promote health and wellbeing. Areas of occupational therapy practice that will continue to be of significance in an Australian context will include:

- Health and occupations of Indigenous Australians;
- Health and occupations of individuals from culturally and linguistically diverse backgrounds including refugees and migrants;

Table 30.2 Books authored by occupational therapists from Australia

- *The work of our hands: A history of the Occupational Therapy School of Victoria* (Sutherland Cameron, 1977)
- *Occupational Therapy: Its place in Australia's history* (Anderson & Bell, 1988)
- *Learn to play* (Stagnitti, 1998)
- *Cognitive and perceptual disorders: A clinical reasoning approach to evaluation and intervention* (Unsworth, 1999)
- *Management of upper limb hypertonicity* (Copley & Kuipers, 1999)
- *Occupation for occupational therapists* (Molineux, 2004)
- *Occupation and context in practice* (Whiteford & Wright St Clair, 2005)
- *Occupational therapy with children: Enabling children's occupational performance and participation* (Rodger & Ziviani, 2006)
- *Client education: A partnership approach for health practitioners* (McKenna & Tooth, 2006)
- *Assistive technology in the workplace* (De Jonge et al., 2007)
- *Play as therapy: Assessment and therapeutic interventions* (Stagnitti & Cooper, 2009)
- *Occupational therapy and physical dysfunction: Enabling occupation* (Curtin et al., 2009)
- *Clinical and fieldwork placement in the health professions* (Stagnitti et al., 2010)
- *Occupation-centred practice with children: A practical guide for occupational therapists* (Rodger, 2010)
- *Using occupational therapy models in practice: A field guide* (Turpin & Iwama, 2010)
- *Physiotherapy and occupational therapy for people with cerebral palsy: A problem-based approach to assessment and management* (Dodd et al., 2010)
- *Raising the best possible child: How to parent happy and successful kids from birth to seven* (Jackson King, 2010)
- *Occupation analysis in practice* (Mackenzie & O'Toole, 2011)
- *Role emerging occupational therapy: Maximising occupation-focused practice* (Thew et al., 2011)
- *Working with parents of a newly diagnosed child with an Autism Spectrum Disorder: A guide for professionals* (Keen & Rodger, 2012)
- *Communication: Core interpersonal skills for health professionals* (O'Toole, 2012)
- *Occupational science: Society, inclusion, participation* (Whiteford & Hocking, 2012)
- *Mental health in Australia: Collaborative community practice* (Meadows et al., 2012)
- *Kids can be kids: A childhood occupations approach* (Lane & Bundy, 2012)
- *The art and science of motivation: A therapist's guide to working with children* (Ziviani et al., 2013)
- *Evidence-based practice across the health professions* (Hoffman et al., 2017)
- *Pain: A textbook for health professionals* (Van Griensven et al., 2014)
- *An occupational perspective of health* (Wilcock & Hocking, 2015)
- *Qualitative research methodologies for occupational science and therapy* (Nayar & Stanley, 2015)
- *Goal setting and motivation in therapy: Engaging children and parents* (Poulsen et al., 2015)
- *Evidence-based education in the health professions: Promoting best practice in the learning and teaching of students* (Brown & Williams, 2015)
- *Lifestyle-integrated Functional Exercise (LiFE) program to prevent falls: Trainer's manual* (Clemson et al., 2016)
- *Bruce & Borg's psychosocial frames of reference: Theories, models and approaches to occupational-based practice* (4th edn) (Krupa et al., 2016)
- *A dictionary of occupational science and occupational therapy* (Molineux, 2017)
- *Occupational therapy for people experiencing illness, injury or impairment: Promoting occupation and participation* (7th edn) (Curtin et al., 2017)
- *Occupation-centred practice with children: A practical guide for occupational therapists* (Rodger & Kennedy-Behr, 2017)
- *Participation: Optimising outcomes in childhood-onset neurodisability* (Imms & Green, 2020)
- *Implementing occupation-centred practice: A practical guide for occupational therapy practice learning* (Dancza & Rodger, 2018)

- Health and occupations of ageing individuals;
- Health and occupations of carers;
- Health and occupations of individuals with chronic diseases and disabilities;
- Promoting environmental fit for persons with special needs;
- Consulting to members of local, state and federal governments;
- Providing services for people with disabilities covered under the National Disability Insurance Scheme (NDIS);
- Providing Medicare-subsidised services for people in the community;
- Becoming occupational consultants and advocates;
- Continuing to expand and develop the body of empirical knowledge about human occupation related to health and the occupational development of humans;
- Continuing the development of the nexus between occupational therapy practice and occupational science;
- Integrating occupational therapy practice into the education sector, private industry (such as natural resources and mining) and community health care;
- Increasing support for therapists and clients in rural and remote regions of Australia;
- Increasing case management roles in community care centres;
- Increasing roles in primary health care; and
- Developing niche practice areas such as providing services for people with cancer, with cognitive impairment or neurological impairment, who require palliative care or driving assessment and rehabilitation or environmental modifications.

Occupational therapy practice in Australia also has several ongoing education, research, practice and policy priorities for the future. These include:

- Continuing with education innovations such as ensuring sufficient practice education placement opportunities for students, increasing use of simulation and use of blended learning strategies;
- Assisting with the ongoing development of occupational therapy practice in Asia Pacific countries where the occupational therapy profession is still evolving and being established (e.g., mainland China, Vietnam);
- Further expansion of the occupational therapy body of empirical knowledge where human occupation is clearly shown to have positive benefits for the health and well-being of citizens;
- Further expansion and refinement of occupational therapy theoretical models and practice frameworks;
- Further expansion of the application of the interaction between the individual and their environment to promote independence and habilitation;
- Further development of the application and integration of technology in the treatment and rehabilitation of clients;
- Further development of lifestyle redesign, health promotion and primary health care roles for occupational therapists;
- Further development of the occupational therapy scope of practice at the population health level of service provision; and
- Consideration of the introduction of the Occupational Therapy Clinical Doctorate (OTD) as an additional entry to practice pathway.

Towards your future career: What will the occupational therapy profession do for you and what can you do for the occupational therapy profession?

Throughout this textbook, the reader has been provided with information from leaders in the occupational therapy profession. From the detailed explanation and discussion of foundational issues, to robust presentation of professional issues and examples of innovative and common practice issues, contributing authors readily and expertly share their knowledge for the benefit of future occupational therapists and their clients.

As a student or a current practising occupational therapist, we encourage you to feel a part of a registered profession with a peak professional body and ever-changing responsive profession that aims to meet the occupational needs of Australians. You may find your place in an established practice area or be an innovator who shapes a new area of practice for the benefit of your community and future occupational therapists. You may find your place in research or knowledge generation that keeps the profession growing with the foundations firmly embedded in evidence. You may find yourself in administration, management and governance roles that directly influence occupational therapy service provision and clients. Wherever you find yourself, make a difference to clients and their families, strengthen the profession through gathering and generating evidence to support practice, and be innovative and responsive to change. As evidenced by the past, the future will bring changes to the Australian population, health, the environment, where and how people live, and what occupations are important to Australians. The systems that support Australians will change and occupational therapists need to help lead positive transformations in health, education, social services and other government level initiatives.

Take some time to reflect on your future. Ask yourself some key questions about the type of profession that you want to contribute to and be part of. Ask yourself how the profession can help you achieve what you wish for and how you can contribute as an occupational therapist. Recording your aspirations and intentions is important because as a lifelong learner it helps you to stay focused and be accountable to your own professional development plan. Consider creating your own six-step professional development plan. We have configured six key questions associated with the steps to build towards your goals. Here are some questions for you. We suggest that you record your answers.

1. Why did I become an occupational therapist?
2. What are my top three professional priorities?
3. What resources and knowledge do I need to build skills in the areas of professional priority?
4. How will I attain sufficient resources and supports to achieve my professional priorities?
5. Who can I learn from and who can I support and mentor as I address my professional priorities?
6. Who can I share my learnings, disseminate the evidence and collaborate with, influence, and educate future occupational therapists who have similar professional priorities to me?

Review your plan in six months. Revise your answers. Keep developing and progressing your career and you will keep contributing to the growth of occupational therapy in Australia. Creating your own professional development plan has multiple benefits.

Meeting the needs of others and making a difference in the lives of occupational therapy clients and their families will have its own reward. All the successes that you experience will have a flow on effect to the development of occupational therapy as a profession in Australia. The profession needs leaders, innovators, advocates, managers, clinicians, researchers, practice educators and others. Help shape the future of the occupational therapy profession in Australia as your professional career develops.

Conclusion

Occupational therapy in the Australian context will continue to make significant progress and innovative developments. With increasing numbers of therapists completing postgraduate degrees and assuming leadership positions, occupational therapists will take up positions of influence. Recognition of the importance of relationships between occupational performance, health and well-being will increase, bringing greater attention to the profession. The number of standardised assessment tools and published books by Australian authors is impressive and well placed. The *Australian Occupational Therapy Journal* and OTseeker continue to grow in stature, rigor and rate of access. Being a member of the occupational therapy profession presents many exciting opportunities for the present and the future. New graduates and currently practising occupational therapists are strongly encouraged to get involved with their local, state or national professional associations. Given that the occupational therapy discipline was only formally established in the 1930s in Australia, the accomplishments of the profession are significant, stellar and inspiring. Occupational therapists may find pride in the profession's past and confidence in its future as the profession is well placed in the Australian context to make significant contributions to the health and well-being of all Australian citizens and the daily occupations they engage in.

Summary

- Occupational therapy is a fairly new profession in the context of Australia.
- Australian occupational therapists have made significant contributions to the field both nationally and internationally.
- Australian occupational therapists have authored several significant assessment tools and books that are used and referred to nationally and internationally.
- There are several areas of future occupational therapy practice that will evolve and develop over the next few decades.
- Create your own professional plan. All of the successes that you experience will have a flow on effect to the continued development of occupational therapy as a profession in Australia.

Review questions

1. What are three significant contributions that Australian occupational therapists have made to the profession internationally?
2. What are three assessment tools that have been authored by Australian occupational therapy authors?
3. Discuss four potential areas for growth in occupational therapy practice in Australia over coming decades.

References

Anderson, B., & Bell, J. (1988). *Occupational therapy: Its place in Australia's history.* N. S. W. Association of Occupational Therapists.

Aplin, T, Chien, C. W., & Gustaffson, L. (2016). Initial validation of the Dimensions of Home Measure. *Australian Occupational Therapy Journal, 63*(1), 47–56. https://doi.org/10.1111/1440-1630.12270

Bourke-Taylor, H. M., Law, M., Howie, L., & Pallant, J. F. (2012). Initial development of the Health Promoting Activities Scale to measure the leisure participation of mothers of children with disabilities. *American Journal of Occupational Therapy, 66*, e1–e10. https://doi.org/10.5014/ajot.2012.000521

Bourke-Taylor, H., & Pallant, J. (2013). The Assistance to Participate Scale to measure play and leisure support for children with developmental disability: Update following Rasch analysis. *Child: Care, Health and Development, 39*(4), 544–551. https://doi.org/10.1111/cch.12047

Bourke-Taylor, H. M., Pallant, J. F., & Law, M. (2014). Update on the Child's Challenging Behaviour Scale following evaluation using Rasch analysis. *Child: Care, Health and Development, 40*(2), 242–249. https://doi.org/10.1111/cch.12035

Bronson, M. R., & Bundy, A. C. (2001). A correlational study of a Test of Playfulness and a Test of Environmental Supportiveness for Play. *Occupational Therapy Journal of Research, 21(4)*, 241–259. https://doi.org/10.1177/153944920102100403

Brown, T., & Williams, B. (Eds.). (2015). *Evidence-based education in the health professions: Promoting best practice in the learning and teaching of students.* Radcliffe Publishing.

Chien, C. W., Brown, T., & McDonald, R. (2012). Examining construct validity of a new naturalistic observational assessment of hand skills for preschool- and school-age children. *Australian Occupational Therapy Journal, 59*(2), 108–120. https://doi.org/10.1111/j.1440-1630.2012.00997.x

Clemson, L., Munro, J., & Fiatarone Singh, M. (2016). *Lifestyle-integrated Functional Exercise (LiFE) program to prevent falls: Trainer's manual.* Sydney University Press.

Cooke, D. M., McKenna, K., & Fleming, J. (2005). Development of a standardized occupational therapy screening tool for visual perception in adults. *Scandinavian Journal of Occupational Therapy, 12*(2), 59–71. https://doi.org/10.1080/11038120410020683-1

Copley, J., & Kuipers, K. (1999). Management of upper limb hypertonicity. Therapy Skill Builders.

Cordier, R., Munro, N., Wilkes-Gillan, S., Speyer, R., & Pearce, W. M. (2014). Reliability and validity of the Pragmatics Observational Measure (POM): A new observational measure of pragmatic language for children. *Research in Developmental Disabilities, 35*(7), 1588–1598. https://doi.org/10.1016/j.ridd.2014.03.050

Cordier, R., Munro, N., Wilkes-Gillan, S., Speyer, R., Parsons, L., & Joosten, A. (2019). Applying item response theory (IRT) modelling to an observational measure of childhood pragmatics: The Pragmatic Observation Meaure-2. *Frontiers in Psychology, 10*(408), 1–17. https://doi.org/10.3389/fpsyg.2019.00408

Curtin, M., Adams, J., & Egan, M. (Eds.). (2017). *Occupational therapy for people experiencing illness, injury or impairment: Promoting occupation and participation (7th edn).* Elsevier.

Curtin, M., Molineux, M., & Supyk-Mellson, J. (Eds.). (2009). *Occupational therapy and physical dysfunction: Enabling occupation.* Churchill Livingstone.

Dancza, K., & Rodger, S. (2018). *Implementing occupation-centred practice: A practical guide for occupational therapy practice learning.* Taylor & Francis.

Darzins, S. W., Imms, C., Di Stefano, M., & Radia-George, C. A. (2016). Personal Care Participation Assessment and Resource Tool: Clinical utility for inpatient rehabilitation. *Canadian Journal of Occupational Therapy, 83(4), 237–248.* https://doi.org/10.1177/0008417416648446

De Jonge, D. M., Scherer, M., & Rodger, S. (2007). *Assistive technology in the workplace.* Mosby Elsevier.

Division of Occupational Therapy, University of Queensland. (2008). Student Practice Evaluation Form-Revised Edition (SPEF-R). In *Student Practice Evaluation Form (SPEF)-Revised Edition Package.* University of Queensland. https://spefr.online/

Dodd, K., Imms, C., & Taylor, N. F. (Eds.). (2010) *Physiotherapy and occupational therapy for people with cerebral palsy: A problem-based approach to assessment and management.* John Wiley & Sons.

Gustafsson, L., De Jonge, D. M., Lai, Y., Muuse, J., Naude, N., & Hoyle, M. (2014). Development of an Activity Card Sort for Australian Adults aged 18–64 years. *Australian Occupational Therapy Journal, 61*(6), 403–414. https://doi.org/10.1111/1440-1630.12145

Hocking, C., & Ness, N. E. (2004). WFOT minimum standards for the education of occupational therapists: Shaping the profession. *World Federation of Occupational Therapists Bulletin, 50*(1), 9–17. https://doi.org/10.1179/otb.2004.50.1.003

Hoffmann, T., Bennett, S., & Del Mar, C. (Eds.). (2017). *Evidence-based practice across the health professions* (3rd edn). Elsevier Australia.

Imms, C., & Green, D. (2020). *Participation: Optimising outcomes in childhood-onset neurodisability.* Mac Keith Press.

Jackson King, J. (2010). *Raising the best possible child: How to parent happy and successful kids from birth to seven.* HarperCollins.

Kay, L. G., Bundy, A. C., & Clemson, L. M. (2009). Predicting fitness to drive in people with cognitive impairments by using DriveSafe and DriveAware. *Archives of Physical Medicine and Rehabilitation, 90*(9), 1514–1522. https://doi.org/10.1016/j.apmr.2009.03.011

Keen, D., & Rodger, S. (2012). *Working with parents of a newly diagnosed child with an Autism Spectrum Disorder: A guide for professionals.* Jessica Kingsley Publishers.

Krupa, T., Kirsh, B., Pitts, D., & Fossey, E. (Eds.). (2016). *Bruce & Borg's psychosocial frames of reference: Theories, models and approaches to occupational-based practice* (4th edn). SLACK Inc.

Lane, S. J., & Bundy, A. C. (2012). *Kids can be kids: A childhood occupations approach.* F. A. Davis Co.

McKenna, K., & Tooth, L. (2006). *Client education:* A partnership approach for health practitioners. Plural Publishing Inc.

Mackenzie, L. A., & O'Toole, G. (Eds.). (2011). *Occupation analysis in practice.* Wiley-Blackwell.

Meadows, G., Farhall, J., Fossey, E., McDermott, F., Grigg, M., & Singh, B. (2012). *Mental health in Australia: Collaborative community practice* (3rd edn). Oxford University Press.

Molineux, M. (Ed.). (2004). *Occupation for occupational therapists.* Blackwell Publishing.

Molineux, M. (2017). *A dictionary of occupational science and occupational therapy.* Oxford University Press.

Nayar, S., & Stanley, M. (2015). *Qualitative research methodologies for occupational science and therapy.* Routledge.

Occupational Therapy Board of Australia/AHPRA. (2020). Occupational Therapy Board of Australia registrant data. https://www.occupationaltherapyboard.gov.au/About/Statistics.aspx

Occupational Therapy Board of Australia. (2018). *Australian occupational therapy competency standards 2018.* https://www.occupationaltherapyboard.gov.au/Codes-Guidelines/Competencies.aspx

O'Toole, G. (2012). *Communication: Core interpersonal skills for health professionals.* Elsevier.

OTSeeker. (2015). *Occupational therapy systematic evaluation of evidence.* http://www.otseeker.com/Info/PDF/OTseeker%20Brochure%20Mar_2015.pdf

Packer, T. L., Boshoff, K., & De Jonge, D. (2008). Development of the Activity Card Sort—Australia. *Australian Occupational Therapy Journal, 55*(3), 199–206. https://doi.org/10.1111/j.1440-1630.2007.00686.x

Poulsen, A. A., Ziviani, J., & Cuskelly, M. (Eds.). (2015). *Goal setting and motivation in therapy: Engaging children and parents.* Jessica Kingsley Publishers.

Randall, M. J., Johnson, L., & Reddihough, D. (2012). *Melbourne Assessment 2: A test of unilateral upper limb function.* The Royal Children's Hospital.

Rodger, S. A. (Ed.). (2010). *Occupation-centred practice with children: A practical guide for occupational therapists.* Wiley-Blackwell.

Rodger, S. A. & Kennedy-Behr, A. (2017). *Occupation-centred practice with children: A practical guide for occupational therapists.* Wiley-Blackwell.

Rodger, S. A., & Ziviani, J. M. (Eds.). (2006). *Occupational therapy with children: Enabling children's occupational performance and participation.* Blackwell Science.

Skard, G., & Bundy, A. (2008). Test of Playfulness. In L. D. Parham & L. S. Fazio (Eds.), *Play in occupational therapy for children* (pp. 71–93). Mosby Elsevier.

Stagnitti, K. (1998). *Learn to play.* Co-ordinates Occupational Therapy Service.

Stagnitti, K. (2007). *The Child Initiated Pretend Play Assessment (ChIPPA).* Co-ordinates Publications.

Stagnitti, K., & Cooper, R. (Eds.). (2009). *Play as therapy: Assessment and therapeutic interventions.* Jessica Kingsley Publishers.

Stagnitti, K., Schoo, A., & Welch, D. (Eds.). (2010). *Clinical and fieldwork placement in the health professions.* Oxford University Press.

Sturgess, J., & Ziviani, J. (1996). Development of a self-report play questionnaire for children aged 5 to 7 years: A preliminary report. *Australian Occupational Therapy Journal, 42*(3), 107–117. https://doi.org/10.1111/j.1440-1630.1995.tb01322.x

Sutherland Cameron, B. (1977). *The work of our hands: A history of the Occupational Therapy School of Victoria.* Gippsland Commercial Times Printing.

Thew, M., Edwards, M., Baptiste, S., & Molineux, M. (2011). *Role emerging occupational therapy: Maximising occupation-focused practice.* Wiley-Blackwell.

Turpin, M. J., & Iwama, M. K. (2010). *Using occupational therapy models in practice: A field guide.* Elsevier.

Unsworth, C. A. (Ed.). (1999). *Cognitive and perceptual disorders: A clinical reasoning approach to evaluation and intervention.* F. A. Davis Co.

Unsworth, C. A., & Duncombe, D. (2014). *AusTOMs for occupational therapy* (3rd edn). La Trobe University.

Unsworth, C. A. (2012). *OT–DORA Battery: Occupational Therapy Driver Off-Road Assessment Battery.* AOTA Press.

Van Griensven, H., Strong, J., & Unruh, A. M. (Eds.). (2014). *Pain: A textbook for health professionals.* Churchill Livingstone.

Wallen, M. A. (1996). *The Handwriting Speed Test.* Helios Art and Book Co.

Whiteford, G., & Hocking, C. (Eds.). (2012). *Occupational science: Society, inclusion, participation.* Wiley-Blackwell.

Whiteford, G., & Wright St Clair, V. (Eds.). (2005). *Occupation and context in practice.* Churchill Livingstone.

Wilcock, A. A., & Hocking, C. (2015). *An occupational perspective of health.* SLACK Inc.

World Federation of Occupational Therapists. (2014a). *List of council meetings and congresses.* https://www.wfot.org/search?q=LIST%20OF%20COUNCIL%20MEETINGS%20AND%20CONGRESSES%20update%20June%202014.pdf

World Federation of Occupational Therapists. (2014b). *Minimum standards for the education of occupational therapists.* https://www.wfot.org/assets/resources/COPYRIGHTED-World-Federation-of-Occupational-Therapists-Minimum-Standards-for-the-Education-of-Occupational-Therapists-2016a.pdf#:~:text=The%20World%20Federation%20of%20Occupational%20Therapists%20%28WFOT%29%20Minimum,quality%20assurance%20for%20development%20beyond%20the%20levels%20specified.

Ziviani, J., Poulsen, A. A., Cuskelly, M., & Hayes, A. (Eds.). (2013). *The art and science of motivation: A therapist's guide to working with children.* Jessica Kingsley Publishers.

Index

Note: **Bold** page numbers refer to tables; *italic* page numbers refer to figures.

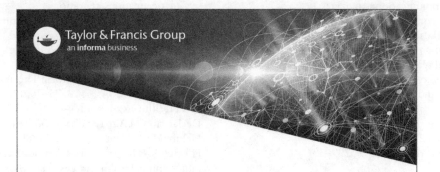